Community Mental Health in Canada

Community Mental Health in Canada

THEORY, POLICY, AND PRACTICE

Simon Davis

UBCPress · Vancouver · Toronto

15 14 13 12 11 10 09 08 07 06   5 4 3 2 1

Printed in Canada on acid-free paper

Library and Archives Canada Cataloguing in Publication

Davis, Simon, 1956-
   Community mental health in Canada : theory, policy and practice / Simon Davis.

Includes bibliographical references and index.
ISBN-13: 978-0-7748-1280-1 (bound); 978-0-7748-1281-8 (pbk.)
ISBN-10: 0-7748-1280-X (bound); 978-0-7748-1281-8 (pbk.)

   1. Community mental health services – Canada. 2. Mental health policy – Canada. 3. Mentally ill – Care – Canada. I. Title.

RA790.7.C3D39 2006   362.2'2'0971   C2006-900160-X

Canadä

UBC Press gratefully acknowledges the financial support for our publishing program of the Government of Canada through the Book Publishing Industry Development Program (BPIDP), and of the Canada Council for the Arts, and the British Columbia Arts Council.

UBC Press
The University of British Columbia
2029 West Mall
Vancouver, BC V6T 1Z2
604-822-5959 / Fax: 604-822-6083
www.ubcpress.ca

For Marta, an unsung hero,

and in memory of Richard N. Davis, MD

The needs of members of the psychiatric community
are not so different, really, from anyone else's needs —
a home, a job, a friend.

– Pat Capponi, *Beyond the Crazy House:
Changing the Future of Madness*

Contents

Introduction

In Canada the field of mental health has seen considerable change in a relatively short period of time. Starting in the 1960s, the locus of treatment shifted from institutions to the community with the downsizing and closure of the "asylums." Around this time pharmacological treatments, promising a breakthrough in the amelioration of psychotic disorders, began their ascendancy, while psychodynamic theories fell from favour. Reflecting a concern with the civil rights of all citizens, laws concerning involuntary detention and treatment were amended to provide persons with mental disorders greater procedural and substantive protections.

Despite these promising developments, problems persisted. It seemed that many mentally disordered persons in the community were not getting treatment; some were homeless, and some wound up in jail. A large number were housed in dingy, custodial-style boarding homes, which in many respects were no improvement over the institutions from which they had been discharged. And these formerly institutionalized persons were now much more visible, with their appearance and behaviour at times frightening members of the public. In response, the pendulum, which had been moving in the direction of greater civil liberties, began to swing back. More coercive, "assertive" approaches to treatment and case management were developed. The legal criteria for involuntary hospitalization, narrowed in the 1970s, were broadened again in a number of jurisdictions, and community treatment orders – akin to probation orders – were developed and increasingly implemented.

Although paternalistic approaches to practice appeared to be reemerging, the vision of empowerment, started with the civil rights movement of the 1960s, persisted. The importance of decent housing, meaningful activity, employment, and friendship – what are now called the "social determinants of health" – were acknowledged. The role of the professional as expert/authority began to be challenged, and articles were written suggesting that treatment should be a collaborative process or even client-driven. People spoke about alternate, nonmedical pathways to healing. Previously ignored, clients were now serving on steering committees and being employed as peer-support workers. Some professionals have adapted to these changes and competing perspectives, while others have not. In short, these have been interesting times for those working in mental health.

Although the field of mental health in Canada continues to evolve, this book is premised on the view that it is worthwhile at this point in the early years of the twenty-first century to take stock of where we are and where we may be heading. To that end, this book offers a critical overview of the provision of services to mentally disordered persons in Canada. The services referred to here are the publicly funded programs mandated to meet the needs of persons suffering from the most disabling disorders – schizophrenia, bipolar disorder, and depression, for example. While some reference is made to children and older adults, the focus here is on adult service recipients.

The intention of this book is to address both the systemic, or "macro," issues (e.g., program philosophies, how services are organized) as well as the clinical aspects of mental health care – that is, the actual interventions that are used. While the notion of covering both systemic and technical concerns in one volume may seem overly ambitious or presumptuous, it has been this author's experience that an appreciation of the political, cultural, and organizational context of mental health care is necessary if clinical interventions are to be effective or if we are to understand why they are less than effective. Readers interested in pursuing subjects in more depth may refer to the other published and Internet sources listed here. Concerning the literature surveyed for this book, an effort was made to use Canadian authors and Canadian data where possible.

Who This Book Is For

This book evolved out of material prepared for an introductory, one-semester course on mental health practice given to senior-level undergraduates. Accordingly, the book is intended in the first instance for those considering or starting a career in health care. The presumed need for this book came from the author's impression that no single text was currently available that addressed both clinical and structural aspects of mental health practice in the Canadian context. While the book is intended for "potential practitioners," it is hoped that others will find it accessible and informative, particularly members of stakeholder groups – that is, service recipients, families, and interested members of the public.

Points of View

Trying to determine how society should respond to people with mental health concerns has produced strong divisions of opinion and heated arguments that, in many instances, remain unresolved. A Health Canada (2002c, 3) document, for example, notes that one of the barriers faced by persons attempting to improve the Canadian mental health system has been the "abundance of ethical dilemmas associated with mental health care that are controversial and actively debated by fractious constituent groups." Examples of questions on which there is still ongoing debate include the following:

- What exactly *is* a mental disorder anyway, and who gets to determine the official categories designating mental disorders?
- What causes mental disorders?
- Are people with mental illnesses really more violent or dangerous than other people?
- What treatments should be offered?
- Should treatment be coerced?
- Is there an overreliance on medication in mental health practice?
- How do we know if any of the treatments being offered are effective (and how is "effective" defined anyway)?
- Are there procedures and approaches used by mental health practitioners that actually create more harm?
- Is there a place for self-help and alternative therapies?
- Is professional involvement always necessary for recovery?
- Are there people out there needing mental health support who are being ignored?
- Are mental health practitioners ethnocentric and sexist in their thinking?
- Is cost containment the overriding concern when determining what constitutes "best practices" in mental health?

The positions taken in responding to these questions are sometimes categorized as, for example, "medical model" or conversely "antipsychiatry." While lumping people together in this fashion is convenient and somewhat reassuring, it results in an oversimplification of a continuum of perspectives – not all psychiatrists, for example, are "medical model" in their orientation – and sometimes in an unthinking dismissal of these competing viewpoints. Adherents of a particular position tend to assume, usually incorrectly, that their opponents' analysis of the issue is uninformed or unsophisticated. Mental health practitioners, for example, may view a service recipient's challenges to treatment approaches as an example of that person's "lack of insight," when in fact the concerns being expressed, which are heartfelt and drawn from considerable personal experience, are legitimate and need to be heard. Thus, in this author's view, it is incumbent upon the different stakeholders – professionals, service recipients, families, advocates – to hear out and seriously consider the positions of others. To that end, when contentious topics are covered in this book, an attempt is made to articulate both (or all) of the competing viewpoints rather than to, in effect, set up "straw persons." Admittedly, one result of this is that at times there may seem to be more questions than answers. In some cases, as readers will be able to judge, the weight of the evidence may favour one position over another; as per Karl Popper, even if the verity of particular theories cannot be ultimately established, some may be shown to be less worthy than others. However, appraisal of competing viewpoints may be compromised by emotional investment and the fallibility of human perception.

While efforts are made here to be balanced in the presentation of competing perspectives, some brief comment must be made on the author's own biases. This book is informed by the author's experiences as a case manager, administrator, and researcher in a large, multisite community mental health service. This experience, along with an undergraduate education concentrated in the biological sciences, has led to an appreciation of the role of medicine and psychiatry in improving the plight of persons with mental health problems. That being said, it is the author's position that our institutional practices have at times been invalidating for service users and consequently that new models – described here – that aim for greater inclusion and empowerment are welcome and overdue.

A Note on Terminology

Because the terms employed in mental health practice have particular connotations – which are not always understood or agreed upon – it is necessary to comment on how they are used in this book. To begin with, there is the book's title: *Community Mental Health in Canada*. "Community mental health" is a phrase often used unthinkingly that, at its narrowest, refers to a *location*: persons with mental disorders are now, unlike during earlier periods, "in the community" in the sense that treatment is provided predominantly in outpatient settings or in the psychiatric units of general hospitals as opposed to in old, remotely located provincial institutions, which have been either downsized or closed altogether.

"Community mental health," however, has a broader and more complex definition, one that has antecedents going back to the "moral treatment" approaches used in late-eighteenth-century Europe, approaches that emphasized human dignity, freedom, and potential. Fast-forwarding to North America in the mid-twentieth century, we see that the "community care" movement was one that looked at environmental factors in mental health, that optimistically spoke about, in the words of President John Kennedy, "the open warmth of community concern and capability," and that emphasized rehabilitation and prevention, beyond simply the management of symptoms (Eaton 2001). This was also a time when people began to speak about consumer rights and empowerment as, in the words of two authors, "part of the seminal ideology of the community care movement" (Scheid and Horwitz 1999, 386). "Community mental health," then, is both a location and a vision, with the former a *fait accompli* and the latter, for reasons explicated in this book, only partially realized.

Also subject to interpretation are the terms that refer to the different players in the mental health system. "Practitioner" will be used here to denote the professionals, such as physicians, nurses, and case managers. A more contentious issue is how to refer to users, or recipients, of mental health services. One of the earliest terms was "patient," which came out of an era when the treatment and containment of mentally disordered persons was largely hospital-based. This term fell out of favour with a number of non-medical disciplines partly because the locale of treatment had shifted to the community and also because of some discomfort with the apparently narrow, symptom-based focus that was implied. During the 1970s and 1980s the designation "**client**" came into more common usage and will be the term used here, except when citing other authors or when referring to hospitalized persons (terms in **bold** can be found defined in the Glossary on p. 316). The use of "client" has in turn been criticized because it would seem to indicate choice or a voluntary relationship, which may not exist in many instances. More recently, "client" has been replaced by "consumer" in a number of mental health programs, although the limitations of the former term would seem to apply to the latter. Most contentious of all is the use of "survivor," a designation that has created some unease and defensiveness among practitioners (e.g., Goldbloom 2003). Some clients and advocacy groups have expanded this into the acronym CSX (consumer, survivor, ex-patient), which one client suggests is "a loose continuum along which most [persons] can locate themselves" (quoted in Brook 2003, H5). In some cases the choices for self-reference may seem politically incorrect or anachronistic – such as the Mental Patients Association in Vancouver – but, as one author points out, this is within the rules in that "the persecuted are allowed to reclaim their own pejoratives" (H5). Although the limitations of the term "client" are acknowledged, its use in this book is not intended to carry any particular symbolic or political connotations, as far as this is possible.

Finally, there is the question of what to call the condition itself. "Mental illness" is still used in many settings and is the term preferred in most instances by physicians. Some have suggested replacing "illness" with "disability" to reflect the impact that mental disorders have on social and vocational functioning and, in the words of one author, "because successful community living requires more than medical care" (Hall 2001, 10). Another term, "mental disorder," is now commonly used in legislation, diagnostic manuals, and other publications, and will be used in this book. Again, possible limitations must be acknowledged, such as the suggestion by the Anxiety Disorders Association of Ontario that "condition" would be a less stigmatizing term than "disorder" (see http://www.anxietyontario.com).

It is important for practitioners to be sensitive about the use of language. At the same time, making the "right" decision is not an easy task: there is no clear consensus among practitioners or clients as to preferred terms (Gibson-Leek 2003; Sharma et al. 2000), and individuals may have different understandings of a particular designation, an example being the woman who told this author that her use of "survivor" referred to surviving depression, not to mistreatment at the hands of the mental health system.

Organization of the Book
Chapters 1 and 2 provide an overview and set the context for what is to follow by examining how mental health programs define their target population, by describing the prevalence and impact of mental disorder in Canada, and by reviewing explanatory models in psychiatry and their implications for treatment.

Chapter 3 is an introduction to diagnosis, with descriptions of the major classes of mental disorder as they are articulated in the *Diagnostic and Statistical Manual (DSM)* of the American Psychiatric Association.

Chapters 4 through 9 look at the organization of mental health services in Canada. Chapter 4 describes the activities and vested interests of stakeholder groups – that is, practitioners, clients, family members, government, and the drug companies. Chapter 5 reviews the major historical shifts in the provision of mental health services, particularly deinstitutionalization and the creation of regional health authorities. Chapter 6 addresses the concept of "best practices." Chapter 7 offers an overview of current community and hospital-based programs. Chapter 8 looks at homelessness and initiatives in the area of housing. And Chapter 9 examines the related phenomena of the "multisystem client" and "transinstitutionalization" as they arise at the interface between the mental health and criminal justice systems.

Chapters 10 through 14 describe in greater detail particular areas and aspects of practice: assessment and medical management; education, skills training, and counselling; rehabilitation; the legal and ethical context of practice; and diversity and cultural competence.

"Boxes" are employed in the text to provide more detail on specific issues and to describe case examples. Terms in bold type are included in the glossary.

Community Mental Health in Canada

The Impact of Psychiatric Disorders

In setting the stage for what is to follow, this chapter provides an overview of the prevalence and impact of mental disorders among the Canadian public. Before we can deal with matters such as prevalence, however, it is necessary to understand *what* is being measured. How do we define mental disorder in the first place? One answer to this question is to look at classification systems, such as the ***Diagnostic and Statistical Manual (DSM)*** of the American Psychiatric Association, which is the subject of a later chapter. Given the length and breadth of the *DSM*, however, a more practical answer is to look at the eligibility criteria used by public mental health programs in Canada.

Defining Mental Disorder: Who Gets Services?
In considering the provision of services to persons with mental health problems, perhaps the most fundamental question of all is: who *are* the "mentally disordered?" Given that there is apparently a wide range of individuals with mental health concerns and that there are limited resources within the health care system, it seems reasonable to suggest that the most severely disabled should be our priority, the group for whom, in the words of two clinicians, "it is medically and morally unjustifiable to limit care" (Satel and Humphreys 2003). This criterion, then, speaks to the importance of being able to identify those most in need; as McEwan and Goldner (2001, 25) note, "accountability within the sphere of publicly funded mental health services and supports is determined, in part, by how well priority populations are served."

Newcomers to the field of mental health may be forgiven for thinking that there is a clear consensus among mental health professionals, if not other groups, as to how the most disabled are identified. Unfortunately, this is not the case. A Health Canada document concludes that "investigations of the usage of the term 'serious mental illness' amongst service providers and administrative organizations have found little consistency and no clear definition" (McEwan and Goldner 2001, 25). Another government document notes that attempts to define the "target population" have been confounded by the fact that inclusion criteria "are either vaguely defined or not defined at all, permitting a wide variation in practice" (British Columbia Ministry of Health 2002c, 33). As acknowledgement of this problem, a recent provincial government report on subsidized housing for persons with mental disorders refers to persons with "serious and persistent mental illness" as being eligible for these programs but adds that "a clear and consistent provincial definition of 'serious and persistent mental illness' will also be required" (British Columbia Ministry of Health 2002d, 20).

So how is "serious" defined in practice? The most common way of defining it is by *diagnosis*. The source used for this purpose in most mental health settings in Canada is, as noted, the *Diagnostic and Statistical Manual* of the American Psychiatric Association. While in theory any of the conditions described therein can be considered mental disorders – such as "caffeine intoxication," for example – only a smaller number of these have come to be considered eligible and appropriate for services in publicly funded community mental health programs (Goodwin and Guze 1996). Of this smaller number, there is general agreement that two, schizophrenia and bipolar disorder (manic-depressive illness), clearly constitute serious conditions. In some schemes the criteria for "serious" or "severe" are limited to these two conditions exclusively. For instance, in a study of substance misuse among mentally disordered persons, Brunette and colleagues regard only those persons diagnosed with schizophrenia spectrum disorders or bipolar disorder as suffering from a "severe mental illness" (Brunette et al. 2003). In another example, in arriving at subcategories of the client population, a Health Canada (2001a) report on concurrent mental health and substance use disorders excludes anxiety disorders, personality disorders, eating disorders, and mood disorders other than bipolar – for example, depression – from the category of **"serious, persistent mental disorders."**

Why are schizophrenia and bipolar disorder considered serious by definition? In looking at the symptoms of these disorders, one can note that in the acute phase of schizophrenia, persons with the disorder may experience delusions, hallucinations, and disordered thinking and may exhibit bizarre speech and behaviour. These individuals may have difficulty maintaining employment, housing, and social relationships because of the impairments caused by the disorder. The symptoms of bipolar disorder include periods of depression as well as mania, the latter typically manifested in the form of excessive energy, racing thoughts, and grandiose plans; when in this speeded-up state, individuals can be very impulsive and engage in overspending or reckless sexual activity.

In considering schizophrenia and bipolar disorder, then, one can draw out several commonalities relevant to understanding how "serious" is defined. First, persons with these conditions can have periods of **psychosis** – by definition, a clear break with reality – manifested by strange beliefs and perceptions. They may at times appear *visibly* different and bizarre, such as the dishevelled man pushing the shopping cart down the middle of the street while angrily talking to himself. Their behaviour is, in short, what the layperson would consider "crazy." Further, their condition is apparently *involuntary* – they have no control over their thoughts and actions. As well, they appear to need and benefit from *medical attention*, for their own safety if nothing else. In particular, we know that in many cases their acute symptoms will respond to medication. If necessary, they may have to be sent to hospital to be stabilized, where they can be medicated involuntarily if they are too unwell to understand the need for treatment. Finally, these two conditions tend to be *enduring* – that is, there may be ongoing disability that lasts for a period of years (Andrews et al. 2000).

However, this raises some questions. For one thing, what happens to individuals who have troubling mental conditions but who appear, outwardly, "normal"? Persons with depression, for example, do not typically act in a bizarre fashion yet may feel profoundly sad and distressed. Their plight, however, is not immediately apparent to others; moreover, they may believe or may have been told – in some cases by a health care provider – that "we all feel this way" at times and that the proper response is to carry on and not dwell on it.[1] Further, not all persons with depression will be similarly impacted; for example, some will experience a "low-grade" form of the disorder known as *dysthymia*. For these reasons, in part, persons with depression may not seek help from mental health professionals. Should the mental health system be more proactive in educating such persons and helping engage them in treatment? While organizations like the Canadian Mental Health Association have attempted to do this, publicly funded treatment programs have not, historically, seen this as their role – despite early visions of community care as looking to prevention (Eaton 2001) – hence the significance of the *visibility* factor in determining "who gets services," a factor that may not be present in the case of depression. As well, the symptoms of depression may not be *persistent;* while some will experience ongoing disability, others will have periods of relatively good remission punctuated by a smaller number of depressive episodes. While recommendations have been made in "best practice" documents that persons with serious but not persistent conditions be accommodated by public treatment programs (British Columbia Ministry of Health 2002e; British Columbia Ministry of Health Services 2003b), the tradition of focusing on persons with enduring disorders such as schizophrenia remains intact in many centres.

What about persons who are evidently experiencing a lot of problems but who seem to have control over their actions – who are apparently being *willful*, in other words? As one author notes, since "acts of will or volition are usually not accepted as diseases" (Campbell 2003, 673), many practitioners have been uncomfortable with the idea that alcoholism and drug addiction, for instance, should be considered mental disorders. But are drug addicts really exercising free will? In a position paper on this topic, a group of psychiatrists notes that, in fact, "the role of biological factors in addiction is supported by increasingly compelling evidence" and that "certain individuals seem more vulnerable to developing alcoholism because of their genetic background" (Committee on Addictions of the Group for the Advancement of Psychiatry 2002, 708). These authors conclude that "if we recognize that an individual with an addiction may not be fully able to exercise free will, then society's obligation to intervene becomes stronger" (712). On the other hand, despite evidence that drug addiction is not a completely voluntary condition, other practitioners have suggested that addicts still have the ability to make choices and should not be given the "illness excuse." A Yale University psychiatrist writes: "To reduce addiction to a slice of deranged brain tissue vastly underplays the reality that much of addictive behavior is voluntary ... During those times [of sobriety] it is the individual's responsibility to make himself [*sic*] less vulnerable to relapse. The person, not his autonomous brain, is the instigator of relapse and the agent of recovery" (Satel 1999, 861). In addressing our confused response to persons with addictions, one author puts it succinctly: "Although we profess support for the disease theory, we continue to believe that addicts are sinful people" (quoted in Priest 2003b, 23).

Another group that creates great ambivalence among mental health practitioners is those who are diagnosed with personality disorders. Rationalizing the eligibility or ineligibility of these individuals for mental health services is a complex matter, having in part to do with the predilections and skill sets of individual clinicians. However, as is the case with drug addicts, clients with diagnoses of personality disorder tend to be seen as willful, as (borrowing the phrase above) the "instigators of relapse," and thus as persons who may not be appropriate for public mental health services. Some public programs do make reference to these diagnoses in their mandates, although usually by adding the adjective "severe" in front of "personality disorder," a qualification that is not necessary in the case of schizophrenia, for example (see Government of Ontario 1999).

Another factor that is taken into account, although not usually spelled out in mandates, is *treatability.*[2] To appreciate what is meant by "treatable," one must understand that a biomedical conceptualization of mental disorder is currently preeminent in most public mental health settings in North America (Boydell, Gladstone, and Crawford 2002; United States Department of Health and Human Services 1999). One of the results of this is that medication now forms the cornerstone of treatment; as a Canadian psychiatrist summarizes, "psychopharmacology has been in the forefront since the introduction of chlorpromazine for schizophrenia" (Rae-Grant 2002, 513). Psychopharmacology has become so dominant, in fact, that decisions about service eligibility sometimes hinge on the question "will this person respond to medication?" As noted, for schizophrenia and bipolar disorder, the answer is probably "yes." Other conditions, however, are ameliorated only partially or not at all by medication. Examples of these are drug addiction, personality disorder, and organic brain disorders, such as fetal alcohol syndrome.

Another group that has historically not been well served by public mental health centres in Canada is those suffering from anxiety disorders – such as agoraphobia, obsessive-compulsive disorder (OCD), and post-traumatic stress disorder (PTSD). A number of individuals and advocacy groups have complained that accessing public mental health programs is difficult for persons with anxiety disorders, even though, in terms of lifetime prevalence rates, these are the most commonly occurring mental disorders in Canada (Antony and Swinson 1996; Hall 2001; see also Chapter 3). To understand this system nonresponse, one must consider several of the eligibility factors referred to already. First, persons with anxiety disorders may not appear to be "visibly different" or display bizarre behaviours. Symptoms may be intermittent or present only in certain situations. Persons seeking treatment for these conditions (previously referred to as *neuroses*) appear to fit the image of the "worried well." In short, there may be some question as to whether the "seriousness" criterion has been met. Second, whether or not a practitioner believes that anxiety disorders are serious, there is the question of treatability, which, as noted, often refers to medication response. Our current understanding is that anxiety disorders respond best to *non*pharmacological interventions, such as education, skills training, and cognitive-behavioural techniques (Andrews et al. 2000; Ehlers et al. 2003; van Minnen et al. 2003). This raises the question: why aren't these approaches offered regularly at public mental health centres? In some cases, they are, and the situation in this regard may be changing. Historically, however, persons employed as case managers in mental health settings, such as nurses and social workers, have not been trained in cognitive-behavioural methods, which have been

seen as the domain of clinical psychology. Further, how the work is organized (read: compressed) at treatment centres – thirty-minute appointments every two to three weeks, for example – does not lend itself to the
more regular, intense contact needed to treat persons with anxiety disorders. Consequently, persons with these problems may be referred for treatment at specialized clinics (which may not exist in all areas or may have
private-pay arrangements).

While diagnosis has been used to identify priority populations in mental
health, critics point out that *DSM* categories do not necessarily speak to the
degree of disability experienced by individuals. McEwan and Goldner (2001,
26) note that "a wide spectrum of symptom severity and functional disability is associated with specific mental disorders; any particular diagnosis ...
does not, in and of itself, provide enough information to make a determina-
tion regarding the presence or absence of serious mental illness." For example, there is, as noted, a tendency to consider, a priori, all persons with a
diagnosis of schizophrenia to be substantially and uniformly disabled, an
assumption that leads to stereotyping and that is not borne out empirically
(Kruger 2000).[3] Conversely, persons referred with a diagnosis of agoraphobia, despite their subjective experiences, may be (as noted above) regarded
as not "really" disabled. For these reasons, assessments should be individualized as much as possible, with functional impairment, apart from diagnosis, being taken into account in decisions about service provision.

We can now summarize what we know about the definition of "serious
mental disorder" – as determined by public treatment programs – and the
answer to the question "who gets services?" Priority populations are defined
to a considerable extent by diagnosis, the paradigmatic examples being
schizophrenia (and related conditions) and bipolar disorder. Persons with
these disorders are known to, at times, experience extremely disordered thinking, exhibit bizarre behaviour, and have deficits with respect to social and
occupational functioning. Persons with other mental conditions are considered eligible to the extent that they meet some or all of the following criteria: (1) the disorder is *persistent*; (2) the disorder causes significant *functional
impairment*; (3) psychotic symptoms and/or bizarre behaviour are manifested;
(4) behavioural problems appear to be *involuntary*, rather than willful; and
(5) the disorder is *treatable* – in particular, responsive to medication. The
first three of these may well be included in agency mandates; the last two are
more likely to be de facto criteria. The reader may also note that criteria are
defined *operationally* rather than by some "objective" standard. "Treatability," for example, is determined by resource availability, practitioner training, and service delivery traditions. On this point it is interesting to note
that, despite concerns about a lack of health care resources in rural areas

(Commission on the Future of Health Care in Canada 2002), mental health centres in these locales may accommodate persons with a wider range of mental health problems than do programs in urban areas *because* there are no other resources to which to refer them.

Finally, it can be seen that some of the factors determining "who gets services" are what might be termed "extraclinical." A key factor in this regard is *visibility* – that is, whether the individual's problems have come to the attention of other persons or the authorities (Mechanic 1999). Arguably, more could be done to reach out to people who are in need but who keep a low profile; it is not the nature of public sector organizations, however, to necessarily seek out new clientele, something that is currently exacerbated by cost pressures in the health care system. Unfortunately, this situation may lead to inequities in service provision, with "squeaky wheels" being accommodated and the quietly unwell being overlooked.

Prevalence and Impact
While there may be some disagreement about how public psychiatric programs define the priority population, there is little debate about the significant effect of mental health problems. Mental disorders have a substantial impact on the quality of life of affected individuals, their families and loved ones, and on society in general because of health care costs as well as lost employment and productivity. The great tragedy is that serious mental disorders interrupt an individual's life trajectory in early adulthood, just when education is being completed, careers are being started, and families and significant attachments are being formed.

The prevalence rates of mental disorder depend, as noted above, on how this term is defined. Based on a more narrow definition that incorporates major depression, bipolar disorder, and schizophrenia – closer to the "serious, persistent" designation – it is estimated that about 4.5 to 5.5 percent of the Canadian population will experience a mental disorder in a twelve-month period; based on a definition that also includes anxiety disorders, eating disorders, personality disorders and suicidal behaviour, this figure reaches one in five (Health Canada 2002b).

While in many cases the impact of a mental disorder will be similar across subsections of the population, there are some notable differences, such as the considerably higher rates of suicide seen in First Nations communities (see Chapter 14). Fairly consistent gender differences have also been seen; for example, depression, eating disorders, and borderline personality disorder are all diagnosed more frequently in women. These differences may reflect the differential impact of socio-cultural factors as well as gender-specific patterns in seeking help (Morrow 2003).

Persons with mental disorders have higher lifetime disability rates than many of those with serious physical illnesses (Bland 1998). For example, a study of the wellbeing of depressed persons found that the social functioning of those surveyed was significantly worse than that of persons with chronic medical conditions such as arthritis, diabetes, and advanced coronary artery disease (Wells, Stewart, and Hays 1989). The World Health Organization estimates that five of the ten leading causes of disability are related to mental disorders and predicts that in less than twenty years depression will be the second-leading cause of disability worldwide and the first-leading cause in developed countries (Desjarlais et al. 1995; Statistics Canada 2003). While depression and anxiety disorders appear to produce less disability than does schizophrenia on an individual basis, they may account for more total disability days when looking at the entire population because they are more common (Andrews et al. 2000; Ustun et al. 2004).[4]

For a variety of reasons – individual and systemic – the unemployment and underemployment rates for persons with mental disorders are very high. As summarized by Rutman (1994, 17), "persons with psychiatric disability often exhibit cognitive, perceptual, affective and interpersonal deficits intrinsic to or resulting from the mental illness" and also "lack [the] normal life experiences and roles that are the foundation of one's vocational identity." Even among those who do find employment, mental health problems can have an impact on productivity: an Ontario report found that workers with a mental condition averaged 7.6 days of diminished or lost productivity per month, about four times that of persons with physical conditions (Stuart et al. 1999). A Health Canada (1997a) report estimated the costs of lost productivity due to long-term mental disability to be $1.6 billion annually, making it the sixth most costly cause of worker disability.

The unemployment and underemployment of mental health clients means that many of these individuals will be living in poverty. Even for those who are able to get disability incomes from the provincial government (an "enhanced" form of income assistance for which persons with mental disorders may apply), their total income is usually still well below the poverty line (National Council of Welfare 2004). On the impact of poverty, interviews conducted with a client group in Hamilton, Ontario, found that the lack of funds affected health and personal empowerment, strained social and family relationships, relegated persons to inner-city environments, and forced them to live in dwellings that could be unsafe and often lacked privacy (Wilton 2003). The author of the study notes how poverty reinforces the stigma of having a mental disorder: "Perceptions of 'bizarre behaviour' and 'poor social skills' may at the very least be exaggerated by poverty where a lack of resources forces consumers to wear old or unmatched clothing, and to do without personal care items. In this sense, the stigmatizing effects of poverty intersect with, and exacerbate, the stigma of mental illness" (151).

Persons with mental disorders have a much higher mortality rate than does the general public due to suicide, accidental overdoses, and premature death from medically treatable conditions (Hall 2001). One in ten persons with schizophrenia will end their lives by suicide, and it is estimated that mortality rates for persons with bipolar disorder are two to three times higher than for the general population due to reckless behaviour, accidents, and suicide (Health Canada 2002b). In British Columbia a study was conducted on the mortality rate of persons discharged from hospitals with psychiatric diagnoses during the fiscal year 1997-98: after this group of 13,476 individuals had been followed for two and a half years, it was determined that the standardized mortality ratio was six times that of the general population (Health Canada 2002b). A provincial government report notes that "higher prevalence of alcohol and substance abuse, poor socioeconomic status and poor health may all have significantly contributed to higher mortality" among this population (British Columbia Ministry of Health Services 2003b, viii). This higher death rate has consistently been found in other settings and at other times partly because, as noted, medical conditions among mentally disordered persons may go undiagnosed and untreated (Felker, Yazel, and Short 1996) or because, if given initial treatment, mental health clients receive poorer follow-up care (Druss et al. 2001).

Concerning the physical health of mental health clients, a review concludes that persons with serious mental illness tend to be in poorer physical health than persons without mental illness, especially in regard to obesity, cardiovascular and gastrointestinal disorders, diabetes, HIV, and both chronic and acute pulmonary disease. The high incidence of substance-use disorders contributes to this overall poor health (Jones et al. 2004).

A number of factors contribute to this poorer health status, including the symptoms of the mental disorder themselves, poverty, medication side effects, lifestyle, and a hypothesized independent association between psychiatric disorders and a tendency toward obesity (Saari et al. 2004; Yager 2004). Persons diagnosed with serious mental disorders have also been found to smoke at much higher rates than the general public (Lawn, Pols, and Barber 2002); for example, an Ontario study determined that over 63 percent of the psychiatric clients surveyed smoked either "daily or occasionally," compared to about 25 percent of the adult Ontario population (Gerber et al. 2003), with another researcher finding that among heavy smokers, cigarettes consumed between one-third and one-half of the clients' incomes (Wilton 2003).

Surveys have determined that persons with mental health problems are overrepresented among homeless populations: about one in three of the nation's homeless have a serious mental disorder and consequently are at greater risk for illness, injury, and exploitation (Allen 2000; Eberle 2001a). Persons with mental disorders are also, for reasons not fully understood, more vulnerable to drug and alcohol misuse and, as a result, have higher rates of illnesses such as HIV and hepatitis B and C (Davis 1998; Rosenberg et al. 2001).

A disproportionate number of persons with mental disorders become involved with the police and wind up in the corrections system: Hall (2001, 16) estimates that 15 percent of the corrections population in British Columbia have a serious mental disorder and observes that "confining disabled persons in jail is a sign of our failed mental health system." This comment relates to the concern expressed by family members that the system will not respond to escalating situations until it is too late, with the result that the loved one is sent to a lock-up rather than to a treatment setting.

The impact of mental disorder can be seen in health care utilization figures. Combined, general hospitals and provincial psychiatric hospitals logged over 10 million hospital bed days for persons with mental disorders in Canada in 2000-01, with the overall average length of a stay being 36 days in general hospitals and 160 days in psychiatric hospitals (although stays in general hospitals are shorter, they represent the majority of admissions) (Canadian Mental Health Association 2003). A survey by the British Columbia government found that, for the period 1997-2000, acute hospital bed utilization by psychiatry patients accounted for 30 percent of all hospital bed days, a figure disproportionate to the number of persons involved (British Columbia Ministry of Health Services 2003a, xvi). In 1998 hospital care costs for mental disorders in Canada totalled $2.7 billion, about one and a half times the hospital care costs for cancer (Health Canada 2000). In 1997 Health Canada estimated that 8 percent of physician care expenditures, 8 percent of drug costs, and 14 percent of hospital costs were associated with mental disorders.

More difficult to quantify, but all too real, is the anguish felt by loved ones involved with a person suffering from a mental disorder. Concerning the situation of family members, a Health Canada (2002b, 20) report notes that "[they] face the anxiety of an uncertain future and the stress of what can be a severe and limiting disability. The heavy demands of care may lead to burnout. Families sometimes fear that they caused the illness. The cost of medication, time off work, and extra support can create a severe financial burden for families. Both the care requirements and the stigma attached to mental illness often lead to isolation of family members from the community and their social support network and may even contribute to the suicide of a family member." In an editorial, a former president of the Canadian Psychiatric Association suggests that the burden of caring for family members "will almost certainly increase over the coming years as the health care system continues to experience financial constraints" (Woodside 2003, 6).

Stigma

Arguably the most difficult aspect of being diagnosed with a mental disorder is the stigma that goes along with it – a "traumatic death sentence" in the words of a recipient of psychiatric services (Capponi 2003, 110) and "social annihilation" in the words of a practitioner (Arboleda-Florez 2003, 635). Two Canadian researchers observe that "schizophrenia sufferers and family members continue to experience social stigma as ... the single most important factor undermining their quality of life" (Stuart and Arboleda-Florez 2001, 251). In reviewing the literature on this subject, Corrigan and colleagues (2003, 1105) conclude that "a majority of [clients] perceive themselves as being stigmatized by others, expect to be treated poorly by the public because of this stigma, and suffer demoralization and low self-esteem

Violence and Mental Disorder

Concerning the purported relationship between mental disorder and violence, American academic John Monahan (1992, 511) notes that "few questions in mental health law are as empirically complex or as politically controversial." He goes on to point out that, notwithstanding its sensitive nature, grappling with this subject is necessary since beliefs about mental disorder drive our informal responses to persons with mental health problems as well as formal laws and policies. For example, prominent psychiatrist and author Edwin Fuller Torrey (1997) has claimed, sensationally, that one thousand homicides a year in the United States are perpetrated by assailants with untreated mental disorders, using this and other assertions to support more coercive modes of treatment, such as outpatient committals.[5] Similarly, high-profile cases have been used as the impetus for new legislation in Canada, such as the Ontario statute providing for involuntary outpatient treatment, which was named "Brian's Law" after a sportscaster killed by an apparently mentally disordered man. While cases like this have given the impression of a clear link between mental disorder and violence, attempts to examine this question more systematically have produced much more equivocal results, in part because of the inherent methodological difficulties (Davis 1991).

That being said, a number of themes can now be identified from an accumulating body of evidence.

First, substance misuse is an important determinant of violent behaviour. This was illustrated by a large-scale study undertaken in Pennsylvania as part of the MacArthur Violence Risk Assessment Study, an ongoing multisite project (Steadman et al. 1998). Researchers followed 1,136 patients discharged from psychiatric wards for one year and found that their risk for violence was no different from the base level in the community, *except* for among those who were found to be abusing drugs or alcohol. Even more compelling numbers come from a twenty-five-year follow-up study of persons diagnosed with schizophrenia in Australia, where it was found that clients with substance abuse problems picked up *six times* the number of criminal convictions as those without substance abuse problems (Wallace, Mullen, and Burgess 2004). The clinical challenge here concerns the finding that persons with mental disorders are unfortunately more vulnerable to substance misuse than members of the general public (Regier et al. 1990).[6]

Second, a few specific symptoms, which have been referred to as TCO (threat control override) (Norko and Baranoski 2005), especially if persistent or untreated, may account for a substantial proportion of violent behaviour among mentally disordered persons. In particular, symptoms reflective of paranoid thinking may be significant, such as beliefs that one is being controlled, followed, or plotted against or that thoughts are being withdrawn from or inserted into one's mind (Arboleda-Florez 1998; Norko and Baranoski 2005; Swanson et al. 1996). More often than not these symptoms are treatable.

Third, environmental factors are significant. One study concludes that "persons with persistent psychiatric disorders may be at increased risk for committing violence because of socioeconomic factors and because of how, where and with whom they live, rather than because of their psychiatric disorders" (Estroff et al. 1994, 670). Persons with serious, persistent mental disorders are overrepresented among homeless populations and in skid-row settings, where day-to-day survival is a difficult challenge.

Fourth, violence by mentally disordered persons is most often directed at intimates, particularly family members, rather than at strangers – the same pattern seen in the general public (Arboleda-Florez 1998; Estroff et al. 1994; Lefley 1997).

Finally, persons with mental disorders are disproportionately victimized themselves, with one study finding the 331 clients in the sample to have experienced two and a half times the general population's rate of violent victimization (Hiday et al. 1999).

due to the internalization of the stigma." Persons identified as mentally disordered can anticipate landlords not wanting to rent to them, employers not wanting to hire them, and potential friends and romantic partners not wanting to associate with them. All of this can create a "why bother even trying?" sort of hopelessness (Barkhimer 2003). A Canadian Mental Health Association publication sums up the devastating psychological impact of stigma: "Discrimination has an all-encompassing, corrosive effect on personhood and citizenship ... the social isolation that results from discrimination impedes recovery and, given that people with mental illnesses are members of the same culture that stigmatizes them, they often internalize negative stereotypes and convert them into self-loathing and self-blame, attitudes that further affect recovery, because people come to expect devaluation and rejection" (Everett et al. 2003, 13).[7]

Stigma is also one of the key reasons why persons with mental health problems may delay or avoid seeking treatment (Arboleda-Florez 2003). For example, a study conducted in Israel found that 80 percent of patients referred to a psychiatrist by their family doctor refused the referral because of the stigma of receiving psychiatric care (Ben Noun 1996). Even mental health professionals may be reluctant to disclose an "in-treatment" status: a survey of psychiatric residents in New York found that while 61 percent stated that they would tell their supervisor that they were in psychotherapy, only 4 percent said that they would disclose being on antipsychotic medication (reported in Barkhimer 2003). Canadian data come from the Canadian Community Health Survey, a study involving 37,000 respondents from all provinces, published by Statistics Canada (2003). It was found that 60 percent of those reporting symptoms of mood, anxiety, or substance-use disorders did not seek treatment. Among this group, those who stated that they *needed* treatment were asked why they didn't seek it: the most common reasons given were that they preferred to manage it themselves (31%), that they did not get around to it (19%), and that they were afraid to ask or were afraid of what others would think (18%) (subjects could choose more than one answer). Readers should bear in mind that this study did not include questions about psychotic conditions – such as schizophrenia – which are arguably the most stigmatizing of all disorders (Arkar and Eker 1992; Capponi 2003; Dinos et al. 2004).

A number of stigmatizing beliefs are known to be associated with public conceptions of mental disorder. A survey by the Canadian Mental Health Association found that the most common of these were that persons with mental disorders (1) are dangerous or violent; (2) lack intelligence or are mentally handicapped; (3) cannot be cured; (4) cannot function or hold a job, having nothing to contribute; (5) lack willpower and are weak or lazy;

(6) are unpredictable and can't be trusted; and (7) are to blame for their illness and should "shape up" (cited in British Columbia Partners for Mental Health and Addictions Information 2003d).

Discriminatory attitudes are sometimes assessed using the concept of "social distance" (Angermeyer, Beck, and Matschinger 2003; Lauber et al. 2004). An example of this comes from a study of 1,653 randomly chosen residents of Calgary, where, by means of a telephone survey, respondents were asked several questions about persons diagnosed with schizophrenia (Stuart and Arboleda-Florez 2001). As the authors note, social distance increased with the level of intimacy required in the relationship; while fewer than 7 percent of subjects said that they would "feel ashamed if people knew someone in [their] family was diagnosed with schizophrenia," one in five (18.1%) said that they would be unable to maintain a friendship with someone with this diagnosis, almost half (47%) said that they would feel "upset or disturbed" about having such a person as a roommate, and over three-quarters (75.2%) said that they would not marry a person diagnosed with schizophrenia. Respondents were asked how they would feel about having a small psychiatric group home in their neighborhood: about 25 percent were in favour, 8 percent opposed, and 67 percent "indifferent."[8]

The association between mental disorder and violence is a particularly strong one in the perception of the public, despite evidence to the contrary (see box). This is illustrated by the results of a large-scale American survey involving 1,444 subjects who were given five vignettes, depicting: (1) a person with schizophrenia, (2) a person with depression, (3) a "troubled person," (4) a person with alcohol dependence, and (5) a person with drug dependence (Link et al. 1999). Respondents were asked how likely they felt it was that the person described in the vignette would do something violent toward others: one-third (33%) indicated that violence was somewhat or very likely in the case of the depressed person, with the figure for the person with schizophrenia being 61 percent, even though there was no mention of violence in any of the vignettes (the figures were somewhat higher for the drug user and alcohol user, and substantially lower for the "troubled person").

One of the most troubling accusations concerns the role that mental health practitioners themselves may play in contributing to stigma. This can occur through an attitude of clinical pessimism that is conveyed directly or indirectly to the client; as a result of medication side effects that impair concentration and work performance and cause the person to look "different"; and through the insensitive use of diagnostic labels. An example of the latter is the term "chronic," which has been used in psychiatry as an adjective ("chronic mental illness," "the chronic wards") and, even worse, as a noun ("the chronics"). This term, while still used, has been dropped from Canadian psychiatric training manuals, although there is always the concern that replacement words such as "persistent" will in time take on the same negative connotation (Lesage and Morissette 2002). A Canadian Mental Health Association (British Columbia Division 1999, 8) publication gives examples of other value-laden terms used by professionals, such as "low/high-functioning," "inappropriate," "non-compliant" and "treatment-resistant." When handling a loaded term like "schizophrenia," practitioners must sometimes walk a very narrow line, dealing with, on the one side, the need to demystify mental disorder and be "up front" with the client about diagnosis and, on the other side, concerns about how psychiatric labels are perceived by others, such as employers and landlords. Kirk and Kutchins (1992) note that in this regard clinicians may deliberately "under-diagnose" to avoid the worst effects of labelling.

Education is clearly crucial in addressing the stigma that is attached to mental disorders. While the public's understanding in this area may not be as unsophisticated as some might think, surveys continue to uncover deficits in knowledge. For example, while 59 percent of respondents in Stuart and Arboleda-Florez's (2001) Alberta study identified the cause of schizophrenia as a "brain disease" or "other biological factor" – consistent with the

Changing Minds: Public Education

Researchers who have implemented and evaluated public education programs have found the process to be more complex than originally anticipated. One example of this comes from a study conducted at the Centre for Addiction and Mental Health in Toronto, where a multimodal program to destigmatize mental disorder, called Beyond the Cuckoo's Nest, was put on for high school students. The study sought to evaluate the impact of a video produced by staff and clients at the centre, which the authors describe as a "powerful and moving portrayal of the challenges facing individuals doubly burdened by mental illness and homelessness" (Tolomiczenko, Goering, and Durbin 2001, 254). It was found, however, that students who *only* saw the video subsequently expressed more negative attitudes toward mental illness and stronger feelings of danger associated with homeless persons than did a control group of students who attended the centre's program without seeing the video. By comparison, the video combined with an audience discussion that included one of the video's subjects was found to *decrease* stigmatizing attitudes, leading the authors to conclude: "These findings point toward a pernicious aspect of stigma attached to mental illness; namely, a tendency to ratchet in a negative direction when emotionally charged material is not grounded or interpreted in the context of either direct discussion or proximate relations [through a friend or family member] with a person or persons living with mental illness" (256; see also Wallach 2004).

The counterintuitive finding of a video (alone) producing negative effects has been observed in other settings in Canada and Europe (Arboleda-Florez 2003; Gaebel and Baumann 2003). The Toronto study did find, however, that greater prior exposure to homeless persons was associated with more tolerant attitudes: subjects with "higher exposure" were less in favour of restrictions being placed on homeless persons and were more inclined to attribute homelessness to economic determinants than to individual pathology.

A second example of an anti-stigma intervention comes from Calgary, the purpose of which was to "assess the extent to which print news about schizophrenia and mental illness could be directly influenced by providing reporters with more accurate background information and by helping them develop more positive story lines" (Stuart 2003, 652). To this end, a senior editor was recruited, newspaper staff were invited to anti-stigma events, and mental health service providers acted as liaison persons and offered expert opinions. Newspaper stories concerning mental illness were analyzed over an eight-month, pre-test baseline period and over a sixteen-month post-test period. It was found that while positive mental health stories increased in number (33%) and length (25%) during the post-test period, *negative* stories also increased in number (25%) and length (100%). In particular, stigmatizing stories about schizophrenia – involving public security concerns linked to people not in treatment – "increased at a faster pace than positive news" (654). Despite these results, the study's author points to the importance of (1) making accurate background briefs available to the media, (2) maintaining a list of local experts for interviews, and (3) maintaining regular contact with key editorial staff. In commenting on this and other studies, Arboleda-Florez (2003, 648) suggests that broad, or "generic," approaches to mental health literacy, particularly among already educated subjects, may not be as effective as the targeting of specific beliefs using "specifically focused interventions among small groups such as high school students ... clinical workers ... [and] ethnic minorities." Corrigan (2004) defines "target-specific" programs as those aimed at the groups that have power in the lives of mental health clients (e.g., landlords, employers, health care providers, criminal justice personnel, policy makers, and the media) and at the specific discriminating behaviours of these groups.

best current evidence – about one-third could not identify a cause, and, further, almost one-half (47.2%) stated that persons with this diagnosis "suffer from split or multiple personalities."

Concerning the genesis of erroneous beliefs, Link and colleagues (2001, 1621) note that people "develop conceptions of mental illness early in life from family lore, personal experience, peer relations, and the media's portrayal of people with mental illnesses." Regarding the media, a relatively recent example that created some controversy was the Jim Carrey motion picture comedy *Me, Myself and Irene* (released in 2000), which featured a split-faced/personalitied Carrey along with the caption "from gentle to mental" on the publicity poster – resulting in justifiable protests by advocacy organizations (see also Wahl 1995). News accounts have also tended to portray mentally disordered persons as dangerous and unpredictable, a reflection of how these sources decontextualize issues and of the maxim that "sensationalism sells" (McIlwraith 1987, 14). Goering, Wasylenki, and Durbin (2000) note that in Canada, when mental health issues are covered at all, the media tend to focus on negative topics such as homelessness and violence.

Historically, advocacy groups such as the Canadian Mental Health Association and the Schizophrenia Society have taken on the role of public education. Increasingly, however, there has been a recognition that clinical staff and indeed all persons working in the larger system have a part to play, given the significance of stigma as a barrier to treatment and **recovery**. Notably, the World Psychiatric Association has launched a campaign – "Open the Doors" – to fight stigma and discrimination resulting from the diagnosis of schizophrenia (Dubey 1999).

Notes

1 For example, in an interview Toronto psychiatrist Marshall Korenblum expresses concern about the "medicalizing of the human condition" and questions whether "doctors are too quick to prescribe drugs for routine sadness and normal existential angst" (Branham 2003, B2; see also Mechanic 1999; Peyser 2004; Ross, Ali, and Toner 2003).

2 Treatability may be referred to, at least indirectly, in the statutory criteria for involuntary hospitalization; in Britich Columbia, for example, the *Mental Health Act* states that persons with mental disorders may be hospitalized against their will if they require "treatment in or through a designated facility."

3 One can take note of the following "diagnostic criteria for identifying persons with highest priority for service," which estimates disability as a function of diagnosis (British Columbia Ministry of Health 2002e, 32): "all schizophrenic and related disorders; all bipolar disorders; 20 percent of major depressive disorders; 20 percent of panic and obsessive-compulsive disorders; 10 percent of social phobia (co-morbid with avoidant personality disorder); and 10 percent of substance-abuse disorders (principally drug dependence)." The figures here presumably have an empirical basis, although the source is not given.

4 Epidemiologists attempt to operationalize the concept of disability by calculating "disability days," which are days when a person is unable to carry out normal activities or to get as

much done as usual because of health problems (expressed as a monthly rate; see Andrews et al. 2000).

5   Torrey is President of the Treatment Advocacy Center, whose mandate is to "eliminate barriers to timely treatment of severe mental illness" (see http://www.psychlaws.org). For a rebuttal of Torrey's claim of "1,000 homicides," see Vine (2001).

6   One study concludes that "treatment non-compliance by persons with co-occurring disorders may not reflect personal motivation for recovery so much as sabotage by others with vested interests in impeding the recovery" (Sells et al. 2003, 1256), a reference to the observation that mentally disordered persons may be more easily exploited by predatory persons, such as drug dealers.

7   Corrigan (2004) distinguishes "public stigma" and "self-stigma," the latter being reactions that individuals turn against themselves; sociology students may note that self-stigma has parallels with the concept of "secondary deviance" (see also Dinos et al. 2004).

8   The likelihood of "social desirability" response bias in telephone interviews means that the negative answers may be underestimates.

Other Resources

- "Open the Doors," an anti-stigma program sponsored by the World Psychiatric Association, has a number of links and downloadable documents at its website (http://www.openthedoors.com).
- A Canadian anti-stigma website run by the Kelty Patrick Dennehy Foundation (http://www.thekeltyfoundation.org) is named after an eighteen year old who committed suicide.

Nature and Nurture:
Explanatory Models in Psychiatry

The preceding chapter considered the question "who gets services?" The next important question is "what *form* do these services take?" For example, will the treatment approach rely mainly on the use of medication as opposed to nonpharmacological interventions? The answer to this depends in part on what technologies we may or may not have at our disposal. The form of the response also depends to a considerable extent on our understanding of the **etiology,** or cause, of mental disorders, an area where, unfortunately, there is still a great deal of uncertainty. As a former president of the Canadian Psychiatric Association observes, "Psychiatry remains a medical discipline long on disorders and short on explanations" (Marie-Albert 2002, 914). On the question of etiology, a Health Canada (2002b, 22) report is appropriately circumspect: "Mental illnesses are the result of a complex interaction of genetic, biological, personality and environmental factors; however, the brain is the final common pathway for the control of behaviour, cognition, mood and anxiety. At this time, the links between specific brain dysfunction and specific mental illnesses are not fully understood."

Some themes have emerged from research conducted in recent years: (1) the evidence for a biological etiology is very strong for conditions such as schizophrenia and bipolar disorder (Kendlar 2003, 2004; Kieseppa et al. 2004; McGuffin et al. 2003); (2) there is increasing evidence that even in the case of (apparently) less "organic-appearing" conditions – such as personality disorders – manifestation of symptoms is mediated by intrinsic vulnerabilities, constitutional and acquired (Paris 1998b); (3) notwithstanding the two preceding points, the expression of symptoms of mental disorders is still influenced to a great extent by environmental stressors; (4) attempts to view biological and environmental determinants in isolation may be misguided, and there is greater utility in viewing mental health problems as the product of a **stress-vulnerability** interaction (Andrews et al. 2000). On this last point, Kiesler (1999, 11) concludes that adherence to *monocausation* models "needs desperately to be abandoned ... available evidence makes it clear that most of the major psychiatric disorders are etiologically heterogeneous."

While mental disorders should thus be seen as "multidetermined" phenomena, it remains the case that individuals, depending on their training and orientation, their experiences in early life and as service recipients, and their personal beliefs, may tend to emphasize one set of etiological factors (e.g., genetics vs. child abuse) over another. While readers may be familiar with "nature vs. nurture" debates from undergraduate psychology courses, it must be stressed that, because of the significant symbolic, political, and practical implications, disagreements about etiology – between clinicians, clients, and family members – are among the most contentious seen in mental health practice and are not easily resolved. To highlight this, biological and psychosocial explanations of mental disorder, and their limitations, are reviewed separately in the following sections, recognizing that this is an artificial dichotomy.

Biological Determinants

Currently, in North America the dominant viewpoint in psychiatry is that conditions such as schizophrenia and bipolar disorder, as noted, are biological in origin and require biological treatments, a position that is supported by substantial empirical and clinical evidence (Dincin 2001; Haynes 2002; Kendlar 2004; Paris 2005). The idea that mental disorders have biological origins – the "somatogenic" viewpoint – is not a new one. In 1872 Dr. John Gray, superintendent of the New York State Asylum and editor of the *American Journal of Insanity,* concluded in a conference presentation that "the causes of insanity, as far as we are able to determine, are physical; that is, no moral or intellectual operations of the mind induce insanity apart from a physical lesion" (quoted in Eaton 2001, 272). Similarly, across the Atlantic, German psychiatrist Emil Kraepelin, one of the first to conduct research on *dementia praecox* (an early name for schizophrenia), published a text in 1883 with a classification system that attempted to establish the organic basis of mental disorders. Biological psychiatry was eventually superseded in North America in the early to mid-1900s by **psychodynamic** approaches (see below), becoming preeminent again in the second half of the century largely as a consequence of the breakthroughs seen with the use of new **psychotropic** medications. Its current preeminence may be judged by unequivocal statements such as the following by a prominent American psychiatrist:

It has now been established that severe mental illnesses, as defined by the National Advisory Mental Health Council, are neurobiological disorders of the brain. These illnesses are thus in the same category as other brain disorders such as Parkinson's disease, Alzheimer's disease, and multiple sclerosis. Like severe mental illnesses, each of these disorders is associated with measurable abnormalities in brain structure and function. And, as with severe mental illnesses, it is not yet known what factors – genes, developmental effects, viruses, toxins, or metabolic defects – contribute to the biological chain of events causing these disorders. (Torrey 1997, 5)

Preeminence may also be judged by the biological model's pervasive, almost hegemonic, influence on how mental health problems are viewed and conceptualized: "This perspective is so ingrained in our thinking as to be almost invisible. We often use it implicitly, without conscious thought, and allow it to shape our research and practice in important ways. Most often, it seems to be the only way to examine the issue of mental illness" (Boydell, Gladstone, and Crawford 2002, 20).

Evidence that mental disorders are biological in origin comes from studies of genetic transmission as well as from structural-imaging techniques. Concerning genetic determinants, researchers have used twins and/or adopted children as subjects to attempt to tease out the separate contributions of environmental and hereditary factors. In the case of bipolar disorder, for example, in a British study involving identical and nonidentical twins (who are, respectively, 100 percent and 50 percent genetically similar), researchers using a variety of mathematical models estimated the heritability of bipolar disorder to be 85 percent, with the remaining 15 percent of the variance in illness risk being attributed to unshared environmental factors (McGuffin et al. 2003). In the case of schizophrenia, Finnish researchers compared 190 adoptees considered a "high risk" for the condition, by virtue of having a biological mother with a schizophrenia spectrum disorder, with 137 "low-risk" adoptees, whose mothers did not have the diagnosis, with subjects being followed to a median age of 44 (Tienari et al. 2003). It was found that the mean, age-corrected morbid risk for a schizophrenia spectrum disorder was over fives time greater for the high-risk group (22.5%) than for the low-risk group (4.4%). While a definitive genetic model has not been found, a 2004 *American Journal of Psychiatry* editorial on the genetics of schizophrenia concludes that research in this area has progressed to the "gene localization" phase – localizing susceptibility genes to specific chromosomal regions – and is now moving into the phase where attempts are being made to identify these specific susceptibility genes (Kendlar 2004).

The biological paradigm is also supported by advances in imaging techniques – positron-emission tomography, magnetic-resonance spectroscopy, and functional magnetic-resonance imaging – that have enabled researchers to examine the physiological substrate of mental activities, leading one observer to speculate that "scientists may [now] venture into the frontier of the neural basis of spirituality and feelings" (Pietrini 2003, 1907). This author notes that imaging techniques have effectively eliminated the distinction between what used to be called "organic" psychiatric disorders (ones where there was a known structural alteration, like dementia) and "functional" disorders (ones like schizophrenia and depression where previously there were no known alterations), a distinction that "reflected our inability to go beyond what could be visible to the naked eye" (1908). Imaging techniques have been able to support "the concept of schizophrenia as a progressive neurodevelopmental disorder with both early and late developmental abnormalities" (Sporn et al. 2003).

Critiques

Not everyone is comfortable with the biomedical viewpoint. Adherents of the "socio-genic" perspective, who may see even psychotic disorders as having psychosocial origins, have argued that judgments about rationality are a function of context: an editorial in a Vancouver, BC, client-run newsletter, for example, speaks about psychosis as *"perfectly understandable emotional behavior under pressure"* (Thor-Larsen 2003, 4, emphasis added), a comment that echoes the views of Scottish psychiatrist R.D. Laing (1969) who, a generation ago, used existentialist philosophy to portray psychotic persons as individuals attempting to live in unlivable situations (see also Breggin 1991). Individuals concerned about the psychological impact and sequelae of child abuse argue that pathologizing and applying a medical label to what are, in their view, trauma-induced conditions is not only a misconception, but also a form of decontextualizing that has the effect of "blaming the victim" (Simmie and Nunes 2001). This critique is often made by feminist writers, such as Lev (1998, 3), who observes that: "The unhealthy ways a woman *copes* with the trauma becomes the avenue for diagnosis, instead of labeling the way she was victimized, or recognizing the healthy ways she has adapted in order to survive."

Other critics of the biomedical perspective take issue not so much with the view that mental disorders have biological origins as with the implications that this holds for treatment, arguing that the medical approach is, at its worst, narrow, reductionistic, and one that fosters excessive dependency, a position summarized by Toronto author and former client Pat Capponi (2003, 4):

If we assume everything is related to physiology then the primary, "sane" response is to treat mental illness with pharmaceuticals – a clean, easy solution, and one we have a lot of comfort with in the twenty-first century. It removes parental guilt and individual responsibility; it pathologizes and medicates behaviours; it elevates a pseudo-science to the big leagues. There is profit in the search for "magic bullets," in the research, development and marketing of newer, better, and costlier medications for the mind. Ultimately, though, this is a soulless and limiting response to pain and distress, however caused. In the rush to study, dissect, and understand the brain, we've forgotten that the whole individual is greater than the sum of her [*sic*] parts.

Sociologists have for some time spoken about how medical practice reinforces the "sick role," a role in which the patient is the passive recipient of professional expertise (e.g., Hewa 2002), which may be contrasted with the current psychiatric rehabilitation literature, where increasing emphasis is being placed on the importance of clients actively collaborating in, if not driving, the treatment and recovery plan (Anthony 2003; Bilsker 2003).

Critics have also argued that the focus on pathology, which is intrinsic to the biomedical model, means that the issue of *prevention* has been neglected or ignored. Even though community programs often have the phrase "mental health" in their titles, it has been observed that the preoccupation in these programs is in fact with illness – symptom management – rather than with health and that this is an approach to service delivery that is inefficient and ineffective. In their submission to the Commission on the Future of Health Care in Canada, the Canadian Mental Health Association (2001, 10) – referring to the high cost of hospital care – argued that the money spent in this area could be reduced by focusing on prevention rather than on "illness paradigms" and by building on determinants of health "such as physical and social environments, personal health practices and coping skills" (see box).

Concerning the definition of mental health, in its constitution the World Health Organization (1994, 1) notes that "health is a state of complete ... well-being and *not merely the absence of disease or infirmity*" (emphasis added). While acknowledging that the concept of mental health "has traditionally eluded definition," Wilson (1996, 70) states that the older, symptom-based definition of this term "has increasingly been challenged by a broader conception of mental health," incorporating interpersonal relationships, opportunities for self-actualization and growth, effective personal adaptation, and quality of life. In this scheme an individual without a mental disorder may still have poor mental health, while conversely someone with a mental illness may enjoy good mental health given the right environmental conditions since mental illness is only one determinant of wellbeing.

Finally, those emphasizing the biological basis of mental disorder have had to face one other, unexpected setback. It had been assumed that establishing a biological etiology would diminish the stigma associated with mental disorders for affected persons as well as their parents since these persons would presumably be considered blameless for their condition (Dincin 2001). This assumption, however, has not necessarily been borne out in surveys of clients or the general public. Service recipients may still find the "socio-genic" position more congenial, an example being the finding of a survey in Toronto of 102 persons diagnosed with depression that "patients did not particularly endorse the dominant biomedical explanation of depression," preferring instead the view that their mood disorder was caused by "stress or negative life events" (Srinivasan, Cohen, and Parikh 2003, 494-95). Concerning the general public, "social distance" surveys have found that blamelessness does not necessarily translate into greater social acceptance: studies conducted in Germany on beliefs about schizophrenia as a brain disease (Angermeyer, Beck, and Matschinger 2003) and in Switzerland on having a medical understanding of mental illness (Lauber et al. 2004) found, in both cases, that adherents of the biological viewpoint tended to express a preference for *greater* social distance from persons diagnosed with a psychiatric disorder.

Psychosocial Determinants

At the other end of the continuum from biological determinism is the view that mental disorders originate in stressful or difficult life experiences. Currently, the strongest expression of this position comes from the work of those involved with the victims of early-childhood abuse.

The socio-genic perspective has antecedents in the work of Durkheim, a late-nineteenth- and early-twentieth-century French sociologist who tried to link higher rates of suicide with industrialization and social upheaval, as well as in the efforts of the early leaders of the "moral treatment" movement, started in late-eighteenth-century Europe. As reviewed by Eaton (2001, 271), reformers such as Pinel (in Paris) and Tuke (in England) "recommended maximum freedom for the mentally ill, normal human dignity, and the stabilizing effects of work and religion ... were optimistic about the possibility of cure ... [and believed] that mental disorder was caused by rapid social change, urbanization, and dislocations in society." Interestingly, research conducted up to the present day continues to support an association between urbanization and increased incidence of mental disorders such as schizophrenia (Peen and Dekker 2004; Sundquist, Frank, and Sundquist 2004), but if urbanization is a risk factor, the interrelations are complicated (Van Os 2004).

The idea that psychiatric disorders can have a nonorganic, psychological basis gained strength with the work of Charcot, a nineteenth-century French neurologist, and the study of *hysteria*, where people would, for example, experience paralysis of part of a limb when there was no possible physical basis for the condition (Gallagher 1995) (in current psychiatric nomenclature, this is referred to as a "conversion disorder"). The work of Charcot and the study of hysteria influenced Sigmund Freud (1856-1939), who began to study the effect of the *unconscious* on the manifestation of mental disorders. Articulated about one hundred years ago, Freud's psychodynamic explanations became very influential in North America and Europe from the early to mid-1900s, determining to a considerable extent the nature of psychiatric practice. From this viewpoint early childhood experiences, rather than biological predisposition, were crucial to understanding the genesis of mental disorders. While Freud is known more for working with persons with neuroses – what we would now call anxiety disorders – protégés such as American psychoanalyst Harry Stack Sullivan applied similar techniques in working with individuals diagnosed with schizophrenia (Sadock and Sadock 2003). Increasing criticism of Freudian psychology, which included concerns about its theoretical validity as well as clinical utility (e.g., Gunderson et al. 1984; Wood 1986), has meant that psychodynamic approaches have now largely fallen out of favour in public mental health settings in North America.

In more recent years, the psychological effects of violence have come to be recognized in military and civilian populations. In the 1970s American psychologist Lenore Walker made some inroads by proposing the concept of "battered woman's syndrome," although this still controversial diagnosis has not been included in the *Diagnostic and Statistical Manual (DSM)* of the American Psychiatric Association (some now consider it to be an implied subcategory of post-traumatic stress disorder, or PTSD) (Walker 1992). Among military personnel, a prominent example of the effects of trauma

Determinants of Health

Listed below are twelve determinants of health, as suggested by Health Canada (2004b). While "biology and genetic endowment" is one of these, it is striking to see how many of the *other* determinants in the list represent deficits as applied to persons with serious mental disorders. By extension, these determinants also suggest target areas with which practitioners can assist. Determinants such as poverty and isolation can be seen as both causes *and* effects of psychiatric symptoms.

(1) *Income and social status,* (2) *education,* and (3) *employment.* As socioeconomic and educational status is strongly associated with better health, it should be noted that persons with serious mental disorders face high rates of unemployment and poverty-level incomes. With the onset of a disorder such as schizophrenia occurring in early adulthood, university education and early career trajectories are cut short in many instances.

(4) *Social support networks* and (5) *social environments.* Social support is associated with better health outcomes, with Health Canada (2004b, 4) noting that "the caring and respect that occurs in social relationships, and the resulting sense of satisfaction and well-being, seem to act as a buffer against health problems." Unfortunately, a large number of those diagnosed with mental disorders face isolation and exclusion, stigma being a major contributing factor. Others face unsafe social environments: frequently residing in poor, inner-city neighbourhoods, psychiatric clients are more likely to be physically and sexually assaulted.

(6) *Physical environments.* Decent, affordable housing is an urgent need for psychiatric clients, who disproportionately face chronic homelessness, which itself is associated with a host of negative health outcomes.

(7) *Coping skills.* This term is defined by Health Canada (2004a, 8) as "actions by which individuals can ... promote self-care, cope with challenges, develop self-reliance, solve problems and make choices that enhance health." Psychiatric clients may have poorer coping skills because of constitutional factors, because the onset of the disorder interrupted the learning process, and unfortunately because of psychiatric practices that have reinforced dependency.

(8) *Healthy child development.* A range of adult mental health problems are the result of childhood trauma.

(9) *Biology and genetic endowment.*

(10) *Health services.* Providing comprehensive, effective, and accessible mental health services continues to be a challenge for governments and health authorities in Canada.

(11) *Gender.* The etiology and expression of mental disorders may differ between the sexes, which has implications for service delivery, one example being the need for programs sensitive to the experiences of sexual assault victims. As the socio-economic status of women remains, on average, lower than that of men, women may be differentially affected by social determinants of health.

(12) *Culture.* The First Nations have poorer health outcomes in many areas, with substance misuse and higher suicide rates being a particular concern for mental health practitioners.

comes from the experiences of Canadians serving as United Nations peace-keepers in the African nation of Rwanda, where, in 1994, some 800,000 Tutsi, an ethnic minority, were slaughtered in a civil war by the majority Hutu. A substantial number of the Canadians who witnessed the atrocities later developed post-traumatic stress disorder, including the mission com-mander General Romeo Dallaire, who subsequently described symptoms such as distress, insomnia, nightmares, and thoughts of suicide in a pub-lished memoir (Dallaire and Beardsley 2003).

It is notable, however, that while evidence of the psychological impact of violence has been documented for some time, including the identification of "shell shock" in the First World War, not until 1980 was post-traumatic stress disorder included in the *Diagnostic and Statistical Manual* – largely as a response to the experiences and lobbying of returning Vietnam War veter-ans in the United States (Yehuda 2002). (The criteria for PTSD in the *DSM* refer to the person experiencing an event "that involved actual or threatened death or serious injury, or a threat to the physical integrity of self or others," where the person's response "involved intense fear, helplessness, or horror" [American Psychiatric Association 2000, 466].)

Notwithstanding the advent of PTSD, it is arguably the case that the psy-chological effects of trauma, and in particular child and spouse abuse, have been overlooked or downplayed in psychiatric practice (Van der Kolk 2002). Notably, Freud himself recognized a connection between childhood sexual abuse and adult mental health problems, but the uproar that this created among his contemporaries led him subsequently to disavow trauma as a causal factor by interpreting patients' accounts of incest as mere sexual fan-tasies (Russell 1986). In an article on "trauma-informed service system(s)," authors Harris and Fallot (2001) talk about the need for a "paradigm shift," arguing that mental health programs still do not adequately screen for trauma histories in new clients given the high rates of abuse seen in this population; as a consequence, these authors note, appropriate referrals are not made, or even worse, insensitive responses may result in the client being retraumatized. Some have also argued that the underrecognition of trauma is reflected in the use and misuse of the borderline personality diagnosis, which has be-come pejorative both in the eyes of clients and clinicians and which some claim is actually a misdiagnosis of persons suffering from PTSD (Briere 2002; Mina and Gallop 1998; Simmie and Nunes 2001).

Critiques
One might assume that the inclusion of post-traumatic stress disorder in the *DSM*, among other things, would have cemented the link between trauma and mental disorder in the minds of psychiatric practitioners. However, some

controversies and disagreements remain. One critique is methodological, with an author noting that most of the research on risk factors has used retrospective designs – interviews of adult clients about their memories of childhood experiences – which "can never establish causality" (Paris 1998a, 150). There is also debate as to whether PTSD can be considered a "trait" or "state" phenomenon – that is, whether the manifestation of a disorder can be attributed largely or wholly to the traumatic event or, in fact, to constitutional vulnerabilities (Briere 2002; Kluft, Bloom, and Kinzie 2000). On this point, a Canadian researcher suggests that individual differences are considerably more significant than the traumatic event itself in understanding client responses (Bowman 1999). Nonetheless, while individuals may differ with respect to vulnerability and resiliency, large-scale research has shown a clear association between early-life trauma and anxiety, personality, and mood disorders (Spataro et al. 2004). A literature review in the *Canadian Journal of Psychiatry* concludes that "despite the methodological limitations of the research in this area, there is strong evidence of a link between childhood sexual and physical abuse and adult self-harm, suicidal ideation and suicidal behaviours" (Mina and Gallop 1998, 793).

The Stress-Vulnerability Model

The preceding leads into a consideration of what has been called the stress-vulnerability (or stress-diathesis) model, which is an acknowledgment that *both* environmental and intrinsic factors (biological and psychological vulnerabilities, constitutional and acquired) contribute to the expression of a mental disorder (Haddock and Tarrier 1998). "Expression" here can mean either the initial onset or the subsequent relapse in persons already diagnosed. As reviewed by Eaton (2001), the assumption here is that more vulnerable individuals – for instance, those with a high degree of "genetic loading" – will manifest symptoms even in conditions of low stress, whereas less vulnerable persons may never meet the criteria for the disorder if they remain within protective environments. Empirical support for the model comes from a long-term follow-up study of 847 New Zealanders (Holden 2003); researchers found that persons with the "short" form of a gene that affects the regulation of serotonin – a neurotransmitter that plays a role in mood disorders – were more likely to report depression in association with an environmental stressor (such as bereavement or job crisis) but no more likely to manifest depression when no stressor was present. Similarly, in a Dutch study that followed 140 teens considered a high risk for bipolar disorder because one parent was so diagnosed, researchers looking at the impact of stressful early life events on the onset of mood disorder found that the risk of mood disorder increased by 10 percent for each "unit" of stressful life event (Hillegers et al. 2004).

In this model, the threshold for a breakthrough of symptoms is lowered by vulnerability factors and environmental factors, examples of the latter being the loss of a job, a relationship break-up, or abuse of street drugs. The threshold is raised by protective factors, which, as per Andrews and colleagues (2000), include medication, social support, stress management, and problem-solving skills. There is thus, at least in theory, the potential for greater personal empowerment in that, notwithstanding predispositions, the client and practitioner can control recovery to a considerable extent by addressing factors such as lifestyle and coping skills.

In describing an education program for clients experiencing a psychotic disorder, the authors of a practice guidelines document emphasize the importance of the stress-vulnerability model as a framework for presenting information:

> Within this [model], one can present both biological and psychosocial strategies to reduce the risk of psychosis and prevent relapse: complying with medications, avoiding substance use, managing interpersonal conflict, making use of peer support, identifying and managing environmental stressors, learning the "early warning signs" of the illness, developing and planning proactive coping and help-seeking strategies. By presenting recovery from a first episode as an active process that occurs in recognizable stages, the educator helps both the individual and family to normalize their own experiences and to recognize the value of their own contribution to the recovery. (Mental Health Evaluation and Community Consultation Unit 2002, 14)

Remaining challenges for the practitioner include the difficulty in mitigating stress in a client population that faces considerable socio-economic disadvantage; as well as the prospect that persons adamantly opposed to medical explanations will still find the stress-vulnerability model to be unpalatable given the emphasis placed on medication as, quoting one text, "the most important protective factor" (Andrews et al. 2000, 339).

Mental Disorders: Classification and Criteria

3

This chapter provides an introduction to diagnosis and a description of the major classes of mental disorder, including schizophrenia, depression, bipolar disorder, anxiety disorders, and disorders first seen in childhood and later life. Readers may also consult standard texts such as the American Psychiatric Association's *Diagnostic and Statistical Manual (DSM)*, the *Merck Manual*, and Sadock and Sadock's *Synopsis of Psychiatry*. As well, a number of websites offer nonspecialists useful information on psychiatric disorders, such as the Report on Mental Illnesses in Canada at Health Canada's website (http://www.hc-sc.gc.ca). The treatment approaches referred to here are discussed in more detail later in the book.

The *DSM*

The psychiatric diagnostic system used in almost all Canadian settings is the *Diagnostic and Statistical Manual*, published by the American Psychiatric Association (2000), which as of this writing was the fourth edition, with text revision (*DSM* IV-TR). The other major system in use is the *International Statistical Classification of Diseases and Related Health Problems (ICD)*, published by the World Health Organization. While attempts have been made to harmonize these two systems, there are differences in the criteria and definitions used, and where diagnostic criteria are used here they will refer to the *DSM*.

The classification system articulated in the *DSM* has been evolving for over fifty years, with ongoing disputes about the validity and reliability of the definitions given in the various revisions of this publication (Genova 2003). A very apparent problem with the early versions of the *DSM* was a lack of clarity in how the disorders were defined, which in turn led to poor interrater agreement when making diagnoses. As reviewed by Eaton (2001), studies on the *DSM*'s diagnostic reliability conducted between 1950 and 1980, using a value of the *kappa* statistic of 0.50 as the minimum acceptable standard,[1] found not one study that was able to attain values above 0.50 for all diagnostic categories; schizophrenia was diagnosed more reliably, relatively speaking, with kappa values above 0.50 being achieved in five of seven studies, while rates of agreement on personality disorders were so low as to be considered unacceptable.

To address problems with reliability, the system changed in 1980 (with the *DSM* III) to a descriptive approach, where clinicians were provided with a "checklist" of operational criteria, which improved diagnostic reliability (Eaton 2001; Grove 1987). As well, later editions of the *DSM* have been deliberately atheoretical, avoiding reference to the etiology of disorders, apparently to obviate disagreements that might arise between different factions in the psychiatric community – although in doing this, the *DSM* ignores one of the purposes of classification (Williams 1994).

Concerning the checklist approach, critics have suggested that the *DSM* still "falls short of using fully operational critieria," pointing out that "terms such as 'often' and 'easily' are used without guidance about the severity of the problems they represent" (Nietzel, Bernstein, and Milich 1998, 367). The checklist approach also means that there is a cut-off (for example, that five of nine criteria must be present) above which a person is said to "have" a disorder and below which he or she doesn't. Some critics have been uncomfortable with this logic, arguing that psychological disorders can be present in varying degrees (Carson 1991). In commenting on the approach used in the *DSM*, Fauman (2002, 11) suggests that differentiation between persons with pathological and mild symptoms is achieved by adhering to the general diagnostic principle that the disorder must be one that causes "clinically significant distress or impairment in social, occupational, or other important areas of functioning."

Historically, criteria have been included in the *DSM* largely on the basis of clinical judgment rather than empirical research. Because of the potential for bias inherent in this approach, starting with the *DSM* IV in 1994, experts were organized into "working groups," which were to incorporate empirical as well as clinical literature and which also conducted field trials using the proposed diagnostic criteria. Despite these efforts, some have expressed concern that there is still too much reliance on consensus in creating diagnostic categories – that is, that the process is more political than scientific. (On this matter, Canadian psychologist Paula Caplan has suggested that the predominantly male caucus that revises the *DSM* has produced a document that manifests a gender bias, among other things [Caplan 1995; Larkin and Caplan 1992; Pantony and Caplan 1991]).

Starting in 1980, the *DSM* introduced the *multiaxial* system, which is intended to (1) give a fuller picture of a client's psychological, physical, and social functioning and (2) enhance diagnostic validity. The five axes currently used are as follows:

- *Axis I:* Clinical disorders and other conditions that may be a focus of clinical attention. This refers to disorders such as schizophrenia, depression, and bipolar disorder and also includes substance-related disorders such as alcohol abuse.
- *Axis II:* Personality disorders and intellectual disability. The rationale for coding these on a separate axis is so that "consideration will be given to the possible presence of personality disorders and mental retardation that would otherwise be overlooked when attention is directed to the usually *more florid* Axis I disorders" (American Psychiatric Association 2000, 28, emphasis added). The *DSM* also offers the option of recording personality *traits* that do not meet the threshold for a personality disorder (687).
- *Axis III:* General medical conditions. This refers to diseases and congenital anomalies that may or may not be related to the mental disorder, such as hyperthyroidism or cancer. It is noted in the *DSM* that this is not meant to imply that mental disorders are unrelated to biological factors or that general medical conditions do not have psychosocial sequelae but to encourage "thoroughness in evaluation" (29).
- *Axis IV:* Psychosocial or environmental problems "that may affect the diagnosis, treatment and prognosis of mental disorders" (31). The *DSM* lists a number of these, such as occupational, housing, and legal difficulties.
- *Axis V:* Global assessment of functioning (GAF), a scale that ranges from 1 to 100, with the highest number indicating "superior functioning in a wide range of activities" (34). Scales of this type can be problematic with respect to their interrater reliability, although guidelines in using the GAF are offered in the *DSM* in an attempt to achieve greater accuracy in application. As an alternative to the GAF, assessors may use the Social and Occupational Functioning and Assessment Scale (SOFAS), which is included as an appendix in the *DSM* IV-TR. The SOFAS is intended to reflect functional ability, which may be more useful with respect to rehabilitation planning than the symptom-based GAF (Hay et al. 2003).

Where no condition is present this is coded as "none" (Axes I to III), and where more information is needed the practitioner may enter "deferred." The formulation created will often include **differential diagnoses** – that is, other conditions that need to be ruled in or out before a more specific diagnosis can be made.

Each diagnostic group also contains a "not otherwise specified" (NOS) option, categories that may serve as "catch-all diagnoses that can be used when a patient does not fit a more specific diagnosis" (Fauman 2002, 12). ("Psychosis NOS" is frequently seen in the case of persons briefly admitted to a hospital emergency where there is little background information available on the client and, presumably, no time to gather this collateral data.) Writing in the *Study Guide to the DSM IV-TR* (Fauman 2002, 12), the author concedes that the NOS option is problematic since persons so diagnosed will be a heterogeneous group and, therefore, the diagnosis will offer "little predictive value for response to treatment or illness prognosis"; he goes on to say that "every effort should be made to gather the necessary clinical information to make a more specific diagnosis" and that the NOS option should be used "as little as possible." Indeed, without detailed historical information and collateral accounts, any diagnosis is necessarily tentative and should be considered a "work in progress."

With mental disorders coded on both of the first two axes, one can ask whether Axis II conditions should be considered qualitatively different from those of Axis I. Among practitioners there is some question as to whether Axis II diagnoses constitute a "serious, persistent mental illness" and, consequently, whether persons so diagnosed should be eligible for services from community mental health programs. While the *DSM* states that coding disorders on Axis II "should not be taken to imply that their pathogenesis or range of appropriate treatment is fundamentally different from Axis I conditions" (American Psychiatric Association 2000, 28), there may be a tendency to regard Axis II conditions as less serious ("florid"). One commentator on this problem observes that, "ironically, whereas a separate axis for personality was created to encourage practitioners to take these forms of pathology into account, it has often led only to their isolation in an Axis II ghetto" (Paris 1998b, 135). Canadian psychiatrist W. John Livesley (1998) has suggested that personality disorders should in fact be coded on the same axis as other mental disorders, and in fact the American Psychiatric Association has started to discuss the possible "merger" of Axis I with Axis II (Peyser 2004).

There are other cautions that should be borne in mind when using the *DSM* or other diagnostic systems:

- Because diagnosis does not speak to the level of disability or ability, other, more *functional* assessments may be necessary. For example, with respect to the assessment of financial competence, a specialist in this area notes that "decisions should be based on function, not diagnosis" (Donnelly 1996, 485).
- While efforts have been made with the *DSM* to improve interrater agreement, the use of some psychiatric categories may still be influenced by local tendencies, influential mentors, or personal idiosyncrasy.[2]

- Attempts to achieve greater diagnostic reliability by using "checklists" do not necessarily result in greater diagnostic *validity*; that is, the diagnosis may still not adequately represent a particular clinical construct. For example, one Canadian psychiatrist argues that the current *DSM* conceptualization of pervasive developmental disorder does not reflect the "true" nature of the phenomenon (Szatmari 2000; see also Hare 1996).
- In a number of instances, clients – particularly victims of trauma – may present with a range of *co-occurring* symptoms, which makes problematic the presumption that clinical entities are separate, or "primary," as implied in a diagnostic formulation (Ballou and Brown 2002; Harris and Fallot 2001).

With these cautions in mind, the remainder of this chapter provides a brief overview of the major mental disorders, their diagnostic criteria as reflected in the *DSM*, and some comments about etiology and treatment.

Schizophrenia

The term "schizophrenia" was coined by Swiss psychiatrist Eugen Bleuler in the early 1900s (replacing an earlier term, "dementia precox"). It means literally "split mind," to denote the schisms between thought, emotion, and behaviour that Bleuler saw in patients with this condition (Sadock and Sadock 2003). Unfortunately, "schizophrenic" is now commonly used in public discourse to refer to, among other things, a "Jekyll and Hyde" personality, disjointed thinking, or contradictory behaviour, which has trivialized the term and contributed to the stigmatizing effect of this diagnosis (Duckworth et al. 2003). Schizophrenia is in fact a serious psychotic disorder that may persist for years and that can cause "marked social, educational or occupational dysfunction" (Health Canada 2002b, 2). Lifetime prevalence rates for this disorder vary from 0.3 to 1.6 percent of the population, depending on the study cited (Goldner et al. 2002).

Symptoms

The symptoms of schizophrenia have been classified in different ways, with a commonly used conceptualization distinguishing *positive* from *negative* features, "positive" denoting a presence and "negative" an absence. The positive signs include:

- *Hallucinations*, that is, false perceptions or sensations. Commonly these are auditory, involving a voice or voices that only the individual can hear. These voices may, in some cases, be simply distracting or can, in other cases, be distressing. Concern may be raised in the case of "command **hallucinations**," where the voices instruct the individual to do something, such as harm him or herself.

- *Delusions,* that is, false beliefs that are held despite contradictory evidence. Often times there is paranoia, an unfounded conviction that the individual is being persecuted. **Delusions** can take various forms, such as the idea that your food is being poisoned, that your mother is really a clone, or that UFOs are sending radio waves into your apartment. Persons with schizophrenia may have "ideas of reference," in which case apparently innocuous objects or symbols take on special meaning for that person; for example, the presence of a man wearing a red tie may be interpreted as a directive or an omen. One important caveat is that "unusual" beliefs may have a cultural basis and so should be viewed through that particular frame of reference.

Negative symptoms, by contrast, refer to apathy, blunted affect or mood, lack of expression, poverty of speech, lack of spontaneity, social withdrawal, lack of attention to personal hygiene, and anhedonia (the inability to derive any enjoyment from life). These symptoms may be part and parcel of the illness itself, reflecting deficits in cognitive functioning, for example, and may also be influenced by social factors such as stigma and rejection by peers. Antipsychotic medications, the primary treatment for schizophrenia, may diminish delusions and hallucinations but typically have much less impact on the negative symptoms. A report by the Schizophrenia Society of Canada (2001, 4) concluded that the negative symptoms were "rated by people with schizophrenia as the most difficult to deal with."

Persons diagnosed with schizophrenia may also manifest thought disorder, referring to thought *form,* apart from content. Thoughts, and speech, may be poorly or loosely connected, causing the individual to go off on tangents or to jump from one thought to another in an incoherent fashion, the most severe manifestation being referred to as a "word salad."

As well, schizophrenia is increasingly being seen as a disorder of information processing and executive functioning, which impacts the individual's ability to properly perceive, acquire, understand, and respond to information (Medalia and Revheim 2003, Bonner-Jackson et al. 2005). Persons with schizophrenia are known to have deficits with respect to concentration, critical thinking, problem solving, and "working memory" – which allows an individual to keep several pieces of information in mind simultaneously – a deficit that appears to be related to structural abnormalities in the prefrontal cortex of the brain (Society for Neuroscience 2004). Recognition of this aspect of the disorder has led to an increased emphasis on *cognitive remediation*, practical techniques to assist clients with deficits in cognitive functioning (Medalia and Revheim 2003).

The *DSM* IV-TR (American Psychiatric Association 2000, 312) requires that "continuous signs of the disturbance persist for at least six months" for a diagnosis of schizophrenia to be made. The *DSM* also lists several subtypes of schizophrenia (such as "paranoid-type"), although the reliability and usefulness of these subcategories have been questioned; in a review of the subject, Helmes and Landmark (2003, 702) conclude that "subtypes may have little utility when the variability of symptoms over the longitudinal course of the illness is considered."

Onset, Course, and Prognosis
Schizophrenia manifests itself in early adulthood, typically late teens to early twenties in men and somewhat later in women. Tragically, the onset occurs at a time when individuals are establishing careers and forming families. Several factors are known to be associated with a better prognosis (outcome), such as an abrupt onset of the illness, onset later in life (e.g., after thirty), and fewer negative symptoms (Menezes and Milovan 2000). In *A Beautiful Mind* (1998), the biography of mathematician John Nash, who developed schizophrenia but went on to win a Nobel Prize in economics, author Sylvia Nasar notes that "someone with Nash's history prior to the onset of his illness – high social class, high IQ, high achievement, with no schizophrenic relatives, who gets the disease relatively late in the third decade, who experiences very acute symptoms early – has the best chance of remission" (353). While some factors associated with better or poorer prognosis can be considered "intrinsic," others have to do with lifestyle and support *after* the onset of the disorder. As reviewed by Liberman and Kopelowicz (2002), more complete recovery is associated with positive family relationships, maintenance treatment with medication and minimizing periods of untreated psychosis, accessible and supportive mental health treatment providers, a repertoire of social skills, and not abusing substances. On this last point, there is evidence that the use of street drugs, marijuana in particular, can negatively influence the onset and severity of psychotic symptoms among adolescents deemed to have a predisposition for schizophrenia (Henquet et al. 2004).

Acute episodes often require hospitalization, with Canadian data showing that frequency of hospitalization is greater in early adulthood, dropping off after individuals reach their mid-forties (Health Canada 2002b). The course of the illness may vary greatly from one individual to the other, and in fact there is evidence that schizophrenia may not be a single disorder but a collection of disorders with similar symptoms that affect the brain differently (Turetsky et al. 2002). It is estimated that about 25 percent of people with this illness will make a complete recovery, that 40 percent will experience recurrent episodes of psychosis, with some impact on social and vocational functioning, and that 35 percent will experience ongoing disability (Andrews et al. 2000). It is an unfortunate fact that persons with schizophrenia have a much higher rate of suicide than other groups, with about one person in ten with this diagnosis ending their lives by suicide (Davis 2000). One story among many is that of Canadian Nobel Prize-winning biochemist Michael Smith, whose son was diagnosed with schizophrenia and died by suicide, and who donated a large portion of his 1993 Nobel Prize winnings to schizophrenia research. Significantly, suicide risk may be greatest not when individuals are acutely psychotic but when they have achieved some "insight" and are presumably aware of the substantial impact that the disorder has had on their independent functioning and life goals (Bourgeois et al. 2004; Keefe and Harvey 1994).

Notwithstanding an appreciation of the potentially serious consequences of schizophrenia, practitioners need to guard against an overly pessimistic attitude concerning outcome and the potential for recovery, a prejudice related to the fact that public mental health programs typically see only the most severely ill (Kruger 2000). Indeed, guidelines concerning practitioner competencies now emphasize the importance of rational optimism and of fostering a sense of hope (Coursey et al. 2000).

Etiology
The best current understanding is that schizophrenia has a biological basis, which was in fact the view of early theorists, such as Kraepelin (Davis 1987a; Turetsky et al. 2002). Theories about social factors, particularly faulty parenting, became more popular in the 1950s and 1960s partly due to the influence of Freudian psychology and its emphasis on early-childhood experiences; however, these have been largely discarded today.

Support for a biological causation of schizophrenia comes from several sources (Sadock and Sadock 2003):

(1) The role of genetics is supported by studies of adoptees and twins that have determined that close relatives of persons with schizophrenia are more likely to have the illness themselves, by a factor of ten in the case of first-degree relatives. More recently researchers at the University of Toronto identified a "risk gene," present more frequently in persons with schizophrenia, that affects normal development of the nervous system ("Risk gene identified," 2003).

(2) Persons with schizophrenia are more likely to show developmental ab-
    normalities from an early age, this apparently being associated with pre-
    natal trauma and illness. A study of Chinese children born to mothers
    exposed to the 1959-61 famine, for example, found significantly higher
    rates of schizophrenia in later life (St. Clair et al. 2005).
(3) In cross-cultural comparisons, it can be seen that symptomatology, age
    of onset, and male-to-female ratio are all similar (Bland 1999; Davis
    1987a).
(4) With the imaging techniques now available, there is increasingly evi-
    dence of brain anatomical and physiological differences between per-
    sons with schizophrenia and comparison groups – in particular, greater
    tissue loss among the former – supporting the hypothesis that schizo-
    phrenia represents a disrupted version of normal brain development
    (Adler 2003).

Concerning the underlying physiological mechanism, the acute symptoms
of schizophrenia are thought to result from faulty regulation of neurotransmitters, particularly dopamine, a hypothesis supported by the known effects of antipsychotic medication.

Other Conditions
There are other conditions, transient or enduring, that may present with
symptoms similar to schizophrenia. *Schizoaffective disorder* may be diagnosed
when "schizophrenic and affective symptoms (depressive or manic) are both
prominent in the same episode of illness, usually simultaneously, but at
least within a few days of each other" (Andrews et al. 2000, 318). *Delusional
disorder* involves beliefs that are nonbizarre and is a condition where hallucinations, especially auditory, are not typically present. According to the *DSM
IV-TR* (American Psychiatric Association 2000, 329), "functioning is not
markedly impaired ... apart from the impact of the delusions." The *DSM*
"Cluster A" personality disorders (paranoid, schizoid, and schizotypal), referring to persons who appear "odd or eccentric" (685), may resemble aspects of schizophrenia but generally do not achieve the degree of impairment
of the Axis I condition; at the same time, they tend to be poorly responsive
to pharmacological interventions.

Psychotic symptoms may also be produced by drugs, both licit and illicit.
For example, stimulants such as amphetamines and cocaine can cause delusions, and marijuana may produce paranoid beliefs in some persons. At the
same time, *withdrawal* from drugs or alcohol, particularly when it is abrupt,
may produce psychotic symptoms. Generally, if a psychosis "clears" quickly,

there may be the suspicion that it was substance-induced, although if a client remains connected with a drug-use environment it will be difficult for a practitioner to clearly establish a causative factor. Where there is insufficient or contradictory information, the *DSM* provides the diagnostic option of "psychotic disorder not otherwise specified."

Treatment and Support
In the first half of the twentieth century, people diagnosed with schizophrenia in North America were often institutionalized for lengthy periods in large psychiatric hospitals. No effective treatment was known at the time, and in some instances the treatments that were offered, such as insulin coma and psychosurgery, were misconceived and potentially harmful. From the 1950s on the primary treatment for schizophrenia has been antipsychotic medication. More recent times have seen the advent of skills training and education, both for clients and family members, vocational programming, and **cognitive-behavioural therapies** (see Chapter 11). In a document on clinical practice guidelines, Bassett et al. (1998) recognized this *range* of services as instrumental for rehabilitation to be successful. In Canada the Schizophrenia Society (http://www.schizophrenia.ca), started as a grass-roots organization, provides advocacy services and support to clients and (especially) family members through its local chapters.

Depression
Depression is a relatively common condition, affecting about 8 percent of Canadians at some point in their lives (Bland 1997). The World Health Organization ranks depression as the leading cause of years of life lived with disability worldwide, and a federal government report concludes that "because of their high prevalence, economic cost, risk of suicide and loss of quality of life, mood disorders represent a serious public health concern in Canada" (Health Canada 2002b, 6).

While depression clearly affects both sexes, it is diagnosed more frequently in women than men, regardless of the setting, by a ratio of about two to one (Sadock and Sadock 2003). Canadian data confirm that women are hospitalized for this disorder at a higher rate than men (Health Canada 2002b). In trying to account for this, it has been hypothesized that women may be more vulnerable to depression, a result of risk and/or protective factors – biological and social – that differ between the sexes; that women are more likely to engage in help-seeking; and that the symptoms manifested by men vs. women may be different or may be *perceived* differently by practitioners (Health Canada 2002b; Rosenfeld 1999).

Symptoms

The most common symptoms of depression include bleak, pessimistic views of the future; disturbed sleep patterns; disturbed appetite; decreased sex drive; reduced energy and activity; reduced concentration; feelings of worthlessness and guilt; reduced self-esteem; loss of interest in various activities; and thoughts of self-harm or suicide. The *DSM* IV-TR provides specifiers for rating the current depressive episode from mild to moderate to severe and for classifying the episode as either with or without psychotic symptoms. Usually the presence of psychotic features, such as delusions or hallucinations, indicates a more severe form of depression. The *DSM* also includes specifiers that may be used to rate the current episode as having catatonic features, atypical features, postpartum onset features, or melancholic features. Postpartum mood changes are not uncommon, and in a smaller number of cases (1 to 2 per 1,000 deliveries) the mood disturbance may reach the proportions of major depression (Sadock and Sadock 2003). Melancholic depression is a severe form characterized by the presence of "somatic" features, such as lack of reactivity and psychomotor retardation.

Onset, Course, and Prognosis

While the onset of depression can be at any age, often it occurs in the mid-twenties (American Psychiatric Association 2000). There is evidence of a delay, in many cases, in seeking treatment, and in a significant number of cases persons suffering from clinical depression never get treated at all. This may be due to the stigma associated with mental illness or to the view that sadness is a normal condition and that attempts to pathologize it indicate a character weakness. Because sadness *is* a normal response to loss and disappointment, the practitioner, in conjunction with the client, needs to determine at what point persistent, distressing feelings of sadness constitute a condition requiring treatment. The concern that depression is being underrecognized has led to the advent in Canada of a National Depression Screening Day each October, which is sponsored by the Canadian Mental Health Association along with other community groups and health authorities.

The course of a depressive illness is variable, although recent psychiatric opinion is that major depression is a *recurrent*, rather than an acute, illness (Angst 1999). The likelihood of having subsequent depressive episodes increases with each episode; following one episode it is estimated that in about one-half of cases individuals will suffer a second, and after three episodes about 90 percent of individuals will suffer a fourth (American Psychiatric Association 2000; Health Canada 2002b). In a majority of cases persons will have a complete remission between episodes, while in about 20 to 30 percent of cases individuals will have some residual symptoms (American Psychiatric Association 2000).

Etiology

Depression appears to be multidetermined, with biological, psychological, and social factors contributing to the onset and outcome of the disorder.

Concerning biological factors, there is evidence of a genetic link in depression: first-degree relatives are two to three times more likely to suffer from major depression, and the concordance rate for major depression in monozygotic (identical) twins is about 50 percent, compared to 10 to 25 percent for dizygotic (nonidentical) twins (Sadock and Sadock 2003). A long-term study of 847 patients found evidence of a gene-environment interaction in persons who experienced a major depressive episode; persons with the "short" form of a gene that affects serotonin metabolism were more likely to report depression in association with an environmental stressor (such as bereavement or job crisis) but no more likely to manifest depression when no stressor was present (Holden 2003).

Evidence of a hormonal effect is seen in the case of postpartum depression, defined as a depressive episode occurring within four weeks of delivery, with prevalence rates ranging from 11 to 15 percent (MacQueen and Chokka 2004). A hormonal effect has also been implicated in a subtype of depression known as seasonal affective disorder (SAD), referred to in the *DSM* as major depression with seasonal pattern. A survey of Toronto residents determined that 11 percent of all subjects with major depression suffered from this seasonal subtype, where symptoms are worse in the winter months (Levitt et al. 2000).

Depression seen in later life is linked to a number of factors, including loss of relationships and declining quality of life. There is also an association between depression and reduced cerebral blood flow, and it may be that declining mood seen later in life is related to the higher rates of cerebrovascular disease evident in older persons (Ruo et al. 2003). Concerning long-term medical conditions, a large-scale survey of the Canadian population concluded that chronic physical illness "may increase the risk of depression or the duration of depressive episodes" (Patten 1999, 151).

The manifestation of depression appears to be influenced by learned responses and preexisting personality. It has been suggested that in some cases persons suffering from depression are experiencing a state of *learned helplessness* and that in these cases therapies that increase the individual's sense of control and mastery will be beneficial (Sadock and Sadock 2003). Depressed persons may also learn or manifest a pessimistic worldview and apply a very negative evaluation of their own activities and relationships;

for these individuals cognitive therapies that challenge these perceptions may be effective (Reesal and Lam 2001). Perfectionism has also been linked to depression and suicidality, notably in younger persons (Hewitt 2000).

Other Conditions
A differential diagnosis that may be considered when assessing for depression is *dysthymia*, which is a chronic, low-grade mood disorder where the individual experiences some but not all of the symptoms of major depression. One text suggests that persons with dysthymia can "almost be regarded as having a depressive 'personality style'" (Andrews et al. 2000, 164). Because depression and suicidal ideation may be exacerbated by depressant substances, individuals using these products – notably alcohol – to cope with a mood disorder may actually be worsening it (Patten and Charney 1998).

Treatment and Support
There are a number of different treatments and supports available for persons suffering from depression, and these include medication, education, skills training, and psychotherapy. The importance of having and applying a range of approaches was emphasized by the Canadian Psychiatric Association in their document "Clinical practice guidelines for the treatment of depressive disorders" (2001). There are also self-help and support groups for clients with depression and family members, such as the Mood Disorders Association (http://www.mooddisorderscanada.ca/links.htm), which has a number of chapters across Canada. Notably, there is evidence that in North America people are increasingly turning to alterative treatment approaches for depression and other disorders, such as acupuncture, herbal remedies, massage, and naturopathy (Eisenberg et al. 1993; Wang, Patten, and Russell 2001). Evaluation of these alternative treatments is lacking in many cases, although this is partly due to debates about appropriate methodology; one review suggests that exercise and hypericum perforatum (St. John's Wort) are effective in cases of less serious depression (Ernst, Rand, and Stevinson 1998).[3]

Bipolar Disorder
Persons with bipolar disorder (previously called manic-depressive illness) experience episodes of *mania* or *hypomania* during which they feel more energetic, creative, and outgoing but at the same time may exhibit poor judgment and engage in a number of risky activities, such as overspending or unsafe sex. Because individuals experiencing a manic episode may feel "on top of the world," they may resent family members and mental health

practitioners who try to redirect them or apply a psychiatric diagnosis to their condition. It is estimated that this illness will affect 0.6 to 2 percent of the population at some point in their lives, with lifetime prevalence rates for men and women being approximately the same (Andrews et al. 2000; Bland 1997). Despite these similar prevalence rates, data from Canadian settings reveal a higher rate of psychiatric hospitalization for women with bipolar disorder than for men, suggesting that the response to this illness involves other, social factors, which are not clearly understood at this point (Health Canada 2002b). It is estimated that mortality rates for persons with bipolar disorder are two to three times that of the general population due to reckless behaviour, accidents, and suicide (Health Canada 2002b; see also Hall 2001).

Symptoms

Symptoms of a manic episode include: elevated mood; grandiosity and inflated self-importance; flight of ideas, racing thoughts, and rapid speech; increased sex drive; decreased sleep; poor concentration; irritability; and impaired judgment and impulsivity, notably in financial decisions. Concerning this last point, there may be a real danger that the individual will overspend and deplete his or her bank account. In more severe episodes the disorder can reach psychotic proportions, with the person experiencing delusions and hallucinations.

The *DSM* makes a number of distinctions to be applied when diagnosing this condition. First, episodes may be characterized as *manic, hypomanic,* or *mixed.* Hypomania, as the name suggests, is less disabling, "not severe enough to cause marked impairment in social or occupational functioning, or to necessitate hospitalization, and there are no psychotic features" (American Psychiatric Association 2000, 368). A hypomanic episode may also be shorter in duration. A mixed episode is distinguished by symptoms of *both* major depression and mania being present nearly every day for at least one week. Second, the disorder may be classified as Bipolar I or Bipolar II, depending on the clinical presentation. Bipolar I refers to the more "classic" conception of the disorder, characterized by one or more episodes of full mania, which may – but not necessarily – be interspersed with at least one episode of major depression. Bipolar II refers to a more primarily depressive condition and is characterized by episodes of depression interspersed with episodes (at least one) of mild manic symptoms, which do not reach the level of full mania.

Onset, Course, and Prognosis

The onset of bipolar disorder is in early adulthood, usually before thirty, with most persons experiencing repeated episodes (manic, depressive, or mixed) throughout their lives. The frequency, duration, and ratio of manic and depressive episodes will vary from one person to the next. Some individuals will experience only a few manic episodes in their lifetime, while others, "rapid cyclers," may experience several episodes a year. There is evidence that the prognosis, with respect to chronicity and length of recovery period, is worse when the course of the illness involves rapid cycling or where the course includes mania and depression as opposed to mania alone (Andrews et al. 2000; Health Canada 2002b).

Etiology
As is the case with schizophrenia, research strongly supports the view that bipolar disorder has a biological basis. As reviewed by Sadock and Sadock (2003, 539), evidence for a "significant genetic factor" being involved in the etiology of bipolar illness includes the finding that first-degree relatives are eight to eighteen times more likely also to have Bipolar I disorder than are first-degree relatives of control subjects and that in about 50 percent of cases persons with Bipolar I disorder have at least one parent with a mood disorder. Studies of twins have shown that the concordance rate for Bipolar I disorder ranges from 33 to 90 percent in monozygotic twins, compared to 5 to 25 percent in dizygotic twins.

Other Conditions
Apart from Bipolar I and II, the *DSM* includes the diagnosis of *cyclothymic disorder*, defined as "the presence of numerous periods with hypomanic symptoms and numerous periods with depressive symptoms" (American Psychiatric Association 2000, 400) that, in the first two years of the disorder, do not meet the threshold of a major depressive or manic episode.

Bipolar disorder may appear at times like schizophrenia or schizoaffective disorder given their common symptoms, such as racing thoughts and (in some cases) delusions and hallucinations, and it is not unusual to find clients who have received both diagnoses. Comparing the course of this illness with schizophrenia reveals that persons with bipolar disorder tend to have good premorbid (pre-illness) functioning and more complete remission of symptoms between episodes (Andrews et al. 2000, 197). Of the two disorders, practitioners may regard schizophrenia as the more pessimistic diagnosis – perhaps unfairly given that there is a range of outcomes in both illnesses.[4]

States resembling mania may be produced by stimulants such as cocaine. As well, being on antidepressant medication may precipitate a manic episode in persons with bipolar disorder. It should also be noted that some medical conditions, such as hyperthyroidism, may produce symptoms similar to hypomania or mania.

Treatment and Support
Persons with bipolar disorder are usually treated with medication, particularly a class of drugs known as mood stabilizers, which includes lithium carbonate (see Chapter 10). Clients may also benefit from education, skills training, and counselling. In some cases arrangements may need to be made to protect the individual from overspending, such as a power of attorney, or "**Ulysses**," contract. There are also support groups for clients and family members, such as the Mood Disorders Association.

Anxiety Disorders
Referred to as "neuroses" in earlier conceptualizations, anxiety disorders manifest as excessive or unrealistic feelings of fear, anxiety, and worry, which an individual may attempt to cope with by avoiding particular situations or by using compulsive rituals. This class of disorders includes generalized anxiety disorder (GAD), phobias, post-traumatic stress disorder (PTSD), obsessive-compulsive disorder (OCD), and panic disorder (which may include agoraphobia as a subtype).

As a group, anxiety disorders are the most common form of mental disorder seen in the Canadian population: it is estimated that the one-year prevalence of any anxiety disorder is about 12 percent, with the lifetime prevalence being as high as 25 percent (Antony and Swinson 1996; Health Canada 2002b). Women report symptoms and receive diagnoses of anxiety disorder more frequently than do men, although there is some question as to whether this represents a true difference in prevalence or, for example, a difference in help-seeking. Canadian data confirm that women are hospitalized more frequently than men for anxiety disorders in all age cohorts and that the highest rates of hospitalization for anxiety disorders occur in adults over sixty-five (Health Canada 2002b). Anxiety disorders have a high rate of co-occurrence with other mental disorders, such as depression, dysthymia, substance misuse, and personality disorder, which makes the correct diagnosis and treatment of the co-morbid anxiety disorder a more difficult enterprise (Health Canada 2002b). Anxiety disorders are more likely to manifest themselves in childhood than are illnesses such as bipolar disorder or schizophrenia.

Anxiety disorders may "markedly compromise quality of life and psychosocial functioning" (Mendlowicz and Stein 2000, 680) and have a major economic impact, taking into account lost productivity, direct treatment costs, and costs of assessment and treatment to rule out somatic causes (Rice and

Miller 1998). Despite this, there is the suggestion that anxiety disorders are underrecognized by practitioners and the public or regarded as less serious conditions (Antony and Swinson 1996). Indeed, it was the case in this author's own experience that anxiety disorders were not necessarily considered to be "serious, persistent" mental disorders – like schizophrenia – and that persons with these conditions were directed more often to specialized clinics (with more limited resources) rather than to community mental health centres. A Health Canada report (Antony and Swinson 1996) concludes that practitioners in many cases simply lack knowledge of the cognitive-behavioural treatments now available for anxiety disorders, which may partly be because these treatments have been seen historically as the exclusive province of clinical psychology.

Panic Disorder and Agoraphobia *SKiP*

Panic attacks are identified by the presence of a number of physical signs, such as sweating, a pounding heart, or shortness of breath, and by altered beliefs, such as a fear of losing control or dying. Agoraphobia is a related condition where the anxiety or panic is particular to "characteristic clusters of situations that include being outside the home alone, being in a crowd, or standing in a line" (American Psychiatric Association 2000, 433). For a diagnosis of panic disorder to be made, the *DSM* IV-TR requires that the course of panic attacks be recurrent and unexpected and that following at least one attack there is a period of residual concerns, such as worrying about the implications of the attack. Diagnosis also requires ruling out immediate physical causes, such as drug effects and medical conditions like hyperthyroidism. The one-year prevalence rate for panic disorder in the Canadian population is estimated to be about 0.7 percent (Health Canada 2002b).

The etiology of this condition and other anxiety disorders is not well understood. Hypotheses include differences in brain structure and autonomic nervous system response, genetic factors, and behaviours learned in the family setting (Sadock and Sadock 1998).

To manage panic attacks, clients should be taught techniques such as relaxation and breathing exercises (Andrews et al. 2000). Treatment of panic disorder may also include medication, such as those antidepressants known as selective serotonin reuptake inhibitors (SSRIs) and, more controversially, benzodizepines; education about the nature of the disorder; and cognitive-behavioural approaches, which may involve challenging irrational beliefs and graduated exposure to stress-inducing situations. It is suggested that avoidance of situations or places, which may be encouraged by the practitioner, in fact "may lead to agoraphobia and increased disability" (Andrews et al. 2000, 248).

Phobias

The *DSM* IV-TR refers to two types of phobia: *social phobia,* also known as social anxiety disorder (a fear of being scrutinized or evaluated negatively by others and hence embarrassed), and *specific phobia* (a persistent and irrational fear and avoidance of a particular object or situation) (Andrews et al. 2000). The one-year prevalence rates for social and specific phobias in the Canadian population are estimated at 6.7 percent and 6.2 to 8 percent, respectively, making these the most commonly occurring anxiety disorders (Health Canada 2002b).

For social phobia, the *DSM* IV-TR specifies that exposure to the feared situation invariably provokes anxiety, which may take the form of a panic attack; that the person recognizes that the fear is unreasonable; that the feared situation is either avoided or endured with intense anxiety; and that the avoidance interferes with the person's normal routine *or* that the person is distressed about having the phobia. Situations that may be commonly feared include public speaking, eating in public, and using public toilets. At first glance, one can see that making this diagnosis is potentially difficult in that fear of public speaking, for example, is quite common. The distinction here is that the response to situations must be seen as excessive and "interfer[ing] with the individual's social or occupational functioning" (Andrews et al. 2000, 259). Social and specific phobias are distinguished from panic disorder in that panic attacks are *unpredictable* and not always in response to specific stimuli.

In the case of specific phobias, the *DSM* IV-TR diagnostic criteria are similar to those for social phobia, with the exception of the source of the fear or avoidance. The *DSM* IV-TR specifies several subtypes of this disorder: animal type, such as fear of insects or snakes; natural environment type, such as fear of heights or water; blood-injection-injury type, such as fear of the sight of blood; situational type, such as fear of elevators or flying, and "other" type. One can note that in some instances these fears do not appear unreasonable, and indeed it is hypothesized that in mammalian evolution a fear of heights, for example, served a protective function for the species. To meet the threshold of a phobia, however, the response is considered to be out of all proportion to the danger.

Hypotheses about the etiology of phobias draw from studies of classical and operant conditioning to explain how a relatively neutral stimulus, such as driving a car, becomes anxiety-producing when paired with an event such as a horrific accident (Sadock and Sadock 2003). It has also been suggested that phobias may be learned in the family context. Genetic factors have not been clearly established, although it is hypothesized that a type of social phobia manifested in early childhood may have a biological basis (Sadock and Sadock 2003). One of the oldest theories about phobias is psycho-analytic; it was proposed by Sigmund Freud that, in trying to repress unconscious drives, underlying conflict could be *displaced* by an individual to an unimportant object or situation, which then became the source of the phobia (Appignanesi 1979).

Treatment of phobias includes antidepressant medication, training in relaxation and breathing exercises, practising conversational and social skills, education, and graduated exposure to feared situations (Andrews et al. 2000).

Obsessive-Compulsive Disorder (OCD)

This disorder is characterized by the presence of *obsessions*, defined as "recurrent and persistent thoughts, impulses or images that are experienced ... as intrusive and inappropriate and that cause marked anxiety" (American Psychiatric Association 2000, 462), and/or *compulsions*, defined as "repetitive behaviors ... or mental acts ... that the person feels driven to perform" (462). The obsessions may involve, for example, fear of becoming infected with a disease by shaking hands, worrying about having left a door unlocked, an impulse to scream an obscenity in church, or a need to arrange household objects in a particular order. Compulsions are repetitive behaviours (such as hand washing) or mental acts (such as counting or repeating words) that are aimed at reducing distress or preventing something from happening *but* that are not connected in a rational way with what they are designed to prevent, or are clearly excessive (American Psychiatric Association 2000). While many persons may have worried about having left a door unlocked, the *DSM* IV-TR diagnosis specifies that these thoughts or behaviours must cause marked distress, be time-consuming (i.e., take more than one hour a day), or significantly interfere with the person's normal activities or relationships. The one-year prevalence rate for obsessive-compulsive disorder in the Canadian population is estimated to be about 1.8 percent (Health Canada 2002b).

The etiology of OCD is not clearly understood, and hypotheses about causation have drawn from behavioural psychology as well as from psychodynamic theories. There is evidence of genetic factors, with higher concordance rates for the disorder being seen in monozygotic twins than in dizygotic twins; as well, family studies have found that up to 35 percent of first-degree relatives of OCD patients are afflicted with the disorder (Sadock and Sadock 2003). At the physiological level, OCD symptoms have been associated with a dysregulation of the neurotransmitter serotonin and respond to serotonergic drugs (such as antidepressants). Sadock and Sadock (2003, 617) note, however, that "whether serotonin is involved in the cause of OCD is not clear."

Treatment for this potentially disabling condition is based on behavioural approaches, with medication being used either as an adjunct or in lieu of behavioural treatments if they are not available (Andrews et al. 2000; van Minnen et al. 2003). As noted, it has been found that antidepressants that inhibit serotonin reuptake may reduce symptoms of this disorder (see Chapter 10) either alone or in combination with other psychotropic agents. In some cases, for treatment-resistant clients, electroconvulsive therapy (ECT) may be considered. Psychological approaches may differ depending on whether obsessions or compulsions are the prominent issue and often involve a planned graduated exposure to anxiety-producing stimuli followed by voluntary response prevention on the part of the client. Other behavioural techniques, such as systematic desensitization, thought-stopping, and flooding may be tried (McLean and Woody 2001; see also Chapter 11).

Post-traumatic Stress Disorder (PTSD)

The *DSM* IV-TR gives six criteria for a diagnosis of PTSD: (1) an individual has been exposed to a traumatic event where the response involved intense fear, helplessness, or horror; (2) the traumatic event is reexperienced – for example, in the form of images or flashbacks – either spontaneously or after cues that resemble an aspect of the original event; (3) there are efforts to avoid reexperiencing the trauma, including mental and emotional detachment; (4) there are symptoms of increased arousal, such as an exaggerated startle response; (5) duration of these symptoms is more than one month; and (6) the disturbance causes significant distress or impairment in daily activities. Events that may lead to PTSD include violent physical or sexual assault, being held hostage or as a prisoner of war, or witnessing the death of a loved one.

As was discussed in the previous chapter, PTSD is a relatively new diagnostic entity, having been included in the *DSM* only in its third edition (1980), even though particular syndromes corresponding to military engagements were identified earlier than this, such as "shell shock" during the First World War[5] and "combat stress reaction" during the Second World War (Hyams, Wignall, and Roswell 1996).[6] A survey of over one thousand residents of New York City following the 11 September 2001 terrorist attacks concluded that 7.5 percent of persons interviewed met the criteria for PTSD as a result of witnessing the catastrophe at the World Trade Center (Galea et al. 2002). More recently, in the aftermath of the devastating tsunami that killed thousands in December 2004, mental health workers in Sri Lanka reported seeing large numbers of people with the symptoms of PTSD (Associated Press 2005). Concerning the effects of war, with the large immigrant population in Canada, it is important for practitioners to be alert to the possibility that refugees from war-torn countries are experiencing post-trauma effects.

The etiology of PTSD appears to be complex. Exposure to traumatic events, by all accounts, is not uncommon: the Badgely Commission reported that 25 percent of children and 40 percent of females had experienced some form of sexual exploitation in their lifetime (Greenberg 1998), and a survey of nearly ten thousand Ontario residents found that 31 percent of males and 21 percent of females reported a history of child physical abuse (MacMillan 2000). In accounting for the finding that not all affected persons will develop PTSD, it is now recognized that manifestations of the disorder are mediated and influenced by a number of factors, including the duration and frequency of the trauma, timing of the trauma in the life cycle, support system, culture, constitutional vulnerability to stress and psychiatric illness, and preexisting differences in personality and belief systems (Bell 2000; Briere 2002; Kluft, Bloom, and Kinzie 2000). One Canadian psychologist has in fact suggested that these individual differences are considerably more significant than the traumatic event itself in understanding client responses, which in turn may have implications for the choice of treatment (Bowman 1999).

PTSD is "a severe disorder that is difficult to treat" (Andrews et al. 2000, 280), and the reader is referred to specialized texts such as Yehuda 2002, Myers et al. 2002, and Bell 2000. Some general points are as follows. The approach may involve "many modalities of treatment [working] in concert" (Kluft, Bloom, and Kinzie, 2000, 88) and usually goes in phases: stabilization, deconditioning of traumatic memories and responses, integration of traumatic personal schemes, reestablishing social connections and personal efficacy, and accumulating restitutive emotional experiences (Van der Kolk 2002). The modalities used include anxiety management (training in relaxation and breathing, positive self-talk, assertiveness, and thought-stopping), cognitive therapy (challenging beliefs such as self-blame), and exposure therapy (confronting situations that remind the person of the trauma, although a high proportion of clients may refuse this). A relatively new therapeutic approach that appears to have some benefit for persons with PTSD is eye movement desensitization and reprocessing (EMDR), although there is some debate over how the effects are achieved (Haynes 2002; Shapiro 2001). EMDR involves a client tracking the rapid movements of a therapist's finger back and forth across an image of a feared scene that is visualized by the client. Skeptics have argued that any effects of the technique are attributable entirely to the exposure component, a form of systematic desensitization, rather than to any novel "reprocessing" mechanism (Antony and Swinson 1996). Antidepressant medication has also been used to treat PTSD.

Concerning therapy with victims of trauma, greater recognition is now being given to the effect that this type of work has on the practitioner and how it may in fact result in secondary or vicarious traumatization (Stamm 1999).

Generalized Anxiety Disorder (GAD)
This disorder is characterized by a tendency to worry excessively about a number of events or activities, such as the possibility of a loved one getting into an accident, financial matters, and work or school performance. For a diagnosis to be made, the *DSM* IV-TR requires that this excessive anxiety be greater than six months in duration, that there be other physical or mental indicators, such as sleep disturbance, muscle tension, or restlessness, that it cause significant distress or functional impairment, and that other anxiety disorders be ruled out. Sadock and Sadock (2003, 632) note that "because a certain degree of anxiety is normal and adaptive, differentiating normal anxiety from pathological anxiety [is] difficult." The one-year prevalence rate for generalized anxiety disorder in the Canadian population is estimated to be about 1 percent (Health Canada 2002b).

The etiology of GAD is not well understood, although it seems likely that both biological and psychological factors contribute to its manifestation. Cognitive-behavioural explanations of the disorder posit that some persons selectively attend to negative details in the environment and may also view their own coping skills in an overly negative fashion.

Treatment for GAD includes education, training in anxiety reduction strategies, and graduated exposure to stress-inducing phenomena. Andrews and colleagues (2000) suggest that a potentially effective approach with GAD is *structured problem solving*, which involves the practitioner and client mutually (1) identifing problems, (2) generating solutions through brainstorming, (3) evaluating the solutions, (4) choosing the optimal solution, (5) planning the actual implementation, and (6) reviewing afterward to see what worked and what didn't. The goal in doing this is to support the client's own efficacy rather than doing everything *for* the individual. Persons with GAD may also be prescribed antidepressants.

Eating Disorders Skip
Eating disorders include anorexia nervosa and bulimia nervosa. The *DSM* IV-TR criteria for anorexia are a refusal to maintain body weight; fear of becoming fat even when manifestly underweight; distorted body image (e.g., viewing oneself as fat despite all evidence to the contrary); and amenorrhea (i.e., a cessation of the menstrual periods). Bulimia is a condition where there is a pattern of binge eating followed by drastic efforts to compensate for the overeating, such as induced vomiting, fasting, exercise, and using

enemas, laxatives, diuretics, and other medication. The *DSM* IV-TR criteria for bulimia are that the amount eaten when bingeing is excessive and that there is a lack of control over eating; that compensatory behaviour follows the binge eating; and that episodes of both eating and compensation occur, on average, at least twice a week for three months (American Psychiatric Association 2000).

Not infrequently, eating disorders co-occur with other conditions, such as depression, anxiety, and substance misuse, which may be independent and/ or premorbid. A further complication is that starvation itself may directly cause psychological symptoms, such as depression, anxiety, poor concentration, and fluctuating mood (Andrews et al. 2000).

Lifetime prevalence rates for eating disorders are estimated to be about 3 percent, with women more likely to be affected than men (Health Canada 2002b). Typically, the disorder starts in adolescence, with later age of onset in fact being associated with a poorer outcome (Andrews et al. 2000). Persons with eating disorders may occasionally be hospitalized to stabilize their condition; Canadian data show that hospitalized persons are predominantly female (93% of admissions) and are most commonly in the fifteen to nineteen age cohort (Health Canada 2002b). These data also show that hospitalization rates have increased somewhat since the mid-1980s, although whether this represents a true increase in incidence of eating disorders is unclear.

Self-starvation may have severe health consequences, such as brittle bones, heart conditions, electrolyte imbalance, kidney failure, and death in some cases. Follow-up studies of persons with anorexia indicate that four years after onset of illness, about 50 percent show a good outcome (weight within normal range), 25 percent an intermediate outcome, and 25 percent a poor outcome (Andrews et al. 2000).

The etiology of eating disorders is complex. Earlier explanations tended to be "unifactorial," falling into conceptions that emphasized either biological, psychodynamic, behavioural, or familial factors. For example, within the field of family therapy, it was proposed that persons with anorexia tended to come out of "psychosomatic families" that had particular transactional patterns, such as enmeshment, overprotectiveness, rigidity, and poor conflict resolution (Minuchin, Rosman, and Baker 1978). Currently, the understanding is that eating disorders result from an interaction of biological, psychological, and social factors, and there is greater recognition, in particular, of the impact of childhood abuse. Young persons with eating disorders may be struggling with developmental issues such as autonomy and identity, have problems with self-image, have poor coping skills, and face teasing and pressure from a peer group that overvalues thinness (Health Canada

2002b). Indeed, the social value placed on thinness in North America, particularly for young women, seems to have only increased over the years.

Concerning the treatment and management of eating disorders, an excellent overview is offered by Andrews et al. 2000, wherein the following points are made:

(1) The intervention should be multidisciplinary and include a physician, a mental health professional, and a dietician.
(2) Psychiatric assessment should include an assessment of eating attitudes and behaviours, which may involve the client keeping a diary of eating patterns.
(3) There should be a thorough physical examination and, in the case of anorexia, weekly measurements of weight and body-mass index (calculated by dividing weight by height squared).
(4) There should be education about the effects of starvation and bingeing and about dieting myths.
(5) Psychological treatment may include cognitive-behavioural approaches, structured problem solving, and training in relaxation and assertiveness.
(6) Treatment may also involve family education and counselling.

Personality Disorders

The *DSM* IV-TR defines a personality disorder as "an enduring pattern of inner experience and behavior that deviates markedly from the expectations of the individual's culture" (American Psychiatric Association 2000, 689). This pattern is "inflexible and pervasive, leads to clinically significant distress or impairment in ... important areas of functioning, [and] is stable and of long duration" (689). In the *DSM*'s conceptualization, personality disorders fall into three categories:

- *Cluster A ("odd-eccentric"):* paranoid personality disorder; schizoid personality disorder; schizotypal personality disorder.
- *Cluster B ("dramatic-emotional"):* antisocial personality disorder; borderline personality disorder; histrionic personality disorder; narcissistic personality disorder.
- *Cluster C ("anxious-fearful"):* avoidant personality disorder; dependent personality disorder; obsessive-compulsive personality disorder.

It is noted that these clusters "may also be viewed as dimensions representing spectra of personality dysfunction on a continuum with Axis I mental disorders" (690). The *DSM* also gives the option of (1) referring to personality *traits* that do not meet the threshold for a disorder or (2) diagnosing *personality disorder not otherwise specified* for a "mixed" presentation.

There have been concerns expressed about the validity, reliability, and utility of the "personality" diagnoses.[7] For instance, a government report suggests that the Axis II categories are largely "arbitrary" (Health Canada 2002b, 70). An editor of the *Canadian Journal of Psychiatry* suggests that "clinicians avoid diagnosing personality disorders [because of] doubts about the validity of the Axis II categories. Although almost every category in our present classification suffers from a lack of precision, Axis II categories seem particularly unclear" (Paris 1998b, 135).

An additional concern is that the presence of these conditions is often seen as an indication of untreatability, which is not surprising given that they are, by the *DSM*'s own definition, "enduring," "inflexible," and "stable" and that, in the words of a Canadian psychiatrist, "personality is stable over time" (Paris 1998a, 149). The author of one text suggests that the "fact that personality disorders ... often are difficult, if not impossible, to treat has become a sobering reality for mental health professionals" (Sperry 1995, ix). While any psychiatric diagnosis can be stigmatizing, the personality diagnoses are particularly so *within the practitioner community* because of the view held by many that the problems seen represent willfulness and consequently that the client in question is (or will be) "difficult" (Lewis and Appleby 1988). On this point, a Canadian woman diagnosed with borderline personality disorder (see below) notes that practitioners may believe, wrongly, that people who fit this diagnosis "enjoy [their situation] and don't want to get well" (Williams 1998, 173). Practitioners may also be reluctant to take on cases that represent a lot of work (persons with Cluster B diagnoses can be very demanding) as well as potential liability concerns (these are clients who may frequently talk about taking their own lives).

At the same time, observers note that personality problems still need to be taken into account since these traits have a considerable influence on the treatment response for Axis I disorders and that "Axis II blindness may lead to ineffective treatment planning" (Paris 1998b, 135). One group of authors suggests that "the concepts under discussion (e.g., paranoia, dependency) might be better viewed as a process and not as a diagnostic label ... [that] can aid the clinician's understanding and management of such individuals" (Andrews et al. 2000, 628). Further, one psychiatrist, in speaking about greater diagnostic clarity, more sophisticated conceptualizations of the different disorders, and the development of a wider range of treatment modalities, offers that "optimism is again mounting about the treatability of personality disorders" (Sperry 1995, ix).

The Axis II category most likely to come to the attention of mental health practitioners (and discussed in more detail here) is borderline personality disorder (BPD). This is the case because individuals with this diagnosis tend to be attention-seeking, to often be in crisis, and to express suicidal thoughts. (The term "borderline" comes from the early view that persons so diagnosed appeared to be on the border between psychosis and neurosis.) It is estimated that 10 percent of psychiatric outpatients have this diagnosis, making it the most common Axis II disorder seen in both public and private practice (Sperry 1995). Because of concerns about suicidality, these individuals may frequently be seen at hospital emergency departments, although there is some debate as to whether hospitalization is an appropriate or useful response (Dawson 1988; Health Canada 2002b; Paris 1993; Williams 1998). The diagnosis of BPD is more frequently given to women than men (Simmie and Nunes 2001).

The *DSM* IV-TR criteria for borderline personality disorder refer to an individual who (1) has unstable and intense relationships (including the one with the practitioner) that alternate between idealization and devaluation (love and hate); (2) makes frantic efforts to avoid real or imagined abandonment; (3) shows impulsivity – for example, in sexual activity, substance abuse, or reckless driving; (4) expresses suicidal thoughts and/or engages in self-harm such as slashing his or her arms or taking overdoses; (5) manifests mood instability, which may include sudden angry outbursts; and (6) under stress may experience brief psychotic states characterized by paranoia or dissociation.

The etiology of borderline personality disorder (and other Axis II categories) is not well understood but appears to involve an interaction of biological, psychological, and social factors and vulnerabilities (Sadock and Sadock 2003; Paris 1998a). Psychologist Marsha Linehan (1993a) has hypothesized that persons with this diagnosis are born with an innate tendency to react more intensely to lower levels of stress and to take longer to recover (although she also incorporates psychosocial factors in her theory). Another hypothesis, articulated by psychoanalyst Otto Kernberg (1984), comes from *object relations* theory. Kernberg notes that persons diagnosed with BPD, who may have had erratic parenting and abusive early relationships, tend to see others as all good one day and all bad the next – that is, they have problems with *object constancy*. Instead, they read each action of people in their lives as if there were no prior context and have a hard time experiencing an absent loved one as a positive presence in their minds.

Discussions of the etiology of BPD have produced some sharp divisions of opinion. In particular, some practitioners and clients place greater emphasis on *trauma* – such as sexual abuse – as a causal factor in BPD, noting parallels in the symptoms of post-traumatic stress disorder and BPD as well as an association between childhood abuse and later-life self-harming behaviour (Briere 2002; Gunderson and Sabo 1993; Mina and Gallop 1998). It has been suggested that what we call BPD is really just an understandable response to trauma rather than a psychopathology (Simmie and Nunes 2001). Author Judith Herman (1992) theorizes that BPD is in fact a form of PTSD, one that manifests primarily in identity and relationship disturbances; when symptoms are more somatic, the presentation is diagnosed as factitious disorder (or hysteria), and when the client manifests dissociative symptoms, the diagnosis may be something different again, such as multiple personality disorder. Other authors and clinicians deemphasize trauma; for example, one Canadian psychiatrist suggests that "the majority of children exposed to trauma are resilient" and that "the symptoms of personality disorders reflect underlying traits, not specific experiences" (Paris 1998a, 151). A study published in the *American Journal of Psychiatry* examining the link between BPD and PTSD found that subjects with BPD, compared to persons with other Axis II diagnoses, had higher rates of early-life abuse and were more likely to develop PTSD. However, the study concluded that the results were not "substantial or distinct enough to support singling out BPD from the other personality disorders as a ... variant of PTSD" (Golier et al. 2003, 2018).

Persons with borderline personality disorder can be very challenging for practitioners partly because they may play one individual off against another ("splitting") and can get different care providers to work at cross-purposes. It has been suggested that despite (or perhaps because of) a genuine desire to help, practitioners may actually make things worse when they attempt to rescue these individuals (Dawson 1988; Williams 1998). It is recommended that practitioners make communications very clear, set clear limits and boundaries, and "establish a protocol with all parties who might be involved so as to clarify the course of action that should be taken when such contact recurs" (Andrews et al. 2000, 643). Sperry (1995, 65-66) reviews what he calls "five points of consensus" in the treatment of persons diagnosed with BPD: (1) that the therapist play an active role in directing the client's behaviours; (2) that there be a stable treatment environment – for example, regarding schedules and role expectations; (3) that connections between the client's actions and feelings in the present be established; (4) that self-destructive behaviour be made ungratifying; and (5) that careful attention be paid to countertransference feelings (negative feelings about the client on the part of the practitioner). Different treatment models have been employed with persons with BPD, including structured problem solving, cognitive-behavioural approaches (Linehan 1993a), and *relationship management*, a "less is more" model that has the practitioner promoting the personal responsibility and efficacy of the client (Dawson 1988). Some have criticized approaches that ignore the traumatic origins of BPD and that focus on symptom stabilization, advocating instead treatments that may be applied with PTSD (Van der Kolk 2002).

As noted, clients with personality problems can provoke strong reactions in the practitioner, and although this is normal, practitioners nevertheless need to be reflective and to avoid ending service with clients simply because of personal animosity (which may be rationalized in clinical terms). As Bachrach (1996, 20) notes, "It is not uncommon for the service system to identify patients whom it will not or cannot serve, or whom it will not or cannot treat, as *difficult* patients and thereby absolve itself of the obligation to care for these individuals" (emphasis added).

Disorders among Young Persons Skip

There has been a rise in the rates of mental disorder seen in young people since the 1950s, especially behaviour disorders, substance abuse, eating disorders, depression, and suicidal behaviour (Andrews et al. 2000). A review in the *Canadian Journal of Psychiatry* concludes that "14 percent of children have clinically important disorders at any given time" (Waddell et al. 2002, 825). A 2003 survey of Ontario students, Grades 7 to 12, found that 11 percent had visited a mental health professional at least once in the preceding twelve months, with females seeking help more frequently than males (14% and 8%, respectively) (Centre for Addiction and Mental Health 2004). The same survey found that the use of psychotropic medication among the student body was not uncommon: about 6 percent of students surveyed (53,900) had used barbiturates, about 6 percent (54,700) had used stimulants, about 3 percent (25,800) had used tranquilizers, and about 2.5 percent (24,400) had used Ritalin.

Young persons in Canada are now considered to be a high-risk group with respect to suicide, with surveys finding one-year prevalence rates for suicidal ideation among teenagers ranging from 12 to 20 percent (Centre for Addiction and Mental Health 2004; McCreary Centre Society 2004; Simmie and Nunes 2001). In British Columbia thirty-one young persons aged twelve to nineteen committed suicide in 2002, with twelve of these individuals being fifteen years old or younger (Zacharias 2003). In Canada, according to a 2004 report, suicide accounted for 24 percent of all deaths among those aged fifteen to twenty-four (CanWest News Services 2004). First Nations youth are at a particularly high risk, with the Inuit having a rate of completed suicide about five times that of non-Aboriginal youth (Kirmayer, Boothroyd, and Hodgins 1998).

While illnesses such as schizophrenia and bipolar disorder typically manifest themselves in early adulthood, premorbid symptoms or indicators may appear earlier in life. In the case of schizophrenia, some persons may start to experience psychosis or become withdrawn and isolated ("schizoid") by their mid-teens. Unfortunately, these signs are difficult to interpret, and the family may assume that the behaviours are a product of youthful rebelliousness, recreational drug use, or "laziness." On this point, two Canadian psychiatrists conclude that "the particular diagnostic complexities of adolescent first episode psychosis, combined with the difficult transition between adolescence and adulthood, imply a need for specialized services for this population" (Menezes and Milovan 2000, 714).

Mood and anxiety disorders may emerge in childhood as well as later in life; these include social and specific phobias, obsessive-compulsive disorder, post-traumatic stress disorder, generalized anxiety disorder, and depression (American Psychiatric Association 2000). Anxiety disorders are the most common mental disorders seen in children (Waddell et al. 2004), with one-year prevalence rates estimated to be 10 percent (Garland 2002; Manassis 2000). A form of anxiety disorder that is peculiar to children and adolescents is *separation anxiety disorder,* characterized by excessive anxiety when the child is away from home or from his or her parents. This condition has a lifetime prevalence rate of about 4 percent and peaks during early adolescence (Andrews et al. 2000).

A condition that has its onset in childhood (before age seven) and that may cause considerable disruption at school and at home is attention-deficit hyperactivity disorder (ADHD). Diagnosis is made on the basis of symptoms of *inattention* (doesn't listen, doesn't follow through on instructions, can't organize tasks, is forgetful and easily distracted) or *hyperactivity-impulsivity* (fidgets, talks excessively, jumps out of his or her seat, can't wait his or her turn). These symptoms must have persisted for at least six months and be considered "maladaptive and inconsistent with developmental level" (American Psychiatric Association 2000, 92). Prevalence rates seen in school range from 3 percent to considerably higher depending on the inclusion criteria used (Rowland et al. 2001). It is estimated that up to 70 percent of persons with ADHD become well-functioning adults but that a smaller number will continue to have problems that may manifest as antisocial behaviour in adulthood (Andrews et al. 2000). The etiology of ADHD is not clearly understood; possible contributing factors are a genetic effect, prenatal insult and toxic exposure, premature birth, and emotional deprivation in early childhood (Sadock and Sadock 2003). Fetal alcohol syndrome has been linked with an early-onset, inattention subtype of ADHD (O'Malley and

Nanson 2002). Treatment approaches with ADHD include stimulant medication (which may need to persist into adulthood), family education and support, and cognitive-behavioural methods that are applied in the family and classroom settings (Weiss, Jain, and Garland 2000).

Having children as clients adds another layer of clinical and ethical complexity to community mental health practice. Practitioners have to wrestle with issues such as the duty to report abuse, informed consent, diagnostic uncertainty, and whether to use pharmacological treatments (Garland 2004). Assessment and treatment approaches may need to be modified to take into account the developmental level of the client (Rapoport and Ismond 1996). Practitioners will typically need to work with other involved systems, such as the family and the school; often practitioners working with children will have training in family therapy. Some childhood disorders, notably the "pervasive developmental disorders" described in the *DSM*, may require that clients receive the services of specialized treatment teams and rehabilitation programs.

Disorders among Older Persons

By the early twenty-first century the number of seniors, particularly those over eighty, had grown dramatically in Canada relative to other age groups, and this trend is expected to continue as the baby-boomer cohort ages (Sullivan et al. 2004). This fact has implications for the incidence of dementia, a progressive impairment of cognitive functioning, since rates of this disorder are directly related to age: while about 5 percent of those over sixty-five will have severe dementia, this figure jumps to 20 percent for persons over eighty (Sadock and Sadock 2003), with a Canadian study determining that 34 percent of those over eighty-five suffer from some form of dementia and that by the year 2031 over 750,000 Canadians will have Alzheimer's disease or a related dementia (Canadian Study of Health and Aging Working Group 1994).

The primary symptom of dementia is memory problems, although affected persons may also manifest mood and behaviour disturbances as well as psychotic symptoms. One great concern is that disoriented persons may wander away from a residence and thereby put themselves at considerable risk. The most common forms of dementia are Alzheimer's-type and vascular dementia, with the latter being caused by strokes (Ivan et al. 2004).

Older adults may experience other mental health problems, such as depression. In some cases (20-30%) depression coexists with dementia, and there is evidence that the onset of depressive symptoms in the year preceding the onset of Alzheimer's disease may represent the early symptoms of this dementia (Butters et al. 2004; Green et al. 2003). An onset of depression in later life may also be influenced by losses of friends and partners and by chronic medical conditions and may be exacerbated by alcohol use. Later-life depression, relative to what is seen in younger persons, is more frequently the melancholic subtype, with somatic symptoms, and may also produce cognitive impairment, which can be confused with true dementia (Sadock and Sadock 1998). Because this form of depression may not respond well to first-line treatments, the use of electroconvulsive therapy (ECT) is not uncommon with elderly patients (see Chapter 7). Older persons, particularly older men, are a higher-risk group for suicide. Apart from gender, suicide risk factors in the elderly include being isolated, living alone, anticipating admission to a nursing home, having financial problems, having a psychiatric illness, and having a serious medical condition such as cancer (Quan and Arboleda-Florez 1999).

For the practitioner, working with elderly clients is particularly challenging because of the interrelated medical, psychiatric, and social concerns. One example is the problem that medication use poses in that older persons may be on a wide range of pharmaceuticals with potentially adverse interactions, the use of which can exacerbate some psychiatric symptoms. At a minimum, the mental health practitioner needs to be in close contact with the family physician (assuming there is one). While prior to the 1980s there was greater reliance on institutionalization of older persons with psychiatric disorders, now interventions are increasingly delivered in the community, which has necessitated the development of interdisciplinary teams with an outreach capacity that provide education and advocacy as well as treatment (Donnelly 2001). Practitioners typically work with a number of allied agencies that provide support to older clients and their families, such as provincial chapters of the Alzheimer's Society (http://www.alzheimer.ca).

Substance Misuse

The *DSM* IV-TR defines substance *abuse* as a pattern of behaviour that negatively impacts on role obligations and relationships, results in substance-related legal problems, or leads to physically hazardous situations (such as drunk driving). A second category, substance *dependence*, is defined by the presence of three of seven criteria, which include: (1) drug tolerance (the need to increase the amount used to achieve the same effect); (2) drug withdrawal (symptoms reflecting the body's adaptation to the absence of a drug on which it is physically dependent – for example, depression, fatigue, agitation, and irritability in the case of cocaine); (3) a persistent desire to reduce intake; (4) a great deal of time spent in obtaining or using the substance or in recovering from its effects; (5) giving up important activities because of the drug-seeking and using behaviours; (6) continued use despite evidence that it is having a detrimental effect on the person's health; or (7) taking the substance in larger quantities or over a longer period than was intended.

One-year prevalence rates for alcohol and drug use disorders in the general population are about 7 percent and 2 percent respectively (Somers et al. 2004). In Canada there is evidence that self-reported rates of illicit drug use are increasing: a study released by the Canadian Centre on Substance Abuse (2004) found that the proportion of Canadians reporting any illicit drug in their lifetime rose from 28.5 percent in 1994 to 45 percent in 2004, with marijuana showing the largest absolute and relative increase. It has been hypothesized that more widespread use of marijuana may be related to more tolerant attitudes in Canada and to the finding that current marijuana products have stronger concentrations of the active compound tetrahydrocannabinol (THC) – making dependency more likely – than was the case previously (Blackwell 2005). Considerable concern has also been expressed about the growing use of methamphetamine in Canada, particularly among younger persons. Practitioners, including this author, have observed that "meth" can produce psychotic states in users that persist longer than the drug-induced psychoses seen with other agents.

Moving from the general public to persons diagnosed with mental disorders, a consistent and significant finding has been that rates of substance misuse are considerably higher for mental health clients in almost all diagnostic categories (psychotic, mood, anxiety, personality, and eating disorders). As reviewed by Minkoff (2001b), studies have found rates of substance dependence among persons with serious, persistent mental disorders ranging from 15 to 40 percent and rates of substance abuse ranging from 32 to 85 percent. A large-scale American survey of persons with schizophrenia found rates of alcohol abuse 3.6 times that of the general public, 5 times that for cannabis, 6.5 times that for opiates, and 13 times that for cocaine (Regier et al. 1990). Staying with schizophrenia as an example, these high rates of co-morbidity are clinically very significant in that co-occurring drug or alcohol abuse is associated with an earlier outbreak of psychotic symptoms, greater severity of these symptoms, and poorer treatment response (Negrette 2003).

In trying to explain the link between mental and addictive disorders, several (overlapping) hypotheses have been proposed:

- Use of alcohol and nonprescription drugs may be a form of self-medication. Persons with serious, persistent mental disorders, such as schizophrenia, can – as noted earlier – suffer from a range of symptoms, both positive (troubling thoughts and perceptions) and negative (dysphoria, anhedonia, and despair), and may be tempted to cope with these by using drugs or alcohol. There tends to be pharmacologic specificity in the drug of choice – that is, substances will be used corresponding to the predominant symptom experienced by the client. As noted, persons with schizophrenia are particularly vulnerable to the stimulant cocaine, which may be an attempt to alleviate the *negative* symptoms being experienced in that users report that the drug helps them with "depression" (Dixon et al. 1991). Drugs may also help clients cope with feelings of boredom, isolation, and loneliness.

- Having a mental disorder may simultaneously predispose an individual to a substance-use disorder – that is, again using the example of schizophrenia, "the inclination to abuse psychoactive substances is an additional symptom of the basic neuropathology underlying schizophrenia itself" (Negrette 2003, 16). Clinicians have observed that persons with psychotic disorders appear to have a more "fragile" (or vulnerable) brain with respect to the effects of street drugs.
- Cognitive impairment caused by the mental disorder may inhibit learning associated with adverse drug experiences, a hypothesis based on the conceptualization of an addictive disorder as "a faulty volitional process caused by a cognitive impairment that prevents the addict from making volitional decisions on the basis of all necessary memory" (Campbell 2003, 672).
- Social factors may be relevant, including (1) the reality that persons with serious mental disorders disproportionately live in poorer urban environments, where there is greater access to drugs and more environmental "triggers" (Phillips and Johnson 2001), and (2) the greater isolation experienced by persons with mental disorders and hence the use of drugs to facilitate interaction and socialization (unfortunately, clients may have to engage in drug use to be accepted as part of a group of peers).
- Persons with serious mental disorders typically have fewer coping resources partly because of their socio-economic status and also because of skill acquisition being interrupted by the course of the disorder.

Considering the complex interplay between mental health and addictive disorders, it can be seen that treatment approaches for persons with co-occurring conditions need to be multimodal, including teaching coping and social skills as well as challenging beliefs that directly or indirectly support the misuse of substances. To this end, cognitive-behavioural therapy, motivational interviewing, and training in relapse prevention have been used with persons with co-occurring conditions.

Clients struggling with co-occurring disorders face a number of treatment barriers. For one thing, mental health practitioners have not traditionally been involved in addictions treatment, which has been seen as a separate specialty. Further, some practitioners may not view drug addiction as a mental disorder at all, seeing it instead as controllable behaviour and an expression of free will, despite evidence of biological vulnerabilities (Committee on Addictions of the Group for the Advancement of Psychiatry 2002; Luchins et al. 2004; Satel 1999). Other potential barriers to treatment include the fact that the prevalence of substance use by persons with mental disorders has historically been underrecognized, and where recognized, used as the basis of *exclusion* from mental health programs. This seems to be changing, however, with greater recognition (finally) of the high rate of co-morbidity and consequently of the need for integrated treatment approaches (Minkoff 2001b).

Notes

1 The *kappa* statistic is used to measure agreement between different raters and runs below zero if agreement is less than would occur by chance, to zero at chance agreement, and to one at perfect agreement.

2 For example, a study of a Canadian forensic psychiatric hospital by this author found that one psychiatrist used the diagnosis "personality disorder not otherwise specified" in 100 percent of his assessments, while the other three psychiatrists in the study did not use it at all (Davis 1994b).

3 There are several caveats concerning the use of herbal remedies. Plants may contain several different compounds in varying concentrations, such that it is difficult to determine what is contributing to the therapeutic effect. There may also be an assumption by the public that "natural" remedies do not have toxic or side effects, which is not true. Further, there is the danger of unrecognized drug interactions.

4 On this point, a document produced by British Columbia Women's Hospital in Vancouver gives a scale that ranks mental disorders, with schizophrenia at the top and bipolar disorder mid-scale (British Columbia Reproductive Care Program, Reproductive Best Practices Working Group 2003).

5 One analyst notes that the First World War's "psychiatric casualties focused attention on the care and treatment of the mentally ill," giving impetus to the development of a mental hygiene movement in Canada (Guest 1980, 220).

6 And, more recently, "Gulf War Syndrome" (Hyams, Wignall, and Roswell 1996).

7 For example, it has been argued that antisocial personality disorder (APD) as a diagnosis is overinclusive and that it does not distinguish cases where socio-cultural factors (such as poverty or gang environment) have led to criminal conduct from cases where individuals' underlying personality traits represent greater clinical and safety concerns. Canadian psychologist Robert Hare (1993, 1996) has suggested that a narrower, more useful clinical entity is *psychopathy*, which is assessed by psychometric instruments and, as a construct, has greater predictive validity.

Other Resources

■ The website of Canadian psychiatrist Phillip Long (http://www.mentalhealth.com) has a large number of links to other websites on specific mental disorders and syndromes.

- The Schizophrenia website (http://www.schizophrenia.com) has many articles and links with information on this disorder for the nonspecialist.
- A handbook for families and clients dealing with the cognitive dysfunction associated with schizophrenia and other mental disorders is available at the website of the New York State Office of Mental Health: http://www.omh.state.ny.us/omhweb/cogdys_manual/ CogDysHndbk.htm.
- The McCreary Centre Society conducts research on health care issues affecting children and adolescents (see http://www.mcs.bc.ca).
- The website of the Soldiers Transition Program (http://www.educ.ubc.ca/faculty/westwood), developed at the University of British Columbia, describes interventions aimed at assisting soldiers returning from overseas who may be experiencing post-traumatic stress reactions or "reverse culture shock."
- The website of the Canadian Centre on Substance Abuse (http://www.ccsa.ca) has a number of research and policy documents related to substance misuse in Canada.
- The Canadian Psychological Association has a webpage with "fact sheets" on anxiety disorders (see http://www.cpa.ca/factsheets/main.htm).

Stakeholders

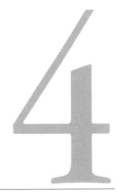

"**Stakeholder**" is a term that refers to individuals or groups who would expect to be consulted, or to have some say, in the development of public mental health policy. Three such groups are practitioners, family members, and clients themselves. While this list may seem unremarkable, the idea that the last two – families and clients – should be included is a relatively new development, since it has been the professionals who, until recently, have driven the policy agenda in Canada (McGrath and Tempier 2003).

Since the 1980s the impact of individuals and organizations representing these other stakeholders has been felt more strongly by service providers. As Curtis and Hodge (1995) note, "We are experiencing significant challenges to the assumptions underlying the balance of power in the service system" (45): "Greater emphasis in weight is [now] given to consumer choice and empowerment in service and supports. Concepts such as recovery, social integration, partnership, satisfaction in life, valued roles and natural support networks are being applied to mental health treatment and support services. Self-help, peer support, and self-advocacy are being recognized as components of wellness, recovery and even treatment" (44). Families as well, represented by organizations such as the Schizophrenia Society and the Mood Disorders Association, are now expecting to be included to a greater extent in treatment planning, policy development, and legislative initiatives. In 1993 the Canadian Mental Health Association published a report, *A New Framework for Support for People with Serious Mental Health Problems* (Trainor, Pomeroy, and Pape 1993, 1), that commented on the emergence of these "new stakeholders." The authors of the document spoke about the need to include all stakeholders in the mental health planning process, challenged the idea of professional expertise as the only legitimate knowledge base, and emphasized the "undeniable importance of personal experience." This theme has been taken up by Health Canada, whose report on best practices in mental health reform (1997b, 112) concluded that "the full range of stakeholders, including consumers and families, [should be] involved in the on-going development and evolution of policy" and that "mental health policy [should be] supported by an explicit vision that the various stakeholders are aware of and in agreement with." The remaining challenge is to make sure that the involvement of other stakeholders is meaningful, not just an exercise in tokenism.

While giving voice to persons not previously heard is almost certainly a positive development, this "new framework" has produced some conflicts of interest for the practitioner since not all stakeholder viewpoints are harmonious. For example, in an article on client empowerment in the *Canadian Journal of Community Mental Health*, the author notes that "the attainment of well-being requires the presence of three key elements: self-determination (sense of control over one's life), equality (respect and recognition of differences), and democratization (participation in decision-making)" (Wilson 1996, 71). This vision, unfortunately, is not easily reconciled with a tradition of hierarchical service delivery where the practitioner role has been that of unchallenged authority/expert. Indeed, since enabling self-determination and democratization has not usually been part of the service delivery tradition in public mental health, practitioners must now deal with the suggestion that the treatment approaches they have traditionally used may have actually fostered *greater* dependence and disability among the client population. A vision of client empowerment is also not easily reconciled with the recent introduction in Canadian jurisdictions of more coercive statutory treatment provisions, such as **community treatment orders**, which were partly the result of lobbying by family support groups – the *other* stakeholder (Davis 2002; Goering, Wasylenki, and Durbin 2000).

While program administrators have incorporated references to other stakeholder groups in their mission statements – at least paid them lip service, in other words – it is not always apparent that the implications of this nominal commitment have been clearly thought through – that is, how in practice these concepts should be operationalized. As one author concludes in reference to client empowerment, professionals "have embraced this ideal, but it may be that we have not really examined the dilemmas that emerge and the choices to be made when a profession adopts empowerment as a mission" (Hartman 1994, 171).

Using client empowerment as an organizing theme, this chapter reviews the "vested interests" of five stakeholder groups: practitioners, clients, family members, government, and (an "unofficial" member of the group) the drug companies. Of particular interest is where these interests are complementary and where they may be conflicting. Before starting, a disclaimer is necessary: while it is useful to comment on themes that appear to be recurring, it is at the same time risky, and presumptuous, to generalize about stakeholders as having one shared voice or one particular agenda. One author notes, for example, that "the psychiatric survivors movement, at least as it has evolved in Canada since the 1970s, is not homogeneous in terms of either membership or ideologies" (Dickinson 2002, 376). Readers should bear in mind, then, that there is disagreement and great diversity of opinion *within* stakeholder groups, let alone between them (Everett 1994; Kaufman 1999; Wilson 1996).

Practitioners
A number of different professionals may be involved in the provision of services to mentally disordered persons. These include:

- *Family physicians.* While general practitioners (GPs) are not considered mental health specialists, they are in fact the main contact point for many clients: surveys have found that 45 to 75 percent of persons requiring mental health care receive this care primarily or exclusively from their family physician (British Columbia Ministry of Health 2002e; Lin and Goering 1998; Watson et al. 2005) and that the majority of prescriptions for psychotropic medications are written by GPs (Lavoie and Fleet 2002). While this arrangement may be workable, specialist care is indicated for more complicated clinical presentations, more disabled clients, special populations (e.g., children, the elderly), and cases that primarily require nonpharmacological interventions. On this point, the fee-for-service billing arrangement means that GPs generally do not have the time to counsel clients with mental health problems (Hermann 2002). At the same time, GPs in remote areas face the additional problem that there may be no psychiatric specialists in their locale to whom they can refer clients.
- *Psychiatrists.* Psychiatrists are physicians who complete an additional period of specialist training (a "residency") that lasts three to five years.[1] Psychiatrists may work in both public and private practice, tending to see less disabled persons in the latter. Psychiatrists in private practice may be "eclectic" with respect to treatment models and the type of clientele seen or may specialize with respect to both. Because of this, it is important for practitioners and clients to have some preliminary, word-of-mouth understanding of whether a referral to a private psychiatrist will produce a "good fit."

    Psychiatrists (and physicians) are given special powers that consequently place them in a prominent position in the mental health system. First, they have the authority to arrange involuntary hospitalization, a procedure known as **certification** or **committal** (only in unusual circumstances can a nonphysician be involved in this process; see Chapter 13). Second, they may prescribe medication, unlike, for example, psychologists (however, see box). The role of psychiatry is distinguished as well by the fact that psychiatric services in both public and private practice are covered by provincial medical plans, meaning that they are effectively free to the client.[2] This is significant in that many persons with serious mental disorders are living in reduced financial circumstances and simply cannot afford private-pay arrangements. (Limited coverage of private-pay counselling is provided in some cases through employee benefit plans, and counselling may also be provided within the organization through "employee assistance" programs.) The undersupply of, and demand for, psychiatric services has meant that many private psychiatrists in Canada have lengthy waiting lists (Canadian Mental Health Association 2001).

- *Psychologists.* For clinical psychologists a PhD is the terminal degree and prerequisite for registration with provincial bodies. Psychology as a discipline is known for its emphasis on **evidence-based** practices in mental health, a stance to which other professions are only just catching up. Psychologists have also been prominent in the development and implementation of cognitive-behavioural therapies, an area of practice that is seen as being of increasing importance in the treatment of a range of mental disorders (see Chapter 11). Psychologists may work in private and public practice. In the public sector they have been used more in a consultative capacity, particularly to clarify diagnosis and treatment options through assessments and the use of a variety of psychometric tests.

  Educational and *counselling* psychologists usually receive training through university faculties of education, with the MEd/MA or EdD/PhD being the qualifying degrees for practitioners. Persons with these credentials often (but not necessarily) work with families and younger clients.

- *Nurses.* Nurses are widely employed in the public mental health system, both in hospital settings and in the community as clinicians and case managers. Their knowledge of medicine and pharmacology is particularly valuable with respect to monitoring medication effects and side effects. Nurses working in mental health may be registered nurses (RNs) or registered psychiatric nurses (RPNs), with these two groups having separate professional associations. RPNs are trained, regulated, and employed only in the four western Canadian provinces (British Columbia, Alberta, Saskatchewan, and Manitoba). Another nursing group is the licensed practical nurses (LPNs), who work primarily in institutional settings.

- *Occupational therapists.* Occupational therapy (OT) is a specialty that focuses on the rehabilitation needs of persons with both physical and psychiatric disabilities. In mental health, OTs may work in hospital and community settings, performing life-skill assessments and developing groups and programs that address social, leisure, and vocational functioning. Training programs in occupational therapy are usually affiliated with university medical or health science faculties, with a master's degree being the qualifying credential.

- *Social workers.* Social workers are employed in hospitals, where they play an important role in discharge planning, as well as community settings, where they often work as case managers. Training is at the baccalaureate or master's level, with most undergraduates receiving a "generalist" education. Most university social-work programs make some reference to social justice, equity, or empowerment in their mission statements. One text notes that with their ecological and systems perspective, "social workers have a unique perspective on the social and familial context of mental health problems, and are uniquely suited to advocate for and link with other systems in which clients are involved" (Sands and Angell 2002, 260).
- *Recreation and leisure therapists.* A relatively new rehabilitation specialty, therapeutic recreation, is provided to persons "who have physical, mental, social or emotional limitations which impact their ability to engage in meaningful leisure experiences" (Canadian Therapeutic Recreation Association 2003, 1). The qualifying credential is usually a college diploma or baccalaureate degree.

For practitioners, the relationship with other stakeholders can be seen in terms of a number of *obligations,* which can be examined, in part, by referring to codes of ethics and practice standards. For the purposes of the discussion here, the *Canadian Medical Association Code of Ethics, Annotated for Psychiatrists (CMA)* (Neilson 1996), will be used as an example. (Ethical guidelines are discussed in more detail in Chapter 13.) Psychiatry is chosen here because of its influential, leading position in interdisciplinary mental health settings.

Prescription Privileges

The idea that physicians should have the exclusive right to prescribe psychotropic medication has been challenged in recent years, primarily in American jurisdictions. In 2002 the State of New Mexico passed legislation granting clinical psychologists qualified prescription privileges, which involves a two-year internship under the supervision of a psychiatrist as a prerequisite to

independent prescribing; similar legislation has also been passed in Louisi-
ana (Yates 2004). While these developments may seem surprising to some,
they were justified on the basis of necessity: the New Mexico state government noted that few psychiatrists were available outside of the major metropolitan areas, that waiting lists were long, and that mental health needs
were high, as evidenced by suicide rates among the populace in more remote areas.

In an article in the *Canadian Journal of Psychiatry,* Lavoie and Fleet (2002)
review the reasons offered by proponents of prescription privileges for psychologists. One argument, consistent with the New Mexico example, is that
this increases public access to treatment. The authors suggest that a shortage of psychiatrists has (in part) resulted in most prescriptions for psychotropic medication being issued by general practitioners, who have limited
training in psychiatry and who may "frequently misdiagnose" their patients
(445). A second argument is that treatment is more coherent and effective
when both counselling and medication are offered by the same party. Finally, there is the "turf-guarding" view: that "psychologists do not and cannot
function as independent professionals because the medical profession places
many restrictions on their practice" (443). Counterarguments include the
position that prescribing would seem inconsistent with the mandate of psychology as well as the concern that nonphysicians would be dealing with
issues such as medication side effects, drug interactions, physical complications, and unrecognized organic causes of psychiatric symptoms (Scully 2004).

The issue of access to treatment has been advanced to support prescription privileges for another, relatively "accessible" professional group: pharmacists. In Canada provincial pharmacy associations, notably in Alberta, have
started to submit proposals to legislators that would see limited prescription
privileges being given to pharmacists, particularly the power to provide refills for long-term patients with already diagnosed conditions or to give out
medications for relatively minor problems, psoriasis being an example
(O'Connor 2003). Physicians have objected to this on the grounds of patient
safety, with the president of the British Columbia Medical Association (BCMA)
stating that while "doctors are not looking for more business, the fact is you've
got to look after some of these people who are on long-term medications
very carefully" (7). In British Columbia in 2001 pharmacists won the right to
give out contraceptive "morning-after" pills without medical authorization;
the mixed feelings that this engendered were reflected by the fact that the
move was opposed by the BCMA but supported by the Society of Gynecolo-
gists and Obstetricians (O'Connor 2003).[3]

Member responsibilities, as articulated in the *CMA* document, are to the *patient*, to *society*, to the *profession*, and to *oneself*. To begin with, it is noteworthy that in the *CMA* guidelines there is no separate section referring to a responsibility to *families* – one of the "new" stakeholder groups. Family involvement is referred to in a single annotation within the section "responsibilities to the patient," as follows: "Be considerate of the patient's family and significant others and cooperate with them in the patient's interest. Psychiatrists recognize well the need to obtain the cooperation of relatives in providing collateral information and supporting treatment plans. They also recognize the need to assuage relative's anxiety about the care of their family member. However, ethical psychiatrists will recognize that *relatives' needs come second to the obligation to maintain confidentiality with the patient*" (Neilson 1996, 5, emphasis added). One can see that in this reference families are apparently placed in a subordinate role, as "providers of information" and "supporters of treatment plans." Crucially, the passage indicates that, in the case of competing interests, family needs come second to the necessity of maintaining a therapeutic alliance with the client (more on this below).

Concerning obligations to clients/patients, the *CMA* document, in brief, notes that services provided should be nondiscriminatory, that whenever possible there should be informed consent given for treatment, that autonomy (e.g., the right of a competent patient to refuse treatment) should be respected, that requests for a second opinion should be adhered to, and that confidentiality should be protected. In the majority of situations psychiatric practitioners strive to achieve these practice standards. At the same time, it must be acknowledged that there are cultural and organizational factors that work against this ideal – in particular, with respect to the ethical ideal of *autonomy* – and thus, ultimately, against a vision of client empowerment.

The first of these is medical authority. One cannot avoid the obvious fact that we – clients and nonclients alike – have been socialized to hold medical professionals in high regard and consequently not to challenge their authority. This authority is based, philosophically and in law, on what has been described as a *fiduciary* relationship between doctor and patient, which refers to a contract wherein "one person (a patient) *entrusts his or her welfare to another* (a physician)" (Gabbard and Nadelson 1995, 1445, emphasis added). One could argue, then, that by this definition – which has the service recipient giving over power to the service provider – the doctor-patient relationship is an inherently paternalistic one. In considering medical authority, a related concept is *collegiality*, which is defined in *Webster's Dictionary* as "cooperative interaction among colleagues" and which can be manifested as the reluctance of one practitioner to criticize another (at least on the record) either because it appears unprofessional or because of the fear that "there but for the grace of God go I." A practical consequence of this conforming tendency is that colleagues may be reticent with respect to second-guessing or – referring to the *CMA* guidelines – volunteering second opinions even when clients may have good reasons for making the request.

A second factor limiting client empowerment is mandated treatment. The nature of psychiatric practice is such that in some cases the relationship with the client is involuntary by definition: examples would be employment in hospital settings with clients who have been certified under mental health legislation; in the field of forensic psychiatry, where client attendance is mandated by court order; or, increasingly, in outpatient settings, where involuntary treatment, not previously an issue, is now made possible with community treatment orders.

A third factor is liability. A key component in practitioner thinking is the perception, held rightly or wrongly, that if a treatment decision turns out poorly, it will come back to haunt the decision maker; at the very least this individual will look bad, and moreover he or she may be disciplined or sued. While fear of litigation may be exaggerated, it can be argued that practitioners nonetheless *should* be aspiring to high standards and – the other way of looking at this issue – be concerned about accountability. At the same time, a consequence of this preoccupation is practitioner decisions that are very cautious or conservative, which may have the effect of working against client autonomy and empowerment. So, for example, a psychiatrist may be reluctant to rescind a community treatment order – permitting an individual to strike out on his or her own – because of a history of self-harming behaviour, even though the last incident occurred quite some time ago. Thus the client is held in an involuntary status longer than is (arguably)

Client Confidentiality vs. Duty to Disclose

One of the most difficult decisions in mental health practice concerns the question of whether information, given in apparent confidence, should be disclosed to a third party, and it is an issue that is a source of tension between practitioners, clients, and family members.[4]

In general, practitioners may not divulge information that they have gathered on a client without that person's written consent. To do otherwise may not only violate agency policy, the common law, and privacy statutes, but could be seen by the client as betrayal and severely damage the therapeutic relationship. Such breaches of confidentiality can be considered professional misconduct and grounds for discipline.

In practice, however, clinicians regularly encounter situations where they may have to consider sharing information with a third party. In many cases, such as communication with another care provider, this is defensible, justified under the principle of *continuity of care*. That being said, a guiding principle is to share only the information deemed necessary to provide the continuity, divulging information only on a "need to know" basis. This becomes more complicated if it is unclear whether the third party is indeed providing care, such as family members who are worried about their mentally disordered relative but who are not living with or looking after the individual.

In some cases, sharing information with another party is legally mandated. Examples of this are when the practitioner is subpoenaed to testify in court or when there is evidence of abuse or neglect concerning a vulnerable individual, such as a child (referring to child protection laws) or a demented older adult (referring to adult guardianship statutes). Since there is no blanket privilege given in law to clinician-client communications in Canada, clients should be told in advance by practitioners that there is no absolute guarantee of confidentiality.

Arguably, the most difficult decision practitioners face in this regard concerns the *duty to warn* since the legal guidelines in this area have not always been clear. The Supreme Court of Canada ruled on this matter in the 1999 *Smith v. Jones* decision, a case where the client, "Jones," had revealed to a psychiatrist detailed plans for the torture and killing of young female prostitutes in a specified area of Vancouver. In this instance, the potential victims were identifiable and in imminent danger of serious bodily harm. In their ruling, the court established a legal test, which, if all three criteria are satisfied, permits a breach of confidentiality on the basis of duty to warn:

1 Is there a clear risk to an identifiable person or group of persons?
2 Is there a risk of serious bodily harm or death?
3 Is the danger imminent (i.e., close at hand or soon to actually happen)?

Unfortunately, actual case scenarios are not usually as clear-cut as the "Jones" example, leaving one analyst to conclude: "Inherent in the *Smith v. Jones* decision is the fact that many ethically challenging scenarios arise in which the law does not provide physicians with the appropriate or necessary legal directives. Absent specific legislative provisions, physicians are left to determine for themselves when disclosure will or will not result in a finding of professional misconduct and/or civil liability for negligence" (Tremayne-Lloyd 2003, 3).

necessary. It should be said that suicide risk is a "red flag" for many clinicians, with attempts and completions becoming a cause for administrative audits in some mental health programs, even though suicidal behaviour in the client population is relatively common and not easy to predict (Davis 2000). Consequently, it is not surprising, nor unreasonable, that practitioners tend to err on the side of caution. Lest some readers find this analysis overly cynical, it is readily acknowledged that clinical cautiousness may also be the result of *best intentions*. Practitioners may simply want to "do good" – that is, to protect the client from harm and look after that person's best interests. In any case, whether driven by benevolence or fear of liability, the consequence can be decisions that some would view as excessively paternalistic.

The other major stakeholder referred to in the *CMA* document is "society." Just as practitioners have a responsibility to consider and mitigate the likelihood of self-harm by clients, there is an obligation to consider the potential of harm coming to others at the hands of their clients, which indeed may form the basis for involuntary hospitalization and treatment of the client. Practitioners have other legal obligations in this regard, one being a *duty to report,* most often applied in the case of information concerning child abuse coming to the attention of the clinician. Further, there is the question of a **duty to warn** (or protect), an area of jurisprudence that has become increasingly prominent since the influential 1974 *Tarasoff* case[5] in the United States, wherein a clinician was found liable for not warning/protecting the intended victim of his client. For a practitioner, breaching the confidentiality and therefore trust of his or her client by reporting to a third party is a very difficult decision, made more complicated by the fact that in most cases references to harm by the client are vague and not necessarily specific to an identifiable individual victim (and not usually carried out in any case). However, it has become clear in the Canadian legal context, following the 1999 Supreme Court of Canada Decision in *Smith v. Jones,*[6] that in the view of the courts, public safety outweighs clinician-client confidentiality (see Chaimowitz and Glancy 2002 and box on previous page). These obligations to mitigate harm to others, as was the case concerning client self-harm, will contribute to caution in clinical decision making and may compromise the goals of achieving trust and collaboration, and of supporting autonomy in the therapeutic relationship.

Apart from safety issues, the *CMA* document notes that psychiatric practitioners have responsibilities to society with respect to "public health, health education ... legislation affecting the health or well-being of the community, and the need for testimony at judicial proceedings" (Neilson 1996, 7). This section of the document also states that members should recognize their responsibility "to promote fair access to health care resources" and to "use health care resources prudently" (8). An annotation adds that "psychiatric administrators have the responsibility to recognize when available resources cannot adequately meet the needs of a population and to determine what constitutes 'fairness of access' in this setting" (8). Here is raised the difficult issue of balancing the needs of individual clients with the need to recognize that "health care resources are finite" (8), an issue that has become more pressing in recent years as health authorities in Canada increasingly emphasize cost containment and "sustainability." The *CMA* document is silent on the question of whether psychiatric practitioners should play a role in advocacy or lobbying for more resources, except for the following annotation, which would appear to separate the clinical from the political: "Psychiatrists may at times feel obliged to comment publicly on certain social issues (for example, on poverty or homelessness) as they may relate to mental health. However, it is important for the profession to state clearly whether the comment or opinion is a personal or professional one and not to use one's professional status to augment the validity of a personal opinion" (7-8).

In summary, it can be said that psychiatrists and other mental health practitioners carry a considerable burden concerning their responsibilities to both clients and society. It can be noted that in many instances these responsibilities to different stakeholders are competing and not easily resolvable: the interests of relatives (see more on this below), the obligation to consider safety and mitigate harm, and the need to "use health resources prudently" all have the potential of compromising the clinical relationship and working against ethical ideals such as client autonomy, particularly with the more recent recognition of client empowerment as a worthwhile goal. While not making excuses for practitioners, it can be argued that the job of dealing with these competing interests is, if anything, underrecognized by others. Indeed, critics of mental health practice – whether clients, family members, advocates, administrators, or academics – need to consider the difficult balancing act that practitioners are asked to perform and the fact that clinicians

Professional Imperialism?

While one way of viewing the actions of mental health practitioners is in terms of a number of obligations to clients and other stakeholders, a different, more skeptical view is to see their group behaviour as reflecting simple self-interest. The idea that organizations act to further their own interests is not particularly remarkable; indeed, one of the key functions of any profession or labour union is to enhance the conditions of employment of its members.

There are, however, several implications that flow from this, one being that professions act to maintain a competitive position in the "marketplace." In looking at the issue of which of these competitors is doing better in this respect, sociologists (e.g., Freidson 1994) point to several attributes that distinguish successful, or higher-status, professions: (1) their ability to claim exclusive domain over an area of knowledge and skill; (2) the political power to control and organize their work, particularly the *content* of the work; and (3) their ability to be self-regulating. Currently, psychiatry is well situated in the mental health marketplace partly because of the preeminence of the biomedical model in mental health. Psychiatric practitioners carry with them the *imprimatur* of medical authority, the ability to admit persons to hospital, the licence to prescribe medication, and the ability to offer services that are covered (with some qualifications) by all provincial health care plans. The advent of apparently effective psychopharmacological treatments, in the words of a former president of the Canadian Psychiatric Association, "confirmed and ratified the psychiatrist in his role of physician as a treater of severe mental disorders" (Marie-Albert 2002, 915). Public funding also gives psychiatry an advantage over other disciplines such as psychology, whose private practitioners generally do not receive Medicare payments, a fact that caused the Ontario Psychological Association (2001) to complain in their report to the Romanow Commission that psychology was being marginalized in the Canadian health care system. (The historically limited role of psychology within mental health prompted the creation of a lobbying group, the Canadian Association for Accessibility to Psychological Services [Rochefort 1992].)

Concerning claims to "knowledge and skill," the skeptical viewpoint is to see mental health professionals overestimating in this regard, claiming broader tracts of psychic territory as a way of maintaining or expanding markets. For evidence of this conduct, critics point, for example, to the increasing number of conditions being defined as mental disorders in successive revisions of diagnostic manuals such as the *Diagnostic and Statistical Manual (DSM)* of the American Psychiatric Association (Kutchins and Kirk 1997; Davis 1997). Noting the expansion from 297 categories in the *DSM* III-R (1987) to 374 in the *DSM* IV (1994), Caplan (1995) suggests that this increasing number is not supportable by the standards of scientific validation and is more a reflection of personal and political agendas. On the tendency of professions to "overreach," Freidson (1994, 69) notes that "professional ideologies are inherently imperialistic, claiming more for the profession's knowledge and skill, and a broader jurisdiction, than can in fact be justified by demonstrable effectiveness. Such imperialism can of course be a function of crude self-interest, but it can as well be seen as a natural outcome of the deep commitment to the value of his [*sic*] work developed by the thoroughly socialized professional who has devoted his entire adult life to it."

On the issue of professional self-regulation, the conventional view is that licensing and regulation are the best means by which accountability is achieved and public safety protected. For instance, in his text *The Regulation of Professions in Canada,* James Casey (1994, 3) notes that "the primary purpose of the establishment of self-governing professions is the protection of the public. This is achieved by ensuring that only the qualified and the competent are permitted to practice and that members of the profession conform to appropriate standards of professional conduct." Similarly, Canadian psychiatrist Jean Marie-Albert (2002, 919) observes that "the three major features of medical professionalism – the ethic of service, clinical autonomy, and self-regulation – benefit patients and society ... Individual psychiatrists should protect ... professionalism in psychiatry ... by contributing to the efforts of organized psychiatry and medicine to maintain and enhance the ethic of service, clinical autonomy, and self-regulation." The skeptical position, on the other hand, is to see self-regulation as a way of demarcating and protecting an area of "turf." By way of example, Dineen (1998) suggests that the establishment of licensing boards by psychologists in the 1950s was a reaction to the threats of psychiatry to designate psychotherapy an exclusively medical procedure.

Another implication of this econometric analysis is to see the need for health care services driven by "supply" (numbers of practitioners) as well as "demand" (number of clients requiring services). Simply put, an increasing number of psychiatrists, psychologists, social workers, and other counsellors will drive the numbers of clientele being seen, although these numbers will ultimately be limited by the caps placed on public and employer funding of treatment services. An argument advanced by University of British Columbia professor Robert Evans (1984) and others in the 1970s and 1980s was that health care costs were fuelled by an overproduction of physicians, leading to a "supply-induced demand" for subsequent medical services and use of hospital beds. One consequence of this was a reduction of medical school places in several Canadian universities in the 1990s, which is now being blamed for an *under*supply of doctors in many areas (Grant and Oertel 1997; Kennedy 2005; Ryten, Thurber, and Buske 1998). Estimating the "right" number of health care workers per capita is currently a matter of some interest for cash-strapped health authorities, which are in the process of arriving at and implementing these "benchmarks."

do not have the luxury of endless rumination and committee work but must *act* – must "do something."

Clients

While clients of the mental health system have for some years spoken and written about their experiences (e.g., Geller and Harris 1994), their opinions have frequently been overlooked, if not disqualified. Sociologist Leona Bachrach (1996, 17) observes that "[clients] are, perforce, experts in the field of mental health program planning, and their products are often frank, articulate, and exceedingly sensitive. In fact, their writings contain important clues and information from which mental health program planners might take direction; yet surprisingly little note has been taken of the patient-authored literature." Disqualification of the views of clients, particularly if these views are hostile to psychiatry, is made easier because their apparent "lack of insight" can be attributed to the disorder itself.[7] As one client notes, "patients have had very little credibility when they do speak, because it's our minds that are in question" (cited in Brook 2003, H5). A Health Canada (2002c, 2) report also notes that having their agenda heard is made difficult because of the socio-economic status of many clients: "[clients may face] difficulties in mounting political lobbying efforts due to the poverty and disability of people affected by mental illness, and their consequent disadvantage in competing with other groups for limited health care services and supports."

Client critiques of the mental health system address several recurring themes. To begin with, there is disagreement over the very fundamental question of our frame of reference: on one side are adherents of a biological model, and on the other side are those clients who see what is called "mental disorder" as a product of "social stigmatization" – that is, as having to do with "the inability of so-called sane members of society to tolerate the emotions and perceptions of others" (Kaufman 1999, 501). Trying to find common ground between these two positions is admittedly a very difficult challenge for all stakeholders.

A second theme has to do with concern about the use of *coercion* in treatment, either in the form of certification or, more recently, with the use of community treatment orders (Hall 2000). In a review of the client-authored literature, Frese (1997, 18-19) concludes that "while not all mentally ill persons are ... strident and ... unappreciative of services received, clearly a substantial segment of those who are willing to share their perspectives voice dissatisfaction, especially with mandated treatment." An example of a client perspective on the issue of enforced treatment comes from Vancouver advocate Jill Stainsby (2000, 155): "I believe that the therapeutic alliance which may be achieved between a patient and a physician or treatment team, which already has been eroded by involuntary committal in the first place, will be further weakened by the practice of [community treatment orders]. People will avoid the mental health system because of its focus on control over individuals with mental health diagnoses ... This approach to care is not a positive step for mental health: it is antagonistic, and it involves the use of threats – mandatory treatment, rehospitalization – in order to maintain individuals in the least expensive treatment regimen."

A third major area of critique concerns the mental health system's apparently narrow focus in responding to the needs of clients – that is, a preoccupation with symptom management to the exclusion of other important domains, such as housing, work, and social relationships (Chamberlin and Rogers 1990). Toronto advocate and author Pat Capponi (2003, xv) puts this quite simply: "The needs of members of the psychiatric community are not so different, really, from anyone else's needs – a home, a job, a friend."

Disagreements about what is important in recovery have been found in a number of surveys. For example, a study on "unmet needs" conducted for the National Alliance for the Mentally Ill in the United States found that while a majority of clients believed they were getting sufficient help with medication support, only 29 percent felt they were getting comparable help in obtaining or keeping a job (Uttaro and Mechanic 1994). Another survey, comparing the priorities of practitioners, family members, and clients diagnosed with schizophrenia, found that housing as an area of need was rated second in importance (out of seven outcome variables) by clients but only sixth by both practitioners and family members (Fischer, Shumway, and Owen 2002). Noting that clients "rarely" agreed with the other two stakeholder groups on the outcome variables, the authors found that practitioners tended to value "control of symptoms" and "medication management" more highly, whereas clients and family members rated social support, housing, and medical and dental services as more important (728). Similarly, a study of 205 clients of a Canadian mental health service found statistically significant differences between the three stakeholders – clients, practitioners, and significant others – among seventeen of twenty-one outcome variables, which referred to "unmet rehabilitation needs" (Calsaferri and Jongbloed 1999). In this survey the proportion of clients expressing an unmet need was compared to the proportion of significant others and practitioners who expressed the same unmet need as it applied, in their view, to that client. It was found, for example, that "job training or education" was seen as an unmet need by 43 percent of significant others, 37 percent of clients, but only 14 percent of practitioners; similarly, the percentages for "making friends" were 45, 32, and 14, respectively.

Regarding social relationships, another area that has been neglected by service providers until more recent times concerns support for clients who are also parents of young children (Lees 2004). Traditionally, the response when there was any concern about parental competence has been child apprehension, and in fact not that long ago mandatory sterilization for persons with mental disabilities was government policy in many jurisdictions. Gradually, more progressive approaches are being implemented, which include support groups, various publications, and the development of *advanced planning agreements*, which give guidelines to a client's support team in the area of child care should the client become unwell due to a mental disorder.

A fourth area of critique concerns access to alternative treatments and applications. For example, one advocate talks about the need to extend "medical coverage [to] non-drug medical support. Massage therapy, reflexology, counseling and 'talk therapy,' yoga and/or vitamin and herbal supplements to strengthen the nervous and immune system are all effective components of a health care regime that lowers stress and can protect any person from the debilitating effects of depression or psychosis" (Thor-Larsen 2002, 4). A spokesperson for the psychiatric survivors movement notes that, despite a lack of ideological unity, "the movement is held together by its common commitment to ... the development of self-help alternatives to professionally provided treatment" (cited in Dickinson 2002, 376). The importance of other, nonmedical pathways to healing is emphasized in the constitution of the Vancouver/Richmond Mental Health Network Society (2004, 16), a consumer-run advocacy and support organization, whose stated purpose is

> to continually advocate for a more integrated, holistic mental health system by encouraging the development of programs and treatments that truly reflect the needs of consumers ... to encourage consumers to become less dependent on the mental health system by educating them about their rights, by sharing information about the availability of alternative programs and treatments, and by supporting the recovery efforts of those who have used the system ... To aid in the promotion and development of alternative mental health treatments, by educating members about such services and by referrals to such practitioners where appropriate; and by lobbying senior governments for inclusion of such services in the mental health funding system.

Efforts to address the deficits in the range of mental health services provided are now being undertaken, driven in part by a new paradigm called the "recovery" model, and the importance of other domains – housing, education, relationships, and work – is now referred to in best practice documents (e.g., British Columbia Ministry of Health 2002b). It is notable, however, that in the early years of the post-deinstitutionalization era – the 1960s and 1970s – gaps in the system were sometimes filled, of necessity, by mutual support efforts among mental health clients themselves. For example, the successful and influential clubhouse program Fountain House, based in New York City, was originally started by a group of ex-hospital patients who formed a mutual-aid organization called WANA (We Are Not Alone). Across the border in Vancouver, British Columbia, the Mental Patients Association (MPA) was formed in the early 1970s by a group of clients who met at an outpatient treatment program and who found "more real support from their informal network than the therapy they received during the hospital hours." The goals of this new organization were to "assist in the rehabilitation and promote the welfare of mental patients and former mental patients" and to "establish and operate social, vocational, recreational, residential and emergency facilities" (Mental Patients Association 2001a, 1).

Nevertheless, it must be emphasized that not all clients of the mental health system are critical of the services they receive and that, most significant, a number have gone on the record to support the use of coercive treatment – that is, involuntary hospitalization – when necessary. For example, an individual diagnosed with schizophrenia summarizes his own experiences as follows: "Although I recognize that some of my fellow mental health consumers are strongly opposed to the concept of forced treatment, I personally feel that I greatly benefited from being forced to accept treatment during periods in which I was incapable of understanding that I needed it. In fact, I sometimes wonder what would have become of me had someone not given me the treatment I so desperately needed but was so opposed to accepting" (Frese 1997, 17).

There is at times an uneasy tension between those clients critical of the system and those more or less satisfied with the services they have received. Capponi (2003, 30) distinguishes the two by referring to the latter as "patients" and the former as "survivors":

Mental health *patients* learn at an early age to trust professional experts, especially those with "doctor" in front of their names ... They are sure the doctors must know, and they must know what's best. *Survivors,* on the other hand, have a jaundiced view of medical models, past and present. They have a strong sense of identity with the patients who have gone before. They understand what these men and women have endured in search of a cure. They understand that they have frightened themselves and others by responding aloud to the voices in their heads and that they have been convicted and incarcerated with no hope of release, simply for being diagnosed as mentally ill. (Emphasis added)

Others take great exception to the implication that one group has a clearer, truer vision, while those who go along with the status quo have evidently been duped or brainwashed. This issue is taken up by a client in an editorial entitled "Client versus client," wherein the author, who states that "treatment by professionals has saved my life" (Gibson-Leek 2003, 1101), criticizes current initiatives that have militant "super clients" being funded by public mental health dollars to be advocates or peer-support workers:

> The *truly mentally ill* are bullied into silence. The "super clients" now speak on my behalf. With their new-found power they abuse the "lesser" client. When I told one of these "leaders" that she did not speak for me and that I benefited from professional treatment, I was told "You have been brainwashed by the system" ... No client should ever be placed above another client or be paid to be a client. Funds that should be going to treat the mentally ill are now squandered on extremists who constantly seek attention, awards, esteem, power and control over others ... I am sure that some people have not had good experiences. This does not mean they control my experiences. Many of these people *were never mentally ill*. They simply couldn't cope unless they were in control, and so they ended up in the mental health system. (1101-2, emphasis added)

While this author may be guilty of rhetorical excess, the words in italics speak to an important and troubling perception: namely that these more strident, critical individuals, whether they are called "survivors" or "super clients," are not representative of the population of persons with mental disorders, not "truly mentally ill," and thus not entitled to speak on their behalf. This is all the more significant when one considers that, while voiced in this case by a client, these same sentiments have been expressed at times by practitioners (although not publicly),[8] who may be used to dealing with quieter, more compliant individuals. While practitioners may be tempted to discount the views of the more strident, they should be alert to the dangers of stereotyping – that is, of holding the view that all clients should behave in a uniform and, in this case, passive manner to qualify as a "real" client. This is similar to the belief that if you recover from a mental disorder or achieve vocational success, you couldn't have really been mentally ill (see Fisher 1999).

The tension between the critical and accepting viewpoints is not easily resolved. Indeed, some observers have suggested that these perspectives represent two separate movements: a "consumer" movement, where the aim is to achieve partnerships with mental health practitioners, and a "survivor" movement, which seeks "complete liberation from psychiatry" (Everett 1994,

63). When receiving conflicting viewpoints in the same setting – for example, in a consumer advisory group meeting with a mental health team – practitioners need to be sensitive and respectful and to ensure that all have an opportunity to contribute to the discussion on the issue. In these situations, coaching, team building, and mediation skills are desirable commodities.

In sum, on the question of consumer involvement, a best practices document (British Columbia Ministry of Health 2002b, 3) talks about the need to offer "advocacy and outreach to give a voice to those without a voice, and to involve more of them meaningfully," as well as the need to put in place "democratic decision-making processes that value and actively include the views and opinions of a variety of consumers."

Families

Trying to support a family member with a serious mental disorder – a child, sibling, or parent – can be a daunting task, a fact not always appreciated by practitioners (see Spaniol et al. 1987). In an article entitled "The family experience of mental illness," Marsh and Johnson (1997) review the challenges faced by families: these include dealing with grief and symbolic loss because of expectations that have been dashed, chronic sorrow (never reaching a stage of acceptance), the emotional roller coaster of not knowing what to expect from one day to the next, the forced return to a parenting role with an adult offspring, stigma, financial burden, self-neglect, and frustrations about dealing with the "system," a lack of support, and an apparent absence of services. On this last point, a review by Calsaferri and Jongbloed (1999, 201) concludes that family members have tended to express "dissatisfaction with professional services for their relatives." Indeed, it is unfortunately the case that the relationship between practitioners and family members is one that, historically, has been characterized by ambivalence, if not mistrust.

Why is this the case? First, one has to consider the unfortunate legacy of etiological theories that implicitly or explicitly blamed family members for contributing to their son's or daughter's mental disorder (see box on next page). Examples of this include the notion of the "schizophrenogenic mother," attributed to German psychoanalyst Frieda Fromm-Reichmann, and the autism-producing "refrigerator mother," an idea proposed by child psychologist Bruno Bettelheim, who drew parallels between the demeanour of mothers with autistic children and guards at Nazi concentration camps – where Bettelheim himself had been imprisoned. These now defunct conceptions were developed in a period when psychiatry was heavily influenced by psychodynamic theories, which sought explanations in early childhood experiences for disorders that are now understood to be more biologically based. While times have changed, an observer notes that practitioners may

Family Theories and Schizophrenia

From the 1940s through the 1970s a number of theories concerning family dynamics were proposed to account for the etiology of schizophrenia, with the role of the mother, in particular, being singled out. As reviewed by Davis (1987a), these included the concept of the cold, rejecting "schizophrenogenic mother," the "double-bind" hypothesis (an investigation of contradictory messages from the parent), the role of marital "schism and skew" in the family of persons with schizophrenia, and an Italian group's findings based on a study of families in "schizophrenic transition" and their use of "paradoxical communications." R.D. Laing, a once influential psychiatrist and author, also implicated the family, notably in his 1964 book *Sanity, Madness and the Family*.

These theories have now, for the most part, been discarded, although it is noteworthy that a text published as recently as 1980 claimed that the "double-bind hypothesis has grown into one of the most scientifically respectable theories of schizophrenia-producing family interaction" (Goldenberg and Goldenberg 1980, 87). Apart from the current research, which increasingly supports a biological conception of schizophrenia, methodological criticisms of these early family studies pointed out that establishing the direction of cause and effect when studying communication patterns is fraught with difficulty and that one could find distorted communications in "normal" families as well. Unfortunately, there has been a legacy of mistrust between family members and practitioners stemming from this perceived tendency to blame the family (Marsh and Johnson 1997).

More recently, researchers have investigated **expressed emotion** (EE) in the social settings of persons with schizophrenia. While not speaking to etiology, researchers have found evidence that in settings and families where there is emotional overinvolvement and excessive negative comments, relapse of persons with the disorder is more likely (Butzlaff and Hooley 1998; Raune, Kuipers, and Bebbington 2004). While this hypothesis seems reasonable – it is, after all, consistent with the stress-vulnerability model discussed earlier – it remains controversial. A guide for the treatment of first-break psychosis from the University of British Columbia offers a dissenting view: while higher EE may develop "over time in families that have difficulties adjusting to the psychotic illness," the authors conclude that "there is little evidence that EE is associated with relapse in early psychosis patients or that family work designed to decrease expressed emotion reduces relapse" (Mental Health Evaluation and Community Consultation Unit 2002, 15). The concept of EE may also create apprehension about the potential for finding fault, with one author suggesting that the conundrum concerning the direction of causality has still not been resolved and that the whole concept "continues to blame families" (Solomon 2001, 68).

still, even if unintentionally, "send the message to struggling parents (whose sensitivity is already heightened to criticism) that they are failing as parents and that their failure is a primary cause of their child's problems" (Duncan 2004, 13).

A second area of potential conflict between families and practitioners has to do with beliefs about "appropriate" family relationships. A clinician's opinion that the client and his family are "enmeshed" may clash with the views of persons from other cultures who value the interconnectedness of families. In an article on the Latin American community in Canada, for example, a clinician notes the fear expressed by parents that their authority will be undermined by mental health professionals who do "not understand the cultural background" (Sanchez 2000, 10).

Finally, there is the perception that a practitioner's involvement with family members will jeopardize the clinical relationship with the client. From this perspective, the primary or sole obligation is to the client alone, and family involvement may be construed as "interference." From the client's point of view, while some will be comfortable with having information shared between the clinician and family members, others will not and may view this sort of collaboration as a betrayal. To understand this reaction, readers should be aware that in many cases persons with serious, persistent mental disorders are estranged from their immediate family, particularly the parents. This happens for a number of reasons. Parents may misunderstand the nature of psychiatric disorders and interpret their child's behaviour as willfulness or laziness, leading to a falling out. A falling out may also occur when parents become involved in evicting the young person from the family home or in arranging an involuntary hospitalization, necessitated by the individual's refusal to get treatment. The dilemma this situation creates for parents is described by Lefley (1997, 9): "Pragmatically and emotionally, family members view the involuntary intervention as an undesirable but essential safety net. Like mental health care consumers and all persons concerned with civil liberties, families would greatly prefer alternatives to involuntary interventions. They are humiliating and painful to all concerned. They not only have an adverse impact on the self-esteem and integrity of the individuals involved but also may generate resentment and alienation against family members faced with impossible choices." Other sources of tension include situations where children have been abused by their parents, or claim abuse. Children may also have the view that not enough financial and material support has been offered to them by family – which is often an issue given the number of persons with serious mental disorders who are on income assistance (Rutman 1994). On some occasions family members may be incorporated into a client's delusional system; in these cases a client may disavow that these persons really *are* his or her parents or perhaps see them as part of some larger conspiracy.

When there is estrangement from family, clients may view the practitioner's contact with these individuals, as noted, as a form of betrayal, particularly when he or she has not given consent. At the same time, family members may be desperate for information on their loved ones – such as where they're living, under what circumstances, and whether they're safe and healthy – and may ask that the clinician or case manager provide this for them. This dilemma may be resolved by strict adherence to confidentiality policies, which in most cases require signed consent by the client before information is shared with a third party. Protecting client confidentiality is supported in some cases by practice guidelines, such as those of the Canadian Psychiatric Association (noted earlier), which stipulate that the obligation to maintain confidentiality supersedes the needs of relatives (Neilson 1996). Similarly, Bogart and Solomon (1999, 1322) conclude that requiring client consent to release information is vital to safeguard clients' trust, promote independence, and "communicate respect and validation of consumers' ability to make decisions in their own best interest." That being said, policies on release of information may still leave room for discretion and uncertainty (Mannion, Solomon, and Steber 2001). For example, in British Columbia, "continuity of care" guidelines permit health care practitioners to release (without consent) information to a third party if that party can be considered a "care provider," leaving open the question of exactly how to define this term. From the perspective of some family members, resorting to confidentiality policies is a "cop-out" on the part of practitioners, a way of avoiding dealing with people who have legitimate needs and interests.

The deliberate or accidental exclusion of family members as a stakeholder group is being challenged, and now agency mandates and best practice documents increasingly speak to the importance of family involvement and support. This move to greater inclusion is supported by evidence that enhancing family knowledge and skills will produce better outcomes for the client, such as lower hospitalization rates (Dixon et al. 2001). A best practices document published by the British Columbia Ministry of Health (2002c) makes the following recommendations concerning family involvement:

- "Families must be informed and aware of the treatment plan and discharge planning should focus not only on the individual's personal functioning, but also on the family's ability to care for the client" (3).
- There should be provision of counselling for family members, which would include provision of information, support, skills teaching, and assistance in accessing services.

- There should be training opportunities and resources to support self-help.
- Support should include diversified respite care.
- Family members should have a role in the planning and evaluation of mental health services.

An appendix in this document contains a "Family Charter of Rights," developed by the Provincial Mental Health Family Advisory Council. The charter goes further than the recommendations contained in the main text, addressing attitudinal barriers encountered by family members. An excerpt is as follows:

Families have a right:
- To explicit information that families do not cause mental illness.
- To respect from professionals for the expertise of the family, as well as the *sharing of power in the therapeutic process.*
- To become appropriately assertive and to *overcome traditional socialization that teaches families not to question authority.* (28, emphasis added)

Some mention must be made of the organizations that work to advance the interests of family members, Canadian examples being the Schizophrenia Society, the Mood Disorders Association, and the Anxiety Disorders Association. Related organizations elsewhere include the National Alliance for the Mentally Ill (NAMI) and the Treatment Advocacy Center in the United States and the Schizophrenia Fellowship in British Commonwealth countries. Organizations like the Schizophrenia Society of Canada (SSC) have a complicated relationship with other stakeholder groups: at times their agendas coincide, and on other occasions they run counter to one another. For example, the SSC strongly supports the medical model with respect to views about etiology and treatment, a position that is congruent with that of many practitioners and practitioner associations. In an SSC position paper (Schizophrenia Society of Canada 1998, vii), the following are articulated as "core values" of the organization: that "schizophrenia is caused by biological factors of the brain," and that "medication is the cornerstone for the treatment of those with schizophrenia." The medical model, however, may be seen as too narrow a focus by those clients and workers who emphasize going beyond symptoms to look at broader existential concerns – although in fairness the SSC does address other aspects of recovery in its publications.

More contentious are the positions taken on coercive practices, an example being community treatment orders, which permit the involuntary treatment of persons outside a hospital setting. While one must be careful about generalizations – recalling the discussion above about parents preferring alternatives to involuntary interventions[9] – it is reasonable to say that the SSC and related organizations have favoured policies and legislation that facilitate access to treatment, and that they have been seen as less supportive of due process protections that might impede this access (Goering, Wasylenki, and Durbin 2000; Hall 2000). One of the baldest statements of the "access to treatment" position comes from an American family support organization, the Treatment Advocacy Center, whose mandate is to "educate policymakers and judges about the true nature of severe brain disorder ... and the necessity of community ordered treatment in some cases" as well as to ensure "that individuals maintain medication compliance upon release from hospital" (quoted in Davis 2002, 243). Client advocacy groups, on the other hand, tend to oppose paternalistic practices, an example being the No Force Coalition in Ontario, which was formed in 1999 specifically to address the stereotype of the "violent mental patient" and to galvanize opposition to community treatment orders (see http://www.qsos.ca/qspc/nfc). A dispute related to this question of "access to treatment," involving practitioners and family organizations on the one side, and civil rights advocates on the other, dragged out the process of amending the British Columbia *Mental Health Act* by several years in the mid-1990s (Davis 1995b). In another example, the Schizophrenia Society of Ontario's appeal to legislators to support the implementation of community treatment orders was strenuously opposed by clients' rights groups (Oakes 2003).

While clinicians may align themselves with support organizations on legislative initiatives, the situation is somewhat different when advocacy activity is directed toward the clinicians themselves. Because of dissatisfaction on the part of family members with the quantity and quality of follow-up offered to their relative/client and because of perceived exclusion (as noted) from the treatment process, organizations such as the SSC have supported family concerns by, for example, requesting and facilitating meetings between relatives and treatment personnel and by drafting checklists of "Questions to ask the psychiatrist" (British Columbia Schizophrenia Society 2000) in order to assist relatives who may be uncertain about what to say in their dealings with professionals. This checklist of questions includes the following:

- How certain are you of this diagnosis? If you are not certain, what other possibilities do you consider most likely, and why?
- Would you advise a second opinion from another psychiatrist at this point?
- What program of treatment do you think will be most helpful? How will it be helpful?
- Who will be able to answer our questions when you are not available?

- What do you expect treatment to accomplish? About how long will it take? How often will you be seeing the patient?
- What do you see as the family's role in the treatment plan? In particular, how much access will the family have to individual treatment providers?
- Are you currently treating other patients with this illness?
- When are the best times, and what are the most dependable ways, to get in touch with you?

One can view this list in different ways. On the one hand, the questions can be seen as reasonable, relevant, and a means to ensuring greater accountability. On the other hand, practitioners may view them as reflecting a somewhat adversarial stance, may feel uncomfortable about what appears to be second-guessing, and more generally, may be unused to this sort of challenge to professional authority. (Responding to a list like this may indeed be the acid test of an agency's nominal commitment to the notion of "consumerism.")

In sum, the practitioner-family relationship is one that has had troubled antecedents and one that continues to challenge both parties, particularly in light of the interest being expressed by health authorities in better accommodating this new stakeholder. That being said, the evidence shows that family support groups have payoffs for both family members and clients and thus deserve to be supported and facilitated by practitioners. As well, through their lobbying efforts, family members have the potential to achieve a better response from the larger service delivery system and are therefore a valuable resource. It is noteworthy, for example, that the British Columbia "Family Charter of Rights," referred to above, states that "families have a right to have a social ethic that is more concerned about the welfare of the person with mental illness, rather than cost-effectiveness" (British Columbia Ministry of Health 2002c, 28).

Government and Policy Makers[10]
Government, for many critics of the mental health system, has been an "absent stakeholder," with one observer noting that "mental illness simply isn't on the government radar screen" (Smiderle 2003, 32). This point was acknowledged in *Building on Values: The Future of Health Care in Canada* (Commission on the Future of Health Care in Canada 2002, 178) – the "Romanow Report" – where the authors spoke about "mental health ... as one of the orphan children of medicare" and the need to "bring mental health into the mainstream of public health care." (Ironically, despite good intentions, mental health remains underrecognized in the report, which devotes only 2 of 357 pages to the topic, slotting it in as a subsection of a chapter on "home

care.") Funding for research on schizophrenia in Canada, for example, remains lower than for other major disorders, even though it occurs more commonly than Alzheimer's, multiple sclerosis, diabetes, or muscular dystrophy (Todd 2004). At the time of writing, Canada remained the only G8 nation without a national action plan on mental health, a fact addressed in a Canadian Senate report released in 2004, the result being, according to one of the report's authors, a "badly organized and under-funded" system (Kennedy 2004, A7).

When governments make mental health policy – for example, by drafting legislation – there is the indication, not surprisingly, that legislators will be influenced by the zeitgeist, particularly by public perceptions about safety and the need to be protected from "dangerous" mentally disordered persons (Corrigan et al. 2004; Monahan 1992). Recent, more coercive legislative provisions, notably community treatment orders, appear to be the product (in part) of this increased preoccupation with "protection of the public," with media accounts of violent behaviour by psychiatric patients playing a role in swaying opinions. This situation is summarized by Goering, Wasylenki, and Durbin (2000, 354):

> Public opinion has somewhat less direct influence on policy-making in a parliamentary system where special interest groups are not as powerful as in the United States and decision making is more centered in the public service bureaucracy ... Still, Canadian provincial and federal politicians are clearly influenced by the opinions of their constituency, and the media is the most common mode of communication between the public and their government. Coverage of mental health issues tends to be centered on a few key topics with homelessness, suicide, and violence receiving the lion's share of attention. At times this coverage influences the development of mental health policy. For example, a number of recent threats and subway pushings by individuals with mental illness (many of whom were not taking prescribed medications) flamed public outrage and supported the efforts of the families of the mentally ill in advocating for a change in legislation to introduce community committal. Shortly afterward, the Ontario government announced its intention to pursue this course of action.

In addition to creating legislation, the other major role for government and senior bureaucrats is in decision making around funding. Currently, the increasing expense of health care as a proportion of provincial budgets has led critics to argue that the system is too expensive, inefficient, and unsustainable (Fuller 1998). The plight of the provinces has been made worse by cuts in transfer payments from the federal government: for example, from 1978 to 1998 the proportion of Medicare paid by the federal government shrank from 27 to 11 percent (Goering, Wasylenki, and Durbin 2000). Hence, in looking at provincial government positions in the last decade or so, it can be seen that the issue of *cost containment* has driven the agenda, which is also the case in the United States, where "managed care" models are employed (Scheid and Horowitz 1999). Cost containment is now explicitly reflected in best practice guidelines; for example, a British Columbia Ministry of Health (2002e, 10) document suggests that, among other objectives, best practice outcomes in mental health should show evidence of "decreased use of more intrusive and/or more costly services."

With respect to mental health, one can point to hospital care as one of the key "cost drivers." For example, an Ontario study found that half of all mental health dollars in the province went to psychiatric and general hospitals, with a third going to physicians and only 10 percent to community mental health programs (Goering and Lin 1996). Reducing hospital bed days is thus a key cost containment strategy.

Another key cost driver is medication, with newer-generation psychotropic agents being considerably more expensive than older products. In Canada almost $15 billion was spent on (all) prescription drugs in 2002, with the cost of public medication coverage programs doubling in the preceding seven years (Thomson 2003); this figure rose to $16 billion the following year, with the relative and absolute amount that is covered by the public sector continuing to increase (Canadian Institute for Health Information 2004). For a provincial example, one can look to British Columbia, where Pharmacare costs relating to the treatment of psychiatric disorders increased by 53 percent during a three-year period in the late 1990s, from $58 million in 1996-97 to $88 million in 1999-2000 (British Columbia Ministry of Health Services 2003a). The huge price increases associated with newer-generation ("atypical") psychotropic drugs has led two American analysts to conclude that public spending in other areas of mental health, such as staffing, "must almost inevitably suffer" (Sernyak and Rosenheck 2004, 1362).

In their submission to the Romanow Commission, the Canadian Mental Health Association (2001) suggested that mental health costs are driven by (1) insufficient attention being paid to *prevention* and the social determinants of health, (2) the lack of attention given to the interaction between physical and mental health, (3) a lack of coordination between family physicians and the rest of the mental health system, and (4) delays in services and treatment – with the result that a problem that could have been treated in a community setting gets worse, requiring more expensive hospital care.

In responding to the costs of hospital care, health authorities have in many cases reduced or privatized services; provincial psychiatric hospitals continue to be downsized, beds have been eliminated in general hospitals, and in some locales, especially rural, entire programs have been closed. Other hospital services have been "out-sourced"; these include housekeeping, laundry, food, and security as well as outpatient programs, such as rehabilitation services, which are increasingly provided by private companies (Fuller 1998). Another cost-saving strategy is the downgrading of staffing complements – for example, by replacing registered nurses with lower-paid licensed practical nurses (Carrigg 2003b).

Concerning privatization, recent years have seen the advent in Canada of the "P3" hospital, which relies on "public-private partnerships" as a way of financing new infrastructures, with officials in Brampton, Ontario, announcing in late 2004 the commencement of construction of Canada's first P3 hospital. The P3 model involves contracts between the public sector and a group of for-profit companies who come together as a single consortium for the purpose of bidding on private hospital contracts. Critics of this development argue that it is not cost effective because public dollars go to fund what is in effect a private building and because there are additional costs related to lost public control and accountability (MacKenzie 2004).

For many practitioners, the concept of cost effectiveness is anathema, an issue either to be avoided or fought against. However, given limited health care resources, and (as noted earlier) codes of ethics that refer to the prudent use of these resources, a commitment to efficiencies by clinicians is not unreasonable. That said, concern remains that cost effectiveness, instead of being one evaluation criterion, will be used as the *sole* determinant of success.

The problem of cost containment has meant that health authorities are increasingly referring to quantitative indicators that show interventions to have some "payoff." On this point, in commenting on future trends in the Canadian mental health system, Goering and colleagues (2000, 356-57) suggest that "there will be more attention paid to utilization review, measurement, and reporting of outcomes, and clearly defining roles and responsibilities between levels of care. [As well] the funding of hospital and community services is likely to be tied more explicitly to performance ... factors." This emphasis on rationalizing services draws its impetus, in part, from American claims that the implementation of "managed care" can achieve cost savings without a major negative impact on clinical outcomes (Mechanic 2003).

Concern about cost containment has driven health authorities, in a number of instances, to justify their actions by revising or altering their mission statements, in turn fuelling public cynicism. For example, authorities explaining the closure of a program may refer to new, or narrowly conceived, "core services," arguing that the care previously provided was outside the mandate or better provided elsewhere. Another example is the emphasis now placed on the benefits of "care at home" – as opposed to care in hospital – whether or not that care actually exists. In British Columbia news releases on mental health planning by the provincial government have often made reference to "Closer to Home" initiatives. Similarly, in Manitoba, to justify time limits on admissions at a Winnipeg general hospital – using a rationale suspiciously similar to American-style managed care guidelines – the hospital CEO was quoted as saying that sending patients home earlier means that they can spend "more time ... recovering with their families," which is superior to being in hospital "because there's a better attitude and support for them at home" (quoted in Fuller 1998, 146). This comment would seem to fly in the face of the reality faced by many family members, namely that providing care for an unwell loved one can be a considerable emotional and financial burden, an obligation that a former president of the Canadian Psychiatric Association suggests is "an invisible subsidy to the healthcare system" (Woodside 2003, 6).

It should be stated at this point that, for mental health clients, the evidence shows that quality of life *can* be better "closer to home," *provided necessary services are in place.* This can also be a cost-effective approach: provision of secure, adequate social housing, for example, can obviate the need for emergency resources, which in the long run are more costly (British Columbia Ministry of Health 2002d). For practitioners, however, past experiences of being let down by funding bodies – experiences that date back to the deinstitutionalization movement of the 1960s – have meant that pronouncements about new initiatives are often greeted with skepticism. As well, even assuming that references to "care at home" are not disingenuous, practitioners are aware, more than policy makers, that families may be unable or unwilling to care for client relatives, or may be absent, and that the notion of "family care" is at least somewhat naive (Davis 1996). There may also be some misunderstanding about a perceived overreliance on hospital resources: policy makers may frame the discussion as home care *instead* of hospital care, while practitioners tend to see inpatient care as part of the *continuum* of services that should be available when necessary.

In confronting the twin issues of underrecognition by government and protection of funding for mental health programs, it has been suggested that lobbying attempts have been ineffective because the different groups involved are either disjointed (Smiderle 2003) or "too often talk primarily to one another and to those already committed to their positions" (Mechanic 2003, 1227). One psychiatrist notes, for example, that allegiances between the professional community and family members are vital since families "are powerful allies when resources are scarce" and "have a most important role in advocating publicly for their affected relatives, whether at a local hospital level or at various levels of government" (Woodside 2003, 6). To present a stronger, more coherent voice, a new umbrella organization, the Canadian Alliance on Mental Illness and Mental Health (CAMIMH), was formed, with representatives from the Canadian Medical Association, the Canadian Psychiatric Association, the Canadian Mental Health Association, the Schizophrenia Society, the Mood Disorders Association, the Canadian Psychological Association, and the Canadian Association for Suicide Prevention. The mandate of CAMIMH is described as follows: "Created in October 1998, the core purpose of the Canadian Alliance on Mental Illness and Mental Health is to put mental illness and mental health on the national health and social policy agendas. It wishes to influence and advise on mental health policy at the national level as a unified voice of consumer, family, community and professional organizations. Its overriding commitment is to improving services and supports for persons facing mental illness and/or mental health obstacles as well as to secure strategies that will enhance the potential for positive mental health among Canadians" (Canadian Psychiatric Association 2003).

In the voluntary/nonprofit sector, a partnership called VOICE (Voluntary Organizations Involved in Collaborative Engagement) in Health Policy was formed in 2001. As described on its website (http://www.projectvoice.ca), this project is about "voluntary organizations working together to build their capacity to affect change in public health policy ... being heard and becoming involved in health policy [and] collaborating with ... peers about how to make your message strong; VOICE reflects a sense that organizations can work together to deliver a unified message." VOICE helps facilitate workshops that, for example, teach participants about how health policy is made, how governments determine priorities, the federal decision-making process, and how to identify "key federal government players," the stated aim being the development of successful strategies to "have your voice heard by government."

The Drug Companies

While recognizing that some would object to including the drug companies in a chapter on "stakeholders," it is undeniable that this industry is an influential player in the mental health system. Medication forms the cornerstone of the treatment offered in most Canadian community mental health settings, and it must be said that, in many cases, these pharmacological agents are effective, notwithstanding expense and side effects. Nonetheless, with the considerable financial resources at their disposal, there is concern that the drug companies wield disproportionate influence with respect to physicians' prescribing practices, research grants, the dissemination of results from drug trials, and the lobbying of politicians.

To begin with, as noted, pharmaceuticals are clearly a profitable industry. Critic Marcia Angell (2004), a former editor of the *New England Journal of Medicine*, notes that in 2002 the combined profits of the ten American drug companies on the "Fortune 500" list ($35.9 billion) were more than the combined profits of the other 490 businesses ($33.7 billion). These profits are based largely on the success of heavily promoted, "newer-generation" products – with prices being in some cases one thousand times the actual cost (Robinson 2001) – many of them psychotropic agents. In Canada, for example, the number of prescriptions for the class of antidepressants known as selective serotonin reuptake inhibitors (SSRIs) – which accounted for $12 billion in sales worldwide in 2002 – grew by 48 percent between 1998 and 2003 (Branham 2003), an increase attributed in part to "effective marketing efforts by pharmaceutical manufacturers" (Priest 2003a, 21).

As we have seen, the relative and absolute amount of these costs being covered by the public sector in Canada has continued to increase: the "Romanow Report" noted that spending on prescription drugs relative to total health care expenses doubled from 5.8 percent in 1980 to 12 percent in 2001 (Commission on the Future of Health Care in Canada 2002). These costs have put enormous pressure on Canada's Pharmacare programs (Thomson 2003). In British Columbia, for example, the Pharmacare budget in recent years has increased by 14 to 17 percent every year, a state of affairs that is unsustainable according to health care economists and that has led to the provincial government's introduction of restraint measures such as means testing, "therapeutic substitution" (for example funding only cheaper versions of acid reflux medications), and requiring special authority for more expensive antipsychotic drugs (Fayerman 2003; Morgan, Bassett, and Mintzes 2004; Priest 2003a). (Lists of preferred drugs are called "formularies.")

The profitability of newer drugs is ensured, to a greater or lesser extent, by **patent protection**, whereby governments legislatively limit the production of cheaper, generic equivalents by rival companies. In Canada *Bill C-22*, enacted in 1987, weakened the licensing arrangement that permitted Canadian-made generic drugs to reach the market before brand-name patents had expired, a move that was purportedly done to gain US approval of the Free Trade Agreement (Fuller 1998). In 1993 *Bill C-91* was enacted, giving twenty-year patent protection to brand-name medications, which one author characterized as a "deregulation of the drug industry [that] led to spectacular increases in the cost of drugs" (191).

Patent protection, and by corollary higher drug costs, is justified primarily by the argument that the research needed to develop newer products is expensive. While this may be true, critics point out that the proportion of revenue spent on research and development – only 14 percent of US sales in 2000, for example – is still much less than that spent on "marketing and administration" (i.e., advertising) (Angell 2004).

An additional argument supporting the high cost of newer drugs is that outpatient treatment with psychotropic medication may obviate the need for other, costly services, particularly hospitalization. This argument is somewhat suspect given that psychotropic medications, especially antidepressants, are being prescribed in Canada much more widely now than was the case previously (Patten and Beck 2004), with one physician suggesting that this may be driven by patients' desire for a quick fix or "an edge" rather than by clinical necessity (Dalrymple 2003; see also Branham 2003). It would seem unlikely that a large number of these new antidepressant users would have previously been at constant risk for hospitalization.

Another concern about the costs of newer, "novel" or "atypical" agents (newer-generation antipsychotics are referred to as "atypicals") is the argument that in many cases these new agents are neither new nor atypical. Angell (2004) notes that, despite claims of innovation by the drug companies, many newer drugs are merely slight variations on older products with, in many instances, no new active ingredients (what she calls "me-too" drugs). An example of this comes from the manufacturer of the antidepressant Prozac, who came out with a "new" form of the drug to be taken weekly, just as the patent on the daily form of the product was about to expire. (In 2005 it was reported that the Federal Ministry of Health would take action to limit this "evergreening" of drug patents [National Union of Public and General Employees 2005]).

As noted, in order to maintain market share, drug companies engage in extensive promotion of their products, the main recipient of this being individual, prescribing physicians. Both private practitioners and public-sector physicians are subject to extensive advertising and frequent visits from "drug reps,"[11] in addition to being offered free medication samples as well as funded trips to holiday venues where "continuing medical education" is offered. The potentially corrupting effect of the large amount of money at stake was evidenced by the example in British Columbia of pharmacies selling doctors' names and prescribing practices to a drug marketing company before the provincial government stepped in to stop it (Robinson 2001).

In addition to physicians, the marketing of pharmaceuticals has for some time included "direct to consumer" (DTC) approaches in the United States, the budget for which more than tripled from 1996 to 2000 (Barer 2004).

While this has been restricted in Canada, more recently the broadcasting and pharmaceutical industries have made proposals that would see DTC advertising being permitted in this country (Smith 2003). Such a move has been strongly opposed by groups such as the National Union of Public and General Employees (2004), who argue that this would be another cost driver for public Medicare programs, that it would provide a greater incentive for drug companies to spend more on advertising and less on research, and that drug company literature is biased, minimizing risks while exaggerating benefits. Concerning the practitioner-client relationship, Hoffman and Wilkes (1999, 1302) suggest that DTC advertising "unreasonably increases consumer expectations, forces doctors to spend time disabusing patients of misinformation, diminishes the doctor-patient relationship because a doctor refuses to prescribe an advertised drug, or results in poor practice if the doctor capitulates and prescribes an inappropriate agent." On the other hand, proponents of DTC advertising suggest that this is a legitimate source of information, that it empowers clients, and that it addresses unmet needs with respect to persons who lack knowledge and who are suffering unnecessarily with an untreated condition (Gilbody, Wilson, and Watt 2004).

To examine the possible influence of DTC advertising, a team of Canadian and American researchers surveyed a group of physicians in both countries, finding that "patients requests' for medicines are a powerful driver of prescribing decisions" in that patients requesting a particular drug in the study were more likely to receive one, even though in about 45 percent of cases the doctor expressed ambivalence about the drug being requested (Mintzes et al. 2002, 279) ("ambivalence" was established by responses to the question "if you were treating another similar patient with the same condition, would you prescribe this drug?"). Researchers from this study group conducted another survey, this time of drug policy experts from Canada, New Zealand, and the United States, asking them about their perceptions of the impact of DTC advertising; it was found that the majority of respondents believed that the quality of information provided through DTC advertising was poor, that there were likely to be negative effects on the appropriateness of care, and that health care costs would increase (Mintzes et al. 2001).

Finally, there is the question of the role of the pharmaceutical industry in sponsoring research trials. Drug companies commonly provide the grants for medical researchers to conduct research on the companies' own products, a conflict of interest that has led some to question whether the results produced can be considered objective or impartial (Bekelman, Li, and Gross 2003; Robinson, 2001). On this matter, the editor of the *Canadian Journal of Psychiatry* suggested that it would be unrealistic to insist that researchers have no attachment to a sponsoring company since "those best able to articulate a review [drug trial] today seem to be involved in funded research of this nature" (Rae-Grant 2002, 513). Indeed, as one author notes, "these days it's nearly impossible to find anybody who doesn't have a conflict of interest, because virtually all the medical experts in every field have taken money from pharmaceutical companies to continue their research" (Branham 2003, B3). Because of this reality, medical journals have been forced to relax their conflict guidelines, with the approach now being that authors of drug trials declare their affiliation and "make presentations as transparent as possible" (Rae-Grant 2002, 513).

A particular concern with the drug companies' involvement in drug trials is the ability of the industry to control the outcome of this research. Clinicians may be required to sign multiyear "nondisclosure" contracts – what some have called "gag orders" – before participating in research sponsored by a drug company, effectively eliminating the dissemination of negative findings (*Canadian Medical Association Journal* 2004). When one medical researcher affiliated with the University of Toronto, Dr. Nancy Olivieri, *did* attempt to publish results of a drug trial showing the product to have unexpected risks, the sponsoring company, Apotex, quickly terminated the trial and threatened Olivieri with legal action (Robinson 2001). The issue of suppressed trial results has become even more prominent with the finding of an increased incidence of suicidal/parasuicidal behaviours among persons using newer-generation antidepressants (Fergusson et al. 2005), particularly with respect to the unapproved use of these products by children and adolescents. This concern led to the office of the Attorney General in New York launching a lawsuit in 2004 against GlaxoSmithKline (GSK), the manufacturer of the antidepressant paroxetine, accusing the company of fraud. This suit was based on the fact that while GSK had conducted five studies on the drug's safety and efficacy, four of them, which showed the product to have mixed or negative results, were suppressed and only one was published. The suit alleged that because the partial information provided by GSK caused doctors to have a biased picture of the drug, they were unable to assess risks and benefits and thus to properly advise their patients about its use (*Lancet* 2004).

Changing Practices

At the beginning of this chapter it was noted that two "new" stakeholders – clients and family members – were asking to be included in the mental health planning and treatment processes. While gains have been made in this regard, it is still not clear – at the time of writing – whether or to what extent the goal of meaningfully incorporating these other viewpoints has been accomplished. Barriers to accommodating the new stakeholders include, as noted, the reluctance of professionals to give up their position of authority as well as what can be termed "institutional inertia." Getting staff to buy in to new collaborative models is difficult, and strategies such as disseminating literature on the effectiveness of client and family initiatives have proven to be uncompelling. When changes start to be implemented, staff may complain, rightly in some instances, that there was no consultation or that the consultation was token or carried a hidden agenda. Some authors appear to question whether staff should be consulted in any case; concerning the tendencies of practitioners, Amenson and Liberman (2001, 589) are blunt in their analysis: "Mental health professionals adopt new services primarily for the same reason that employees of any firm change their work practices – namely, because the authority structure and contingencies of reinforcement that impinge on their daily activities are altered in a direction favoring change." They go on to conclude that "administrative clout must be brought to bear" in order to ensure that change happens. Notwithstanding this viewpoint, the perception of staff that their administration is being sensitive and supportive in a time of change is important and can only help morale.

Without diminishing all the difficulties, some suggestions can be made to assist the process of formalizing the involvement of clients and family members in service planning (Mueser and Fox 2000; Reidy 1992; Treherne and Calsaferri 2002):

- There needs to be commitment from senior management, with a clear vision and mission statement expressed.
- Staff should be allowed to express concerns and reservations, and any change should be gradual.
- Family and client advisory committees should be established to oversee the implementation of the plan.
- With respect to the client and/or family initiatives, coordinator positions should be created, thus acknowledging the importance of the initiative and building in greater accountability.
- The coordinator should collaborate with staff educators, senior clinical staff, and existing stakeholder groups.
- One to three staff should be identified on each mental health team to receive further training and to act as "cheerleaders" for client and/or family involvement at the local level; staff who have worked successfully with, for example, client peer-support workers may be able to provide valuable testimonials.
- An orientation training module should be designed and implemented to ensure that all staff have sufficient knowledge and skills to educate,

support, and collaborate with clients and families in each program unit. Consideration should be given to "cross-training," meaning that all stakeholders participate and share experiences in these sessions.

Notes

1 Subspecialties, such as geriatric psychiatry, have longer residency periods.
2 Provincial medical plans may limit the amount that private psychiatrists can bill: in British Columbia, for example, a psychiatrist cannot bill more than two hours per week for an individual client.
3 On the question of nurses prescribing, see Bailey (2004).
4 A poignant example of this is the case of Stephanie James, an eighteen-year-old University of British Columbia student who committed suicide in February 2004 after a previous documented attempt one month earlier. Stephanie's mother, living in Oregon, was upset that university officials had not notified her about the earlier attempt, but in a report on the incident, officials from the university and health authority, as well as an ethicist, defended the lack of notification as consistent with legal and ethical guidelines (O'Brian 2004b).
5 *Tarasoff v. Regents of the University of California* (1974), 188 California Reporter 129, 529 P2d 533.
6 *Smith v. Jones* (1999), 169 Dominion Law Reports (4th) 385 (SCC).
7 In the classic Freudian conceptualization, psychic conflicts are unconscious and thus by definition inaccessible to the patient/client.
8 This claim is based on the author's own practice experience.
9 See also the "family member's perspective" on the website of the No Force Coalition: http://www.qsos.ca/qspc/nfc/mpp.html#1.
10 "Policy makers" here refers to senior bureaucrats and health authority officers.
11 More recently, the pharmaceutical conglomerate Lily changed the job title of drug salespersons to "neuroscience nurse representatives."

Other Resources

- A number of Canadian family/client support organizations have websites. These include the Schizophrenia Society (http://www.schizophrenia.ca), Mood Disorders Association/Society (http://www.mooddisorderscanada.ca), Anxiety Disorders Association (http://www.anxietycanada.ca), and Canadian Network Around Disordered Eating (http://www3.telus.net/anad01/network.shtml).
- Canadian groups critical of psychiatric practices, especially the use of coercion, have established a number of websites. These include the No Force Coalition in Ontario, described as a "group of individuals and organizations against force in psychiatry" (http://www.qsos.ca/qspc/nfc); and the Psychiatric Survivors Archives of Toronto at http://www.psychiatricsurvivorarchives.com.
- The Alberta Mental Health Self-Help Network has a website at http://www.selfhelpnetwork.org.
- At the website of the American Self-Help Group Clearinghouse (http://www.mentalhelp.net/selfhelp), there are links to clearinghouses in the United States and other countries, including Canada.
- A "family toolkit," with five learning modules on mental disorders, can be accessed at http://www.heretohelp.bc.ca/helpmewith/ftoolkit.shtml.
- "Parenting Well" is a website with resource information for parents with mental health problems and their supporters (see http://www.parentingwell.org).
- "Healthy Skepticism" is a website whose aim is "improving health by reducing harm from misleading drug promotion" (see http://www.healthyskepticism.org).

Deinstitutionalization and Regionalization

Since Canadian confederation there have been two major shifts with respect to the care and containment of mentally disordered persons. The first of these began in the mid to late 1800s, with the building of large, long-stay psychiatric hospitals – the "asylums" – the first being built in New Brunswick in 1836 (Rochefort 1992). From the late nineteenth century to the mid-twentieth, mentally disordered persons considered unmanageable in the community could expect to be housed in the high-ceilinged dormitories of these often remotely located institutions, sometimes for many years.

Then, starting in the 1960s, concomitant with development of new psychiatric medications, the second shift – the move away from the institutions – began. Institutional stays became shorter, and the asylums were downsized and in some cases closed altogether. Practitioners and policy makers were buoyed by the promise of *community* mental health, even though a clear conceptualization of the term appeared to be lacking. However, the promise of the 1960s gave way to the gradual realization in the 1970s that there were still many unresolved problems: mentally disordered person were not "connecting" with care providers and with their communities, the latter of which did not appear to be welcoming in any case. Many were homeless or in jails. Practitioners began to write about a "new chronic" population, which in a number of respects resembled the "old chronic" population despite the apparently harmful effects of institutionalization being removed (Davis 1985). Health authorities began to rethink, and are still rethinking, what they were/are doing. Attempts were made to reform or "redesign" the system, some of these being at the program level, others at the level of governance. During the 1990s, with the spiralling costs of health care becoming a pressing concern, the issues of *efficacy* and *efficiency* became paramount for policy makers, which meant that mental health systems now had to accommodate the concept of *evidence-based* practices in their redesign.

To set the context for a description of Canadian mental health programs in Chapter 7, this chapter provides an overview of these policy shifts, from deinstitutionalization to regionalization, before looking at the development of the concept of an evidence base for interventions and at the principle of "best practices" in Chapter 6.

Deinstitutionalization

In Canada the asylum movement started in the middle part of the nineteenth century, with provincial institutions being opened in Quebec, New Brunswick, Ontario, Newfoundland, Nova Scotia, British Columbia, Prince Edward Island, and Manitoba during this period; in Saskatchewan and Alberta psychiatric hospitals were opened in 1911 and 1914 respectively (Sussman 1998). By many accounts, the move to asylums represented a progressive shift, one that would "provide safe settings for physical and spiritual care and ... shield residents from the harm and peril that commonly befell people with mental illnesses in cities and towns" (Health Canada 2002c, 1). Similarly, Sussman (1998, 260) notes that the policy of housing people in asylums in Canada "began with humane intentions as a part of a progressive and reformist movement, which attempted to overcome neglect and suffering in the community, jails and poorhouses." A survey in Halifax from the mid-1840s, for example, determined that "lunatics" made up 20 percent of the population housed in the city poorhouse (Rochefort 1992). Later accounts of the asylum movement were more skeptical and identified "less humanitarian motivations for asylum development: the segregation of those with mental illness from a society that did not want the discomfort of eccentric behaviour in its midst, and the self-interests of health professionals" (Health Canada 2002c, 1).

Regardless of intentions, the asylums ultimately became overcrowded and understaffed facilities, which, in the absence of any effective methods of treating psychotic disorders, were vast warehouses providing "custodial care." Further, as a Canadian psychiatrist observes, "the custodial, institution-based model of care for those with mental illness contributed to their stigmatization by segregation" as well as to "the banishment of mental illness, and also of psychiatry, from the general stream of medicine" (Arboleda-Florez 2003, 646). The patient census for these facilities peaked in Canada in the early 1960s (Dickinson and Andre 1988).[1] At this time, for example, about 5,000 persons were housed at the Essondale mental hospital near Vancouver, British Columbia, while in Saskatchewan 3,500 persons were kept in two large institutions near Saskatoon and Regina (Gray, Shone, and Liddle 2000).

The 1960s saw a major shift in mental health policy, a shift fuelled by what one author describes as the "widespread belief that community-based care would be more humane and more therapeutic than hospital-based care" (Bachrach 1994, 24). American President John F. Kennedy, referring to new legislation that was to encourage the replacement of asylums by community clinics, proclaimed in a passage from a 1963 speech that "reliance on the cold mercy of custodial isolation will be supplanted by the open warmth of community concern and capability."

In Canada, starting in the 1960s and continuing through the 1970s and 1980s, there was a drastic downsizing of many of the old provincial psychiatric hospitals, a process referred to as **deinstitutionalization,** which Bachrach (1994, 24) defines as "the replacement of long-stay psychiatric hospitals with smaller, less isolated community-based service alternatives for the care of individuals with schizophrenia and other major mental illnesses." This author notes that "deinstitutionalization, in theory, was to consist of three component processes: the release of patients residing in psychiatric hospitals to alternative facilities in the community; the diversion of potential new admissions into those alternative facilities; and the development of special community-based programs, combining psychiatric and support services, for the care of a noninstitutionalized patient population." It can be argued, then, that by this definition "deinstitutionalization" refers more to a theoretical ideal than to what was actually accomplished, at least initially. What *was* accomplished was a considerable reduction in the inpatient census, done by increasing the number of discharges (opening the back door) and limiting new admissions (closing the front door), the latter being achieved in part by narrowing the legal criteria for certification (involuntary admission). Other legal changes provided for more procedural protections for individuals detained under provincial mental health acts and for shortening periods of mandatory detention.

From 1960 to 1976 there was a reduction in capacity in Canadian psychiatric hospitals from 47,633 to 15,011 beds, with general psychiatric hospital beds increasing from 844 to 5,836 over the same period (Goering, Wasylenki, and Durbin 2000). Regional examples include Greater Toronto, where the number of long-stay psychiatric beds fell from 3,857 to 761 between 1960 and 1994 (Eberle 2001c), and Saskatchewan, where the psychiatric hospital bed count dropped from 3,500 in the mid-1950s to about 200 in the year 2000 (Gray, Shone, and Liddle 2000). Not all provinces have downsized at the same pace, although the ultimate goal is the same; in surveying data from the different provinces, Sealey and Whitehead (2004, 249) conclude that there was "tremendous variation among the provinces in the timing and intensity of deinstitutionalization," with percentage decreases in provincial hospital bed capacity from 1965 to 1981 ranging from a low of 34 percent in Prince Edward Island to a high of 84 percent in Quebec. Despite these differences, a much greater proportion of persons with serious mental disorders were now, clearly, "in the community," particularly when one considered increases in the general population and the fact that people who previously would have been, in all likelihood, long-term residents of psychiatric hospitals were no longer being admitted.[2]

It became evident in the aftermath of this wave of hospital bed closures that many problems still remained, notwithstanding optimistic beliefs about community care. Indeed, whether formerly institutionalized clients were achieving reintegration – were *really* "in the community" – seemed questionable. The situation is summarized in a Canadian Mental Health Association (2001, 5) document:

> By the mid 1970s, however, it was becoming clear that the realization of this vision (deinstitutionalization) was flawed. For many former hospital residents the new system meant either abandonment, demonstrated by the increasing numbers of homeless mentally ill people; "transinstitutionalization": living in grim institution-like conditions such as those found in the large psychiatric boarding homes; or a return to family who suddenly had to cope with an enormous burden of care but with very little support. In addition, fears and prejudices about mental illness, in part responsible for the long history of segregation in institutions, compounded the problems in the community. These attitudes increased the barriers to access to community life in areas such as employment, education and housing.

How did this state of affairs come about? In attempting to answer this question, one needs to look at the factors that originally influenced the deinstitutionalization movement, of which three are generally recognized as being significant: (1) new treatments, (2) changing ideologies and attitudes, and (3) economics.[3]

New Medications
Concerning new treatments, the 1950s saw the first psychiatric use of two drugs that would radically alter mental health practice: *chlorpromazine*, used as a treatment for psychosis, and *lithium*, used for manic depression. Prior to the discovery of the antipsychotic properties of chlorpromazine, treatments for schizophrenia – which included **electroconvulsive therapy** (ECT), insulin coma, and psychosurgery – were found to be of questionable efficacy, if not harmful. Now, with the advent of an oral medication that patients would presumably take voluntarily, there was the promise that individuals would not require containment in hospitals but instead could

be treated on an outpatient basis in community settings. Whether the community programs offering these new medications would be coordinated and accessible and whether all persons would agree to take these drugs were issues that would be struggled with subsequently; it soon became apparent, in the post-institutionalization era, that continuity of care would be a more pressing concern than the availability of medication (Eaton 2001).

Changing Attitudes

In the post-Second World War era a number of critiques, some popular, some academic, were levelled at the practice of "warehousing" huge numbers of patients in psychiatric hospitals. While many of these critiques came from the American context, they also proved to be very influential among Canadian academics, policy makers, and the public (Gray, Shone, and Liddle 2000). Examples include:

- *The Shame of the States,* a journalistic account of the living conditions in American psychiatric hospitals by Albert Deutsch (1948).
- *The Snake Pit* (1948), an Academy Award-nominated film that, while at least somewhat sympathetic toward psychiatry, led a number of American state governments to amend their legislation concerning the hospitalization of mentally disordered persons.
- *One Flew over the Cuckoo's Nest,* Ken Kesey's 1962 novel, and subsequently an Academy Award-winning film (1975), wherein the protagonist is first given ECT, then lobotomized, in apparent efforts to quell his anti-authoritarian behaviour. To this day the phrase "cuckoo's nest" is used to refer to psychiatric hospitals.
- *Titicut's Follies,* a once-banned 1967 documentary film that is a genuinely horrifying account of life in a Massachusetts psychiatric hospital, where patients are verbally abused, force-fed, and paraded about naked.
- *Asylums* (1961), an ethnography of life in a Washington, DC, psychiatric hospital by Canadian sociologist Erving Goffman. The thesis of this very influential book was that institutionalism not only stripped away individual dignity, but actually *fostered* many of the regressive behaviours and symptoms seen among the patients.
- "On being sane in insane places," a controversial study by David Rosenhan (1973), published in the journal *Science,* which detailed the experiences of "fake" patients who had surreptitiously gained admission to psychiatric hospitals and who were never distinguished from the "real" patients by the professional staff. Among other things, Rosenhan spoke about the invisibility and *depersonalization* experienced by institutionalized persons.

These critiques of the policy and effects of institutionalization coincided with a burgeoning civil rights movement that now incorporated the patients' rights agenda along with women's rights and minority rights. Based on the work of Goffman, Rosenhan, and others, it was now asserted that institutionalization not only didn't help persons with mental disorders, but seemed to make them *worse* – that is, exacerbate regressive behaviours – in a number of instances. The concept of "chronicity" as it was applied to mental disorders was attributed to the effects of institutionalization rather than to a disease process. Following from this, it seemed reasonable to suggest that being in the community, in and of itself, would have major therapeutic benefits for persons with mental disorders. While none of these assertions is necessarily wrong, the realization of this vision was compromised by several factors:

(1) The persistence of negative public attitudes toward persons with mental health problems, manifested by the **"not in my back yard" (NIMBY)** syndrome.

(2) The need for more than simply a release from institutional confinement – that is, the provision of respectful, accessible, and comprehensive community support services. Putting it a different way, the provision of civil liberties – "negative" freedoms – did not obviate the need for positive care and support.

(3) The reality that persistence of symptoms may be related to intrinsic factors and is not simply a product of institutionalization.[4]

The overoptimism of the 1960s is summarized by Bachrach (1994, 26): "Early advocates were so completely certain of the curative powers of community-based care that they sometimes elected to understate both the seriousness and chronicity that are part of long-term mental illness. Indeed, they were sometimes so expansive in their optimism that they chose to think in terms of mental health, and effectively to ignore the existence of mental illness."

While some of the criticisms of the asylums – no effective treatment, overcrowding, and degrading, inhumane conditions – seem less relevant today, concern about the possible **iatrogenic** effects of institutionalization, and rhetoric to this effect, remain in force. For example, a Health Canada (2002b, 25) report suggests that, "although hospitalization provides important short-term respite and care, prolonged periods in hospital remove individuals from their normal environment and can weaken social connections, making reintegration into community living more challenging."

Economic Factors

A third factor associated with the downsizing of psychiatric hospitals had to do with the cost of maintaining these facilities, which by the 1960s were, in many cases, outdated and in poor repair. Concerning economic factors, a critical thesis attempting to explain what he referred to as the "decarceration" movement was advanced by sociologist Andrew Scull (1977). In this account it was argued that, by the 1970s, Western governments were facing a "fiscal crisis" and saw an opportunity to offload costs by closing hospital wards and discharging patients, who by the post-Second World War era, were eligible for new subsistence-level welfare and income assistance programs and new privatized services in the community. As summarized by Cohen (1985, 104), "money [could be] saved, and benevolent intentions proclaimed." Scull downplayed the idea that deinstitutionalization came about as a result of progressive reform and critiques of the asylums, arguing that similar critiques had been made in earlier historical periods. Similarly, according to this perspective, abstract references to "community care" and "family care" were smokescreens obscuring the reality that little or no care was in fact being provided.

Scull's thesis has been attacked on a number of points (Cohen 1985). It was noted, for example, that what appeared to be happening in North America was not necessarily applicable to other countries – for instance, in Europe. Further, the time sequence seemed questionable: the census reduction in psychiatric hospitals had been well underway *before* the downturn in the North American economy of the 1970s. Arguments have also arisen over intentions – that is, can it be said that community programs, in the immediate post-deinstitutionalization period, were *deliberately* neglected and underfunded, or were problems encountered during this time "unintended consequences," the result of (as noted earlier) overoptimism?

Finally, should we have assumed that community-based care *would* be less expensive? This question is still relevant since cost containment is a current priority for Canadian health authorities and since cost effectiveness is addressed primarily by making comparisons with the expense of inpatient care. Latimer (1999, 452) notes that "there is no inherent reason for community-based services to be necessarily cheaper than hospital-based ones" since "their relative prices [can] be attributed to historical factors related to reimbursement policies." Bachrach (1994, 29) concludes that community-based care is "probably not" less expensive than hospital-based care, "when we consider all the hidden costs associated with simultaneously running what is, in effect, a two-tiered system covering both hospital- and community-based care"; she points out, however, that determining the "success" of deinstitution-alization depends on what yardsticks are used: "the imputed cost savings" or "the more humanistic elements of the policy."

Recent Policy Concerns and Initiatives

The struggle to establish an effective, comprehensive, and responsive system of mental health care in the post-deinstitutionalization era has been com-plicated by the different and sometimes competing interests of different stake-holder groups. Client representatives have spoken to issues such as choice, empowerment, and civil liberties, while some clinicians, members of the public, and expedient politicians have sought stricter controls on mentally disordered persons deemed to be "noncompliant" and dangerous. At the same time, families have asked for greater support and greater input into the treatment process. Overriding all of this, government officials have increas-ingly emphasized efficiencies, cost containment, and evidence of efficacy. One can get a sense of the number of unresolved policy questions from the following "partial list" of "policy issues relevant to mental health system reform" provided by Health Canada (2002c, 3):

- continuity of care across time, place and providers
- efficiency and rationalized allocation of resources
- effectiveness of services and supports
- acceptability of services to full range of stakeholders
- accountability structures
- appropriateness of services and ability to meet expected standards
- competence of service providers
- safety and risk minimization
- accessibility of services and supports
- shift from institutional to community-based programs
- addressing the broad determinants of health
- devolving governance to regional authorities
- coordination with other policy and service sectors
- consumer involvement in shaping policies and practices
- fiscal models and their impact on health services and systems
- addressing conflict between evidence and values
- complementary or alternative medicine
- sharing of information between agencies
- ensuring access to services by people with severe mental illness
- physician funding mechanisms and integration with other mental health service providers.

In sum, concerns have been voiced by a range of stakeholders relating to questions such as service effectiveness, the underfunding of mental health programs, the lack of coordination of services, the limited range of services offered, and the philosophy underlying the approach to service delivery. Some comment is offered here on the nature of these concerns and proposed responses.

Concerning program philosophy, dissatisfaction has been expressed with (1) a treatment approach that focuses narrowly on symptom management to the exclusion of other existential concerns and (2) the idea of the client as a passive recipient of professional expertise rather than as a collaborator in the rehabilitation process. By contrast, a discussion paper on mental health reform notes that two "critical cornerstones" of reform are "recognition that mental health care should not be limited to formal mental health supports" and "acknowledgment of consumers and families as critical partners in planning, delivering and evaluating mental health care delivery" (Clarke Institute of Psychiatry 1997, 1). In response to these concerns, an approach that incorporates a broader vision of rehabilitation, known as the *recovery* model, has been articulated and (to a lesser extent) implemented in mental health programs. A related development has been the wider use of skills teaching with clients and concomitantly an emphasis on greater self-reliance in contending with symptoms of mental disorder, an approach referred to as *self-management*. Recovery and self-management are described in greater detail in later chapters in the book.

Concerning the range of services offered, earlier community programs were office-based, offering little in the way of outreach support to persons struggling to manage activities of daily living. The housing options offered to clients leaving psychiatric hospitals were limited, consisting mostly of drab boarding homes run for profit by private operators. There was also limited consultation or support offered to family members. Rehabilitation services were in their infancy, with vocational programs mostly taking the form of "sheltered workshops," while education was hardly discussed at all. Prevention and health promotion were not usually on the agenda of community treatment services, with nonprofit programs such as the Canadian Mental Health Association being left to attempt to address these issues. Now the need for a "comprehensive range of services" is recognized, services that include treatment, rehabilitation, prevention, and promotion (Clarke Institute of Psychiatry 1997, 1). Different jurisdictions are now implementing these initiatives by offering, for example, outreach programs to complement office-based case management, a wider range of housing alternatives, early detection programs for persons suffering from psychosis and depression, and more varied rehabilitation programs that include supported employment in competitive settings and peer-support work with other mental health clients. These initiatives are discussed in the chapters that follow.

Apart from the nature and range of programs offered, concern has been expressed about the poor integration of services (Latimer 2005). Goering, Wasylenki, and Durbin (2000, 347) note that "until very recently the provision of mental health services in Canada has been characterized by fragmentation, lack of mechanisms to coordinate or integrate services, and little accountability." These authors go on to describe the "four solitudes" of the mental health system: provincial psychiatric hospitals, general hospital psychiatric units, "overburdened" community mental health programs, and private practitioners, each operating in relative isolation. Another policy document speaks about "the historical imbalance between institutional and community-based care" (Clarke Institute of Psychiatry 1997, 1). To remedy this, it has been suggested that programs be integrated and in particular that "hospital and community services [be] unified into a single system within a local mental health area" (British Columbia Ministry of Health 2002e, 8). To this end, the approach used in most Canadian jurisdictions has been decentralization and the devolution of mental health services from provincial administration by establishing regional health authorities, with these authorities now having "responsibility for the planning and operation of all health, including mental health, services for a defined population" (Goering, Wasylenki, and Durbin 2000, 347). Provincial psychiatric hospitals are now either under the aegis of the health authorities or have autonomous incorporation. An alternative approach, implemented in the province of New Brunswick, is the establishment of a provincial authority or commission specifically devoted to mental health, with regional mental health boards operating locally. Having a single regional health budget (as opposed to separate budgets for hospitals and the community) enables better integration and comprehensiveness of services, it is suggested, "by discouraging cost shifting and by localizing, within one body, the full consequences of decision making" (Clarke Institute of Psychiatry 1997, 23).

There is also greater recognition now of the need to incorporate addiction services within the health authorities and to have persons with co-occurring disorders (psychiatric and addictions) treated in the mental health system (British Columbia Ministry of Health 2002e). It has unfortunately been the case that persons with co-occurring disorders – representing a large proportion of the mental health client population – have in many instances had their concerns dealt with by separate programs, in separate locations, with different treatment philosophies, and operating under separate ministries. In British Columbia, for example, addiction services were part of the Ministry for Children and Families in the 1990s, being moved to the Ministry of Health Services (with services devolved to the regional health authorities) following the election in 2001 of a new government, which nonetheless decided to put addiction *prevention* in a different ministry (Health Planning) while moving services for gambling addiction to the Ministry of Public Safety and Solicitor General. Increasingly, however, both at the level of governance and service delivery, there is a move to integrating operations. In this respect, it is noteworthy that one of Canada's leading mental health services, Toronto's Centre for Addiction and Mental Health, was created (in 1998) by the amalgamation of two addictions programs (the Addiction Research Foundation and the Donwood Institute) and two mental health programs (the Clarke Institute of Psychiatry and the Queen Street Mental Health Centre).

In addition to better integration of services, an apparent benefit of regionalization is that the system becomes more responsive to local needs (Clarke Institute of Psychiatry 1997; Wilson 2005). On this point Dickinson (2002, 383) notes that "the anticipated advantages of decentralization and regionalization are twofold: It is hoped that they will enable the identification of location-specific service delivery needs, and that they will facilitate the creation of local commitment to the mobilization and reallocation of resources in the communities most directly affected. This last point is particularly important in light of the commitment to self-care and mutual aid as essential elements in the health promotion framework." In British Columbia, following the establishment of five regional health authorities in 2001, work to "redesign" and devolve the one provincial psychiatric hospital to the regions has been supported by memos that speak to the benefits of local services – for example: "The Riverview Hospital Redevelopment Project decentralizes tertiary mental health care currently located at Riverview Hospital to the five regional health authorities. Best practices indicate that better mental health outcomes can be achieved in smaller community settings. By building tertiary mental health capacity in the regions, each health authority can provide a more complete continuum of mental health services and families and patients will be able to access these services closer to home." A subsequent memo notes that this process will "enable regional self-sufficiency."[5]

Whether the anticipated benefits of integrated care and regionalization are achieved remains to be seen in many cases. It is noted that barriers to implementation include the different cultures existing within, and the historical lack of trust between, the hospital and community sectors (British Columbia Ministry of Health 2002e).

Finally, with respect to stakeholder concerns, there is the question of service *effectiveness*, which has become a very prominent issue in an era of cost containment and limited resources. In addressing this concern, health authorities are increasingly emphasizing *evidence-based* interventions and what are called "best practices." These concepts – their strengths and limitations – are discussed in greater detail in the following chapter.

Notes

1 Deinstitutionalization in Canada lagged behind the same process in the United States by several years: in the US state psychiatric hospital censuses peaked in the mid-1950s.

2 In British Columbia, for example, the province's population nearly tripled (1.1 to 3.2 million) in the same period that the bed count at the provincial institution fell by over 80 percent (from around 5,000 in the 1950s to just over 900 in 1993) (Mental Health Evaluation and Community Consultation Unit 2000).

3 As was the case with the asylum movement, there have been more skeptical accounts of the deinstitutionalization movement, accounts that are dismissive of "best intentions" viewpoints. French social theorist Michel Foucault (1965, 1977) has suggested that systems of "care" evolve but don't necessarily progress – that is, that coercion/control of clients continues to be practised, although in new forms.

4 During the 1970s and early 1980s, in recognition of the persistence of symptoms among mentally disordered persons who were too young to have experienced long-term hospitalization, researchers began referring to a group called the "young adult chronics" or "new young chronics" (Davis 1985).

5 This comes from "Vancouver Coastal Health Riverview Redesign Project Update #3," 25 June 2003.

"Best Practices" and Evidence-Based Interventions

6

Historically, it has largely been taken on faith that the mental health services offered to clients and their significant others were beneficial – and were what they wanted. Decisions about psychiatric interventions were driven more by theory, conjecture, and practitioner idiosyncrasy than by systematic empirical support. Increasingly, however, in attempting to accommodate the interests of stakeholders such as clients, families, and funding bodies, there is the recognition that mental health practice should be evidence-based (Garfinkel and Goldbloom 2000). Evidence-based practices are defined by one group of authors as an integration of "individual clinical expertise with the best available external clinical evidence from systematic research" (Sackett et al. 1996, 71) and by another group as "interventions for which there is consistent scientific evidence showing that they improve client outcomes" (Drake et al. 2001, 180). In a Canadian Psychiatric Association position paper on this topic, the authors explain why evidence-based practice is an important concept:

> The most compelling reason to adopt an evidence-based approach is an ethical obligation to support patients and families in making informed choices about medical decisions. This is a central tenet of medical codes of ethics such as that of the Canadian Medical Association. It is reasonable for patients and families to expect the best available information about the efficacy of various treatments and their potential risks and side effects. Correspondingly, physicians have an obligation to provide high-quality information to their patients and to assist in summarizing and interpreting the research literature so that patients, incorporating their values and preferences, can make informed decisions ... Evidence-based information helps patients and families to counter popular misconceptions regarding diagnoses and treatments. Further, the level of credibility of the information

that the physician provides may be a critical element in the subsequent acceptance of and compliance with treatment. (Goldner et al. 2000)

That clients now have greater access to information on mental health from sources such as the Internet also underlines the importance of practitioners being current and conversant with the evidence base (Marie-Albert 2002).

A concept related to "evidence-based" interventions is **"best practices,"** which is defined in a government document as follows:

Best practice means that mental health programs and initiatives for care are based on evidence that they will achieve the outcomes government, clinicians and consumers want, specifically:

- reduction of symptoms
- decreased use of more intrusive and/or more costly services
- improved functioning in various areas of clients' lives
- enhanced quality of clients' and their families' lives, and
- consumer and provider satisfaction with mental health services. (British Columbia Ministry of Health 2002e, 10)

"Best practices," then, refers to the *outcomes* that are deemed desirable by different stakeholders. However, this raises a number of issues. For one thing, if governments, clinicians, and consumers disagree about outcomes, how does one reconcile these competing interests? For example, community treatment orders – where clients are under a legal order to take medication and report to a treatment team – have been shown to reduce rates of rehospitalization but are still regarded with ambivalence (at least) by many clients because of the coercive aspects (Davis 2002). As well, invoking the term "best practices" often raises the fear of program cutbacks or closures, of the "program evaluator as hatchet-person" – a not unreasonable inference given the references, as above, to "decreased use of costly services" – notwithstanding the need to consider cost pressures on the health care system. Jaded practitioners may come to see phrases such as "least intrusive services" as code words for "*no* services." Clients, similarly, may worry about a loss of choice when restraint measures are brought in, as one author suggests: "Consumers [may] perceive a loss of empowerment as evidence-based practices are implemented. The loss of empowerment could result in a new polarization of consumers and mental health professionals just when collaboration between the two was beginning to seem the norm" (Tracy 2003, 1437).[1] On a more positive note, the last three bullets in the definition above are apparently a reflection of a broader conceptualization of mental health, focused on client satisfaction and quality of life rather than primarily on symptomatology. Still, when considering "outcomes" in mental health, the practitioner needs to ask the question "*whose* outcomes?"[2]

Quantitative Methods and Experimental Design

One may ask, concerning the "evidence" in evidence-based practices: where does it come from and what form does it take? A Canadian document on best practices suggests the following:

> Evidence on which to base program design and clinical care is available
> from different sources and in different forms. Common sources include
> clinical trials, consumer reference groups, outcomes research and evaluation,
> expert consensus and, finally, clinical practice guidelines (CPG). The purpose
> of CPGs is to bridge the gap between producers of health care research and
> the providers who wish to use that research in their clinical decision-
> making and care. Effective guidelines promote informed decision-making
> by providers and clients and are flexible enough to allow both groups some
> choices in individualizing care. They reduce the variance between practice
> known to be effective according to the best evidence available and the actual
> practice taking place. (British Columbia Ministry of Health 2002e, 10)

In considering this passage, it is noteworthy that reference is now being made to consumer reference groups; as we have seen, consumer contributions to the knowledge base have tended to be overlooked until recent times (Bachrach 1996).

While evidence may come from different sources, medical publications speak about a hierarchy where the highest level of evidence – the "gold standard" – is that produced by randomized clinical trials (Sackett et al. 2000), referring to studies where (1) subjects are randomly assigned to treatment and control groups, (2) the researcher has the ability to manipulate a particular intervention, (3) neither the person scoring the results nor the subject knows who received what (termed "double-blind," which presumably eliminates the expectation effect), (4) the treatment environment is controlled, and (5) data are analyzed with inferential statistics. The argument here is that only by ensuring initial group equivalency (through randomization) and isolating the independent variable (the presumed cause) can one rule out confounding factors and make causal inferences. The strength of the evidence is increased when multiple trials produce similar results; *meta-analysis* is a statistical method of pooling such results.

Below the true **experimental design** are evidence sources considered not as strong or unequivocal, including quasi-experimental designs (no true control group), and at the lowest level "expert consensus," which Health

Canada (2001a, 24) suggests may be used "to fill the gaps in the scientific literature." "Consensus" in the absence of systematic validating research has historically had its limitations, as evidenced by concerns about bias in the creation of diagnostic categories in early versions of the *Diagnostic and Statistical Manual (DSM)* of the American Psychiatric Association (Caplan 1995; Larkin and Caplan 1992). Health Canada (2001a, 24) notes that "criticisms of this [expert consensus] approach often centre on the fact that the process of selecting experts is often a reflection of professional hierarchies which may result in no more than a group guess."

Inherent in the experimental approach is a bias in favour of quantifiable indicators when researching outcomes in mental health. The reasons for this have to do with research traditions – for example, a view that qualitative research is not "real" science – as well as with pragmatic considerations: quantitative measures of hospital utilization patterns, for example, are favoured by health authorities because they are fairly easily accessed, have "face validity," and address cost issues. In a recent *Canadian Journal of Psychiatry* review paper on "quality management," the authors state that "for usefulness and consensus ... outcome measures should have established psychometric properties. These include high reliability (both internal and test-retest) and validity. Only then can one confidently base decisions on results obtained from outcome measures. [Further] data obtained from a particular outcome measure should be amenable to statistical analyses. This will allow for accurate interpretation of outcome data" (McGrath and Tempier 2003, 471). Consistent with this approach, in workshops on program evaluation and goal setting, practitioners are taught the acronym "SMART" – that is, that outcomes should preferably be:

- *Specific:* detailed enough that a third party would be able to tell when it had been achieved.
- *Measurable:* subject to client self-report, staff report, or third party objective appraisal.
- *Attainable:* within the capabilities of the client and staff (program) to achieve.
- *Relevant:* currently either a genuine need of or a challenge for the client.
- *Time-bound:* achievable within a stipulated, finite period of time.[3]

An example of a goal-setting and tracking sheet, where goals are to be SMART, is given in the box opposite.[4] The form can be used, for example, in case management planning.

A wide range of quantitative indicators have been used to evaluate mental health practice. Sometimes structured psychometric instruments are used,

Goal-setting and Tracking Sheet

Goal areas:
(1) Mental health	(5) Housing	(9) Leisure
(2) Physical health	(6) Finance	(10) Education/work
(3) Spiritual health	(7) Living skills	(11) Legal issues
(4) Substance use	(8) Interpersonal relationships	

Area	Date set	Goal description	Target date	Outcome (A/P/N)*	Review date
_____	_____	_____	_____	_____	_____
		_____			
		_____			
		_____			
_____	_____	_____	_____	_____	_____
		_____			
		_____			
		_____			
_____	_____	_____	_____	_____	_____
		_____			
		_____			
		_____			
_____	_____	_____	_____	_____	_____
		_____			
		_____			
		_____			
_____	_____	_____	_____	_____	_____
		_____			
		_____			
		_____			
_____	_____	_____	_____	_____	_____
		_____			
		_____			
		_____			
_____	_____	_____	_____	_____	_____
		_____			
		_____			
		_____			
_____	_____	_____	_____	_____	_____
		_____			
		_____			
		_____			

* *Note:* A = achieved, P = partially achieved, N = not achieved.

such as psychological tests, symptom rating scales, and self-report surveys like the Beck Depression Inventory. Clinicians may also use indicators such as number of hospital admissions, number of evictions or admissions to emergency shelters, number of calls to the crisis line, number of missed appointments, time on and off the job, and so on. As noted above, utilization patterns are commonly used by health authorities as indicators of success or failure: both hospital stays beyond a certain length and readmissions before a certain period of time may be counted as negative outcomes. For example, a document produced by the British Columbia Ministry of Health Services (2003b) proposes that a hospital admission for psychiatric reasons within thirty days of a previous discharge be counted, for evaluation purposes, as a negative outcome. Authorities may also look at assessing quality of care based on quantitative indicators, such as length of time from referral to initial assessment as a measure of system responsiveness. To appraise these data, benchmarks are applied; an example, concerning waiting times, comes from a government document stipulating that urgent community mental health referrals should be seen "within 72 hours, others within 10 days" (British Columbia Ministry of Health 2002e, 5). In practice, benchmarks such as these may be hard to achieve because of resource limitations.[5] (For a comprehensive overview of quantitative indicators used to evaluate mental health practice, the reader is directed to McEwan and Goldner 2001.)

The emphasis on quantifiable outcomes has been criticized by some clinicians partly because of concerns about their validity. Some would suggest, for example, that using quantitative indicators to capture a concept such as "quality of life" is a crass, insensitive approach. On this point, William Anthony and colleagues observe that "simple dichotomous counts of ... hospitalization are an enormous conceptual distance from what might be described as recovery outcomes" (Anthony, Rogers, and Farkas 2003, 105). An additional concern, for instance with the use of utilization data, is that the real issue and overriding consideration is *cost*. An American psychiatrist decries the idea that outcome indicators should refer "only to observable, and possibly measurable, characteristics of a patient," noting that this "seems to fit the focus of managed care – that functioning, not internal suffering, is the most important issue for insurance coverage" (Moffic 2003, 1063).

Experimental designs use a particular type of data analysis, which deserves some comment. Statistical significance, a *sine qua non* for study credibility and "publishability," allows researchers to have greater confidence in their conclusions but provides only general guidance to practitioners. For example, given that drug response is idiosyncratic, practitioners still need to use good clinical judgment when employing research evidence as a guide to choice of medications in individual cases; on this, Kravitz, Duan, and Braslow (2004) note the difficulty in applying global evidence – "average effects" – to individual clients or groups who may depart from the population average.

One should also bear in mind that statistical significance is to a great extent a function of sample size: a large enough sample will achieve the "alpha" cutoff of 0.05 even if the effect size is weak.[6] To take one example among many, a large-scale study comparing newer- and older-generation antipsychotic medications, published in the *American Journal of Psychiatry*, found rates of relapse that "were *modestly but significantly* lower with the newer drugs" (Leucht et al. 2003, 1209, emphasis added). Significance levels, then, must be placed in the context of effect sizes.

A type of study that addresses the issue of effect size and that is commonly seen in psychiatric publications is the *meta-analysis*, which involves the calculation of an average effect size across several previously completed studies on a particular topic. Meta-analyses offer several benefits, such as providing the benchmarks used when considering the relative strengths of different interventions as well as showing how mean effect size varies by different clinical or methodological factors (Rubin and Babbie 2001). Meta-analyses have some limitations, however, particularly the danger of skewed results due to the inclusion of methodologically weak studies with stronger ones. As well, reviewers may miss important studies for inclusion, either by chance or because they were not published.

Unpublished Research

The issue of unpublished research deserves at least some brief comment since there is evidence that it is not a random occurrence but rather dictated by the commercial interests of either drug companies, which do not want bad reports on a new product, or universities, which do not want to lose sponsors' contracts (Bekelman, Li, and Gross 2003; *Canadian Medical Association Journal* 2004). Additionally, medical journals may prefer to publish exciting new findings rather than "boring, negative results" (Bekelman, Li, and Gross 2003, 463). Health Canada (2001a, 24) notes that the evidence-based approach relies "on a body of literature that is subject to pervasive publication bias." A disturbing example of this concerns the unapproved use of antidepressant medication in children, particularly the class of drugs known as selective serotonin reuptake inhibitors (SSRIs). In 2003 regulatory bodies in Britain and Canada started issuing advisories to physicians concerning the use of these drugs with patients under eighteen since evidence of adverse effects appeared to outweigh evidence of therapeutic benefit. In looking at the evidence base to support the "off-label," or nondesignated, prescribing of SSRIs, it was noted that fifteen clinical trials had been conducted with young people but only three published – because the results of the other trials showed that the medication didn't work (Branham 2004). For example, an internal document obtained by the *Canadian Medical Association Journal* advised staff at the multinational drug company GlaxoSmithKline "to withhold clinical trial findings in 1998 that indicated the [SSRI] antidepressant paroxetine had no beneficial effect in treating adolescents" (Kondro and Sibbald 2004, 783).

In a report on the limitations of the clinical trial process for evaluating the efficacy of psychiatric medications, doctors interviewed by a Vancouver journalist expressed the need for an independent research body in Canada, akin to a national institute of health, and for the reporting of *all* trial data, positive and negative (Branham 2003). Similarly, in an editorial on this subject, the *Canadian Medical Association Journal* (2004, 437) concluded that "the behaviour of industry, government and investigators must change. Investigators must demand access to all the data collected in clinical trials in which they participate and to suitably anonymized [sic] aggregate information from adverse drug reaction reports. Investigators should be at liberty and even encouraged to provide alternate analyses and interpretations of clinical trial results and adverse event reporting and to publish these. Physicians, research subjects and the public should demand no less."

Nonexperimental Methods
In reality, the standards of the true experimental design are very difficult to achieve in mental health research or in social science in general (Anthony, Rogers, and Farkas 2003). Coming closest is the drug trial, where one group of subjects is given a new medication and one or more control groups are given either a placebo or an older medication. Even with drug trials, there has been debate about whether the "gold standard" is being achieved: critics have argued that drug manufacturers' claims that newer-generation antipsychotic medications have fewer side effects are based on trial comparisons with control groups that were given older medications in disproportionately high, "nonoptimized" doses – violating *ceteris paribus,* the "initial group equivalency" requirement – that spuriously made the new products better by comparison (Whitaker 2002; see also Rosenheck et al. 2003).

In speaking about the difficulty of using experimental designs in a field such as occupational therapy, University of Toronto professor Susan Rappolt (2003, 589) notes that "even in the much larger, and relatively more quantifiable and controllable field of medical research, there is a shortage of coherent, consistent scientific evidence. How much more difficult is it, then, to produce research evidence on the effectiveness of occupational therapy practices, when occupational therapy focuses on the complexities of individuals in their occupational contexts rather than on their cells or biological subsystems?"

Mental health researchers investigating nonpharmacological interventions must contend with issues such as not having a true control group, self-selection of subjects, subject drop-out, inconsistent application of protocols and procedures ("low fidelity") between settings, and an absence of "discrete and controllable variables" ready-made for analysis (Rappolt 2003, 590). In these instances researchers may adopt quasi-experimental designs, from which reasonable inferences may still be drawn provided that guidelines are conscientiously applied,[7] as well as *qualitative* research methods, which may be better suited "to access and analyze complex and abstract phenomena and relationships" (590). Anthony, Rogers, and Farkas (2003, 107) conclude that "correlational and quasi-experimental research are excellent sources of information for the development of evidence-based practices and can guide the development of appropriate studies of effectiveness."

Concerning qualitative approaches, researchers in this tradition must contend with prejudice in the psychiatric community against the use of "anecdotal" sources of information, which unfortunately may be applied in the case of the subjective experiences of clients themselves. As noted earlier, first person accounts have historically not been included in the practitioner knowledge base. Boydell, Gladstone, and Crawford (2002, 21) note that "experiential knowledge – the direct experience of a mental illness and the intimate knowledge of what it means in a human life – traditionally has been devalued in psychiatry." Even when included, client accounts may be regarded as tentative, if not suspect, requiring further corroboration. For example, McGrath and Tempier (2003, 469) suggest that "[while] assessing patient satisfaction provides a particularly valuable reflection of the consumer perspective on quality of care ... it would be wrong to conclude that individuals perceiving treatment more positively necessarily show better outcomes. Thus, it is important to assess not only patients' subjective perceptions of treatment progress and outcome but also more *objective* perceptions" (emphasis added). Even when written by practitioners, anecdotal accounts – case studies – have an inferior status in publications like the *Canadian Journal of Psychiatry*, being placed in the back end of the journal under "brief reports" rather than in the front under "original research."[8]

This situation may be changing. Boydell, Gladstone, and Crawford (2002, 22) suggest that "the experiential component has resurfaced in research with the burgeoning interest in the use of qualitative methods in tandem with the development of consumer/survivor initiatives and a growing consumer/survivor-authored literature." Students in the social sciences are now exposed to approaches such as participatory action research, a vision of the research enterprise that emphasizes practical payoffs and subject-driven designs. As well, prominent mental health journals such as *Schizophrenia Bulletin* and *Psychiatric Services* regularly publish client "personal accounts." However, while case studies and qualitative research methods are used prominently in disciplines such as nursing and social work, medicine and psychiatry still rely on large scale, quantitative designs. For this reason, clients and practitioners interested in giving voice to the recipients of mental health services, if not already doing so, may need to incorporate quantitative methods into their research repertoires. At the same time, it should be stressed that quantitative and qualitative methods can be complementary rather than conflicting; knowledge gained through personal accounts, clinical work, content analysis, and case studies – inductive methods – can form the hypotheses that are subsequently tested and analyzed through quantitative designs (e.g., see Hilty et al. 2003). Anthony and colleagues conclude that "at this point in time, the knowledge underlying evidence-based practices must be derived from a variety of methodologies" (Anthony, Rogers, and Farkas 2003, 111).

The Role of the Practitioner
Finally, what is the position of the clinician in contributing to the knowledge base in mental health? While at university, students in a number of disciplines – medicine, nursing, psychology, occupational therapy, social work – will be told about their potentially important role as producers and disseminators of knowledge ("scientist-practitioners"). In reality, once they graduate, most of these same people will have little or nothing to do with research for a number of reasons – one being simple lack of interest. For those who would like to participate in the research enterprise, however, there are a number of barriers. Most significant, there is usually neither the time, resources, nor mandate to do research. Further, practitioner research will tend to be small-scale, not "real research" – an exception being trials sponsored by drug companies. (In addressing the "small-scale" issue, *single case designs* – a quasi-experimental method – were touted in the 1980s as a way of applying a more rigorous, quasi-experimental methodology to clinical research [Barlow and Hersen 1984]; despite the promise of this approach, studies of this sort are not often seen in mental health publications.) Persons who *are* able to conduct projects "off the sides of their desks" may be regarded with a certain degree of suspicion by administrators as to their real intentions. Another barrier faced by practitioner-researchers is the prospect that the final product will either be shelved or evaluated on the basis of political criteria rather than its own merits. That practitioners interested in carrying out research should be deterred from doing so is unfortunate in

that they have a valuable insider perspective. Notwithstanding the barriers, practitioners may support the research enterprise indirectly by mentoring students and clients and facilitating their projects, by participating as subjects in focus groups and surveys, and by creating and disseminating topics for research in committees and other forums.

Notes

1 This author suggests that evidence-based services need to be complemented with "value-based" services, which he defines as "practices that have limited scientific evidence supporting their efficacy but that have high consumer satisfaction" (Tracy 2003, 1437).
2 Cohen and colleagues observe that "notions of mental illness and treatment outcomes depend on social norms and values," the conundrum being that "there *are* no universally acceptable psychological norms" (Cohen et al. 2003, 462, emphasis added).
3 This comes from a "guidelines and definitions" sheet, which is attached to goal-setting and tracking forms used in the author's agency. There are variations on SMART – for example, "appropriate" rather than "attainable," "realistic" or "results-oriented" rather than "relevant," and "trackable" rather than "time-bound."
4 This is a modification of a form used in the author's agency, Vancouver Community Mental Health Services.
5 In the case of "waiting time until initial assessment," the limiting factor is often physician availability, particularly since a longer period of time must normally be blocked off in the schedule to do an initial assessment.
6 For further discussion of the misapplication of statistics to the social and psychological realms, see for example, Best (2001) or Uttal (2003).
7 On this topic, interested readers are directed to the work of Donald Campbell, Thomas Cook, and colleagues (e.g., Cook and Campbell 1979).
8 Concerning the use of case studies in psychological research, one author notes that "many ... consider these individual cases to be outside the pale of good science – the pejorative 'anecdote' all too often being quite appropriately applied to such singular observations" (Uttal 2003, 122).

The System:
Mental Health Programs in Canada

While the creation of regional health authorities was intended to lead to more comprehensive and better coordinated services, at the time of writing it was evident that these goals had not been fully realized. Hospital resources are overstretched partly because of restraint measures and partly because complementary community-based housing and support programs are insufficient, meaning that psychiatric crises cannot be "headed off" before inpatient care is required. Other concerns include the fact that a disproportionate number of mental health clients are treated by general practitioners alone and that persons with co-occurring disorders – psychiatric and addictions – continue to be a "poor fit" with existing services.

This chapter offers an overview of mental health programs in Canada, including programs that have been regarded as core services, such as hospital care and community-based case management, as well as newer developments, which include shared care, home-based treatment and crisis services, assertive outreach, early intervention programs, programs for persons with co-occurring disorders, and telepsychiatry, although it should be noted that these newer programs have not been implemented in all settings. Where relevant, reference is made to best-practice guidelines.

Centralized Intake

Accessing community mental health services can be a confusing ordeal for clients and loved ones, with the resultant delays in getting services meaning that manageable problems may become crises (Hall 2001). One way of addressing this is through the use of a centralized intake process – that is, a single contact point and phone number for all mental health services within a region. Such an arrangement is easier for clients to follow, and there is also evidence that accessibility and accountability are improved given that local responses to referrals can be idiosyncratic (British Columbia Ministry of Health 2002e). Centralized intake has been implemented in a number of other British Commonwealth countries and is becoming more commonly used in Canadian jurisdictions. A 2003 news release from Calgary, for example, noting the over 800 mental health programs in the region, speaks about the need for "one stop shopping" and the consequent value of their single information line, which would become a full intake and triage service by 2004 (Calgary Health Region 2003). In another example, a toll-free 1-800-SUICIDE line has been set up in British Columbia, a pilot project that will likely be expanded across the country (Thomas 2004).

Hospitals and Hospital-Based Programs

Hospital Utilization
With the downsizing of provincial psychiatric hospitals, the inpatient care of persons with mental disorders now takes place predominantly in general hospital psychiatric units (GHPUs).[1] For example, data from the period 2000-01 showed that 87 percent of hospital separations related to mental disorder were from GHPUs, while only 13 percent were from provincial psychiatric hospitals (Canadian Institute for Health Information 2003). (A "separation" is defined as a discharge or death, so a person being admitted and discharged on three separate occasions in a reporting period would be counted as three separations.) This same data source found that persons leaving GHPUs had considerably shorter average lengths of stay (36 days) compared to those leaving provincial institutions (160 days). It is noteworthy that separation rate and average length of stay varied considerably from one province and territory to the next, with the northern territories having the fastest "turnover," which may be a reflection of differences in "the health of the population, mental health service delivery models, and variations between jurisdictions in the availability and accessibility of ... community-based health services" (2). Variations are seen within provinces as well: in British Columbia, for example, during the period 1997-2000, the average length of GHPU stay for persons diagnosed with schizophrenia was 19 days, with regional averages ranging from 9.2 days in a more rural locale (the Kootenays) to 30.6 days in the Victoria metropolitan area (British Columbia Ministry of Health Services 2003b). A Health Canada (1997b) report notes that length of hospital stay will also be determined by the tendencies of the individual physicians involved.

Notwithstanding fluctuations over time and between jurisdictions, the general trend through the latter part of the twentieth century was a shortening of the average length of stay in both GHPUs and provincial psychiatric hospitals. In provincial institutions, the average length of stay decreased from 250 days in 1994-95 to 160 days in 2000-1. Data from GHPUs covering the period from 1987 to 1999 show that the length of stay fell 20 percent for persons diagnosed with depression, to 15 days on average, 27 percent for those diagnosed with bipolar disorder, to an average of 20 days, and 26 percent for persons diagnosed with schizophrenia, to 27 days on average (Health Canada 2002b).

This trend toward briefer hospitalization is influenced by both (1) cost containment and the relative scarcity of inpatient resources and (2) changing philosophies with respect to treatment, the role of the hospital, and the psychosocial impact of institutionalization. Concerning changing philosophies, different reports have concluded, for example, that "best practices in this area will contribute to reducing hospital average lengths of stay and hospital bed utilization rates" (British Columbia Ministry of Health 2002e, 17) and that "inpatient stays [should be] kept as short as possible without harming patient outcomes" (McEwan and Goldner 2001, 33). In support of this position is evidence that a large proportion of mentally ill persons presenting for admission to hospital, as many as 40 percent according to one report, "can be managed in alternative care settings, including ... day hospital or intensive ambulatory care facilities" (Gordon 1997, 1). It can also be pointed out that long-stay hospitalization may place in jeopardy a client's housing arrangements – for example, in the situation where provincial income assistance policies do not permit continuing payment of rent when the individual remains in hospital. Attempts to empirically examine the relative benefits of short vs. long-stay hospitalization have not been conclusive and are made difficult because of methodological issues (Health Canada 1997b).

The current emphasis on early discharge has at times created tensions between hospital and community-based practitioners, with the latter group complaining about "premature" discharges and arguing for the benefits of longer inpatient stay. While the actions of both parties may to some extent be guided by expedience, community-based practitioners may justifiably point to the fact that community alternatives that are supportive yet "less restrictive" – such as "step-down" facilities, outreach programs, or the availability of friends and family – either do not exist or have lengthy waiting lists; for their part, hospital practitioners may argue that it is not their role to make up for all the deficiencies on the community side of the system. Regardless of these differences of opinion, it is important that both groups come together at time of discharge so that there is effective linkage and continuity of care for clients leaving the hospital.

With a reduction in the total number of psychiatric hospital beds and the consequent pressure on general hospital resources, attempts have been made to arrive at *benchmarks* for appropriate bed levels in the mental health system. Not surprisingly, there are some discrepancies in the literature. For example, a report from a group of Quebec authors comes to a figure of 20 long-stay beds per 100,000 population as an "ideal ratio" (Lesage et al. 2003, 485), while the figure produced by the Ontario Health Services Restructuring Commission is 14 per 100,000 (Goering, Wasylenki, and Durbin 2000), with Toronto-based researchers suggesting that this figure could be closer to 10 or even 7 provided adequate outreach and residential programs were in place (Wasylenki et al. 2000). With respect to acute care psychiatric beds, the Ontario commission set a target of 21 per 100,000 population (Goering, Wasylenki, and Durbin 2000), whereas a position paper by the Canadian Psychiatric Association (CPA) concludes that 50 beds per 100,000 is a more appropriate figure (Gordon 1997). The CPA suggests that there is "little evidence that psychiatric services can manage at the lower [bed] levels ... and advises caution in setting these low targets," adding that they would "emphasize the importance of taking into account the local situation using sound criteria and methods in assessing needs, including local prevalence and incidence as well as the availability of appropriate community resources and alternative care settings" (1).

General Hospital Inpatient Programs

Most community hospitals will have only one psychiatric unit, and some hospitals, unfortunately, may lack even this. Inner-city hospitals typically have busy emergency departments and may at times be on "diversion," meaning that mental health clients being sent in ambulances are diverted to other, outlying hospitals. Alternately, and unfortunately, clients with psychiatric crises may be backed up into the regular emergency department or may be held with paramedics in other waiting areas, including hallways, all of which can mean a more traumatic experience for the clients involved. While direct admission to psychiatric wards may be possible, often times incoming certified patients have to be medically cleared first through the hospital's regular emergency department.

Larger centres, in addition to general psychiatric units, may have other, specialized programs. These include:

- *A short-stay assessment unit*, where admissions are typically under fifteen days (Goering, Wasylenki, and Durbin 2000).
- *A psychiatric intensive care unit*, defined as a "secure unit for patients requiring the highest level of observation and containment" (British Columbia Ministry of Health 2002e, 20).
- *An adolescent inpatient unit*. The previously cited best practices report notes that "adult ... inpatient units are not ideal for children and adolescents" and that each region should have a "residential assessment and treatment

unit exclusive to adolescents and with programming specifically tailored to their developmental needs" (British Columbia Ministry of Health 2002e, 22). In some cases adolescent units will be located within hospitals, either general or children's, although separate, smaller-scale residential settings may be preferable.

- *Geriatric units.* The admission criteria, clinical issues, and care needs are usually quite different with respect to the psychogeriatric population, underlining the need for a separate unit with specialized staff. Best practices standards emphasize the importance of integrated care with an elderly population, meaning that continuity should be maintained with family, general practitioners (GPs), psychiatrists, mental health teams, and the community long-term care system while the individual is in hospital, which may be achieved in part with joint care rounds. Geriatric hospital units often have an outreach component (Donnelly 2001).

Outpatient Programs

Hospital outpatient programs go by different names, including "ambulatory care" and "partial hospitalization." Such programs, where patients go home at night, "combine the advantages of intensive treatment with the advantages of keeping individuals in the home environment" (Clarke Institute of Psychiatry 1997, 60). Similarly, Briggs and colleagues note that the benefits of this approach include the client being able to "maintain contact with their family and peers, thus facilitating reintegration into the community following their treatment," as well as the fact that "costs of treatment are greatly reduced" (Briggs, Choptiany, and Steinberg 1997, 79).

A review by the Clarke Institute of Psychiatry (1997, 60) describes the different categories of outpatient programs:

- *Day hospitals,* which "diagnose and treat acutely ill individuals who would otherwise be inpatients, and provide intensive rehabilitation for those who need more treatment than can be supplied by outpatient service."
- *Day treatment* programs, which serve diverse functions and which may have specific target groups such as adolescents or persons with substance misuse issues.
- *Day care* programs, which "focus on longer-term maintenance and rehabilitation of those with chronic, disabling disorders."

Hospital outpatient programs may also include clinics that provide assessment and consultation services for community practitioners. Treatment programs often utilize group modalities and may involve graduate students or postgraduate fellows in disciplines such as psychology.

Tertiary Care

"**Tertiary care**" is distinguished from "**secondary care**," with the latter term applying to services provided in a general hospital psychiatric unit. Tertiary care has been used to refer to (1) inpatient programs that accept admissions only from other hospitals, (2) long-stay inpatient programs, and (3) most commonly, *specialized* inpatient programs for persons whose needs are more complex (Goering, Wasylenki, and Durbin 2000). Examples of populations with specialized needs that may require tertiary resources include: persons with eating disorders, persons with treatment-resistant psychosis who may also have aggressive behaviours, persons with neurological complications, persons with co-occurring intellectual handicaps, persons with co-occurring substance misuse issues, elderly persons, and children and adolescents (British Columbia Ministry of Health 2002e). Apart from inpatient treatment, the goals of tertiary services may include consultation, education, outreach support, and research. Goering and colleagues note that "the availability of tertiary care back-up often results in greater willingness among primary and secondary care providers to accept individuals with difficult conditions and behaviors" (Goering, Wasylenki, and Durbin 2000, 352).

With aging provincial psychiatric hospitals effectively becoming tertiary care facilities, the need for smaller, more homelike settings has become apparent. One group of authors speak about the "increasing interest in portable and community-based tertiary care models to delink delivery of tertiary care from particular settings or time frames" (Goering, Wasylenki, and Durbin 2000, 352). Concerning the evolution of tertiary care resources, a British Columbia report concludes that these services have developed "unsystematically" (British Columbia Ministry of Health 2002e, 45) and recommends that advisory boards be established at both the provincial and regional levels, with representatives from the primary and secondary care systems present to ensure that the needs of these stakeholders are addressed.

Case Management

Case management is recognized as a crucial component of the service delivery system; the authors of a best-practices document observe that "among the core services and supports within a reformed system of care, case management and assertive community treatment [see below] have the most relevance to the creation of an integrated system of care" (Clarke Institute of Psychiatry 1997, 20). Case management is usually provided by nonphysician practitioners at community mental health clinics; family physicians and psychiatrists generally do not have the time, knowledge of resources, or mandate to perform this function.

While recognized as important, "case management" is not easily defined or conceptualized, with Health Canada (1997b, 4) concluding that there is "no standard definition" of this term.[2] That being said, there is some consensus that it refers to a role – rather than to a particular professional background or discipline – where the focus is on *linkage* with resources and *coordination of care*, not necessarily on direct provision of services (Commission on the Future of Health Care in Canada 2002; Maguire 2002). The importance of case management becomes apparent when one considers the complaint, expressed by clients and family members, that negotiating "the system" is a difficult, bewildering ordeal, where information does not seem to be readily available and where at every turn the individual must deal with gatekeepers whose job seems to be finding reasons for *not* providing assistance. For example, the mental health advocate of British Columbia reported in 2001 that the issue generating the most calls to her office (44%) was "difficulties with accessing the health care system" (Hall 2001, 18). Similarly, a survey by the provincial government found that "consumers are quite dissatisfied with the level of information they receive regarding programs and services that are available to them" (British Columbia Ministry of Health 2003b, vii). In an article describing twelve core competencies that mental health practitioners should possess, the authors speak about the ability to "effectively access and employ community resources" – that is, to "develop and maintain good links with a wide range of community resources," to "know about entitlement and benefit programs," and to "integrate community resources and entitlement programs into service planning and delivery" (Coursey et al. 2000, 374). An effective case manager, then, is one who is knowledgeable about resources, who is able to provide a single point of accountability, who will advocate for the client, who will hang in for the long haul, and who will not "pass the buck." The importance of case management was recognized in the "Romanow Report" on the future of health care in Canada as one of the key services that should be available for persons with mental disorders to "ensure both continuity and coordination of care" (Commission on the Future of Health Care in Canada 2002, 179).

There are variations within the case management approach that relate to the degree of direct service provision, staff specialization, and worker "assertiveness." One distinction that can be made is between *brokerage*, where linkages are made but no direct services are provided, and a full support model, where the client attends a program offering a range of services, such as medication management, counselling, and rehabilitation. A second distinction is between generalist and specialist models. The generalist case manager is someone who in theory provides assistance in a wide range of goal areas, such as counselling around drug addiction, vocational planning, and healthier lifestyles, while the specialist team provides a primary worker who focuses on medical management and otherwise refers (and defers) to team colleagues from other disciplines, such as occupational therapy. There is greater recognition now of the need for generalist knowledge among case managers. For example, findings that physical illness is underrecognized and undertreated in persons with serious mental disorders has placed a greater onus on practitioners to be knowledgeable of and alert to the medical conditions of their clients (Davis 1998; Hall 2001). There is also greater expectation that case managers will know a range of psychological interventions, such as cognitive-behavioural therapy (Coursey et al. 2000; see also Chapter 11). At the same time, it may be unrealistic to expect that an individual practitioner will possess the requisite knowledge, skills, and interest to be able to expertly perform all manner of duties. In many cases the practitioner's role will fall somewhere between these two "types," with services being provided directly in some areas and referrals being made in others.

Finally, a distinction can be made between "regular" case management and *assertive* or *intensive* case management. Assertive case management, described in more detail below, differs from other approaches in that it targets the most disabled clients, is outreach-based, involves more frequent and prolonged contact with clients, has a lower client-to-staff ratio, and focuses on the "nitty-gritty" activities of daily living that are apparently causing difficulties for the client (Davis, Eaves, and Wilson 1999). An Ontario report estimates that about 25 percent of individuals with severe, persistent mental disorders require an "assertive" treatment approach (Goering et al. 1994).

There are several assumptions underlying the presumed need for case management (Maguire 2002). One, as noted, is that coordination of care is required. A second is that services will be required for the *long term*. And a third is that, because of the degree of functional impairment, clients will need assistance in *a number of areas*, such as mental health, physical health, housing, finances, substance misuse, leisure, education, work, interpersonal relationships, and life skills. Although case management is potentially an effective model for assisting persons with mental disorders, it must be acknowledged that this approach comes from a tradition where mental disorders were viewed as poor-prognosis illnesses, which could only be "managed" and not successfully treated, and is an approach that some clients may view as overly paternalistic and controlling (Davis 2002). One author observes that "it is easy to see why some consumers and professionals find the term 'case manager' distasteful, and antithetical to empowerment and strengths models of practice" (Sullivan and Rapp 2002, 182). Practitioners should be aware of these concerns, and in their role as case managers should carefully assess the level of functional impairment in their clients, emphasize and build on client strengths, and not continue to do for clients what they could potentially do for themselves.

Assertive Community Treatment

The service delivery approach known as **assertive community treatment** (ACT) evolved in response to the recognition that, in the aftermath of deinstitutionalization, a number of clients in the community were not "connecting," either with treatment programs or with other community resources, and also appeared to lack the skills necessary to manage activities of daily living, skills that either had not been learned or practised or were not transferable from institutional to community settings. Unlike traditional, office-based case management, assertive community treatment is delivered *in situ* – on an outreach basis – and emphasizes the acquisition of life skills in addition to the clinical management function (Health Canada 1997b, 5). The first version of ACT, and the model that has most strongly influenced subsequent programs, was the Training in Community Living Program, developed in the 1970s in Madison, Wisconsin, by Stein and Test (1980). As summarized by Drake and colleagues (2003, 45), in this program outreach teams were formed "to teach skills and provide supports in natural environments such as the client's home, neighborhood, or work setting. These approaches initially focused on teaching basic living skills, e.g., helping people learn the necessary skills for cooking, cleaning their apartments, and using public transportation, but they also began to focus on jobs, social relationships, housing and leisure activities." In addition to North America, ACT programs have been implemented in Europe and the British Commonwealth (Phillips et al. 2001). In Canada, ACT programs have become more widespread (although do not exist in all regions) and in best practices documents are referred to as an integral part of a comprehensive mental health service (McEwan and Goldner 2001). In Ontario, for example, forty-four such teams were operating by 2003 (White et al. 2003).

Given that ACT is a labour-intensive model of service delivery, some efforts have been made toward determining and delimiting the target population. One best-practices document concludes that clients of ACT programs should (1) have a serious, persistent mental illness, (2) exhibit functional impairment, and (3) be "intensive users of the system of care" (British Columbia Ministry of Health 2002a, 6). Examples of functional impairment would include poor hygiene, poor budgeting, inability to meet nutritional needs, transiency, poor problem-solving skills, and inability to develop or maintain a support system (British Columbia Ministry of Health 2002a). Given that most users of the public mental health system have a serious, persistent disorder and some functional deficits, the third criterion – "intensive system use" – would appear to be the main distinguishing factor for potential ACT clients. While "system use" may refer to other community agencies or to the criminal justice system (Wilson, Tien, and Eaves 1995), for the most part, in the conceptualization and evaluation of ACT programs, it refers to use of *hospital* resources. For example, a best-practices report (British Columbia Ministry of Health 2002a, 7) states that the first objective of assertive community treatment is "to reduce the need for hospitalization, and improve community tenure." "Need for hospitalization" in this context can mean: (1) frequent hospitalizations, which, while an arbitrary figure, is defined as two or more per year by one report (British Columbia Ministry of Health 2002e); (2) being at risk for rehospitalization without additional supports; and (3) being detained as an inpatient when intensive outpatient services, if available, would make discharge a more viable option. Often rehospitalization is the result of treatment noncompliance – that is, an inability or unwillingness to come in for appointments or to take medication. Thus a core function of the ACT model is to address the "compliance" issue.

In describing the service delivery approach and roles within an ACT program, it should be said at the outset that there are a number of "ACT-like" programs in existence that do not achieve complete adherence or fidelity to the model as it is delineated in policy documents. For instance, having a psychiatrist on staff is made difficult by the shortage of these specialists, particularly in outlying areas (Latimer 1999; McGrew, Pescosolido, and Wright 2003). In another example, a survey of Ontario ACT programs found that not all were employing a peer-support worker, as stipulated by Ministry of Health guidelines; the reasons for this included a lack of enhanced funding, no guidelines concerning the role of peer-support workers, and "hesitancy to create the position because of worry of losing a clinical staff member to fund a peer support position" (White et al. 2003, 270). In fact, a survey of seventy-three ACT programs found that "several important ingredients [program components] appear to be consistently underimplemented" (McGrew, Pescosolido, and Wright 2003, 370).

A Health Canada (1997b, 5) report notes that the literature on case management reflects "considerable confusion" when making distinctions between ACT and other case management models; the report concludes that "in practice ... differences are often blurred" and that "most programs are hybrids which do not always fit into neat definitional packages." This is further complicated by the fact that these various "assertive" programs are known by a variety of different names (Witheridge 1989). Concerning the question of program fidelity, while closer adherence to standards is associated with better outcomes (Latimer 1999; McGrew, Pescosolido, and Wright 2003), exact replication of models may be extremely difficult given that local contingencies will affect the implementation and eventual shape of a new program (Rapp 1998). This issue is addressed as follows by the director of an ACT program in Chicago: "Although its inspiration came straight from Madison, the Chicago project took shape in a vastly different urban environment, under different agency auspices, with different funding circumstances, and with a different target population. Thus, a literal replication of the Madison model was not possible" (Witheridge 1991, 49).

While there may be variations in the shape of ACT programs and while more research needs to be done on the key "active ingredients" of this model, the following service components are considered "vital to successful implementation" (British Columbia Ministry of Health 2002a, 9):

- A *low client-to-staff ratio*, typically around 10:1. This is necessary to sustain the frequent (several times per week) client contact characteristic of this type of program. Through frequent contact and more intimate knowledge of clients, the hope is that crises can be headed off (Witheridge 1989). Concerning staff attributes, there is some suggestion that "street smarts," pragmatism, initiative, and nonjudgmental attitudes among ACT workers are at least as important as formal credentials (Phillips et al. 2001; Witheridge 1989).
- A *shared caseload*, meaning that clients are rotated among the different case managers. As reviewed by Rapp (1998, 366), the purported advantages of this are reduced worker burnout, better continuity of care, increased availability of someone who knows the client, and "more creative service planning." There are, on the other hand, a number of limitations of this team approach: (1) it goes against the "single point of accountability" tenet; (2) it can be confusing and frustrating for clients, who have to develop relationships with several workers or who may be getting the message that they are "so abnormal, bad or different that a whole team of people is needed to work with them" (Spindel and Nugent 1999, 7); and (3) it necessitates detailed information sharing among staff and frequent (daily) case management meetings to bring everyone "up to speed," all of which can be time-consuming.
- *Assertive outreach*. Most of the staff time in ACT programs is spent out of the office, which is seen as "home base ... rather than a primary treatment site." "Providing services in the environment of the consumer's choice enables the team to assess the consumer's needs in the real world and to provide support and teaching in daily living skills. Assertive outreach is the key to engaging clients who do not connect with traditional office or institution-based approaches" (British Columbia Ministry of Health 2002a, 15).

■ *Continuous services.* Working in conjunction with other services, ACT programs aim at providing comprehensive coverage, including during after-hours emergencies. Also key to this model is that service is indefinite, if necessary. This aspect is important when one considers that the target population is a group that others may have given up on, if not avoided, meaning that perseverance is important in order to establish trust and to make gains that are sometimes incremental. Workers may have to make repeated attempts to engage clients in the program, unlike a conventional service where the file may be closed after a single failed appointment.

Evaluations of ACT and ACT-like programs have generally found them to be effective in reducing client rehospitalization and in maintaining housing stability partly because these programs are superior to other services at retaining clients in treatment (Health Canada 1997b; Phillips et al. 2001). For example, in an Ontario study, investigators found that clients randomly assigned to an assertive outreach program spent only 39 days in hospital during a follow-up period of one year, compared to 256 days for the control group, who were followed by a hospital outpatient program (Lafave, deSouza, and Gerber 1996).

Surveys of clients of ACT programs have also in many instances found user satisfaction to be high (Burns and Santos 1995; Chue et al. 2004; Phillips et al. 2001), which may be related to the fact that clients gain access to more resources and services. When dissatisfaction with the ACT model has been expressed, it often relates to the more coercive, or intrusive, aspects of service delivery, the view that "assertive community treatment is paternalistic and has a tendency to overuse social and monetary behavioural controls, and to overemphasize the role of medications" (McGrew, Wilson, and Bond 2002, 761; see also Davis 2002; Gomoroy 2001; Spindel and Nugent 1999). A Canadian user satisfaction survey by Gerber and Prince (1999, 549) found that substantial minorities of ACT clients expressed dissatisfaction with respect to "demands in treatment" (31%), "extent of clients' influence over treatment" (30%), and "whether their opinion was considered in treatment planning" (23%).

While ACT programs are labour-intensive and have relatively small caseloads, this concentration of resources has been justified by the argument that by preventing the rehospitalization of a targeted, high-risk group, the intervention is still cost effective. Research has tended to support this hypothesis – that is, that ACT will be cost effective if the comparison group, or target group, has had "extensive previous hospitalization" (Barry et al. 2003, 269) and thus can be considered at high risk for relapse (Essock, Frisman, and Kontos 1998; Lehman et al. 1999). In a literature review by

McGill University researcher Eric Latimer (1999, 443), the conclusion was that, using the costs of hospitalization in Quebec as a reference, ACT programs would need to enrol people with prior hospital use of about fifty days yearly, on average, to "break even." Given current hospital utilization patterns in Canadian community mental health programs, a figure of fifty-plus inpatient days per year would be considered quite high,[3] underlining again the need for ACT to be a carefully "targeted" program. Latimer (1999, 443) suggests that, since the fifty-day reference point will become increasingly difficult to achieve "as care systems evolve to reduce their reliance on hospitalization as a care modality with or without ACT," "the primary justification for implementing ACT services will then become their clinical benefits."

Primary Care and Shared Care

"**Primary care**" is defined as the first and most frequent point of contact with the health care system. For many persons this will mean care provided by their family physician. Primary *mental health* care may be provided through private psychiatrists or through community mental health clinics, which typically provide multidisciplinary programs where the client is assigned a case manager and a consultant physician/psychiatrist. For example, in Vancouver, British Columbia, there are eight geographically based community mental health teams, with individual team caseloads ranging from about four hundred to one thousand and with individual worker caseloads ranging from fifty to sixty adult clients per case manager.

In many if not most cases, however, primary mental health care in Canada is provided by general practitioners. For example, an Ontario survey found that fully three-quarters of those using physician mental health services received this care from GPs alone (Lin and Goering 1998). Similarly, it has been found that most prescriptions for psychotropic medications are written by family physicians (Lavoie and Fleet 2002).

While this arrangement may be workable, particularly for those with less disabling mental disorders, that such a large proportion of clients are not receiving specialized care is a cause for concern. That clients may not be receiving optimal mental health care in this arrangement is supported by findings that sessions with GPs "tend to be shorter in duration, less often include therapeutic listening, and more commonly result in prescription of medication" (Clarke Institute of Psychiatry 1997, 64). Conversely, there is evidence that, when psychotherapy can be provided concomitantly, reliance on and possible overuse of medication diminishes (Wiggins and Cummings 1998). There is also evidence that, when dealing with the initial onset of a psychotic disorder, involvement with a GP – rather than with a mental health specialist – may actually result in delays in receiving appropriate treatment (Birchwood and Brunet 2004).

In short, despite good intentions, GPs may lack the expertise or, more often than not, the *time* to deal with psychiatric concerns since most provincial fee schedules do not provide any incentive to spend additional time counselling patients (Branham 2003). In such an arrangement there is as noted a greater possibility of misdiagnosis, particularly given that clients with mental health concerns may in a significant proportion of cases present with somatization – apparent physical manifestations – which in turn may have a cultural basis. Family doctors also do not have the same access to resources: McEwan and Goldner (2001, 32) note that "many physicians work in isolation from community mental health providers who frequently are the gatekeepers to the array of services and supports required by those with serious mental disorders."

GPs wishing to refer clients to specialist care may face various barriers. One may be a lack of knowledge of the resources. A second is that, particularly in remote or rural areas, specialized mental health care, either through private psychiatry or public clinics, may be unavailable or may involve waiting lists – which is not helpful when a client is in crisis. A third factor is the stigma associated with being referred to a mental health specialist (Ben Noun 1996). And there is the problem that eligibility criteria for mental health clinics are relatively narrow, at least in the perception of many attempting to make referrals. In particular, clients whose diagnoses stray outside the locally defined parameters of "serious and persistent" may be deflected; this fact, along with the increased promotion and greater public acceptance of antidepressant use, may help account for the fact that a larger number of persons with depressive and anxiety disorders are now being treated by family physicians (see also Olfson et al. 2002).

Because of the potential difficulties associated with GPs working in isolation, there has been increasing interest in models of **shared care**, which has been defined as "collaborative activities between family physicians and psychiatric services designed to improve mental health care for clients" (British Columbia Ministry of Health 2002e, 48). One can note, for example, how important it is for GPs and specialists to be on the "same page" when working with a geriatric population given the potential for problematic drug interactions and side effects. Shared care may involve telephone access to psychiatrists by GPs to discuss mental health issues or psychiatrists working, at least part time, at primary care clinics (Goering, Wasylenki, and Durbin 2000, 350).

Acute Home Treatment and Crisis Response

Acute home treatment is defined as "acute care provided in the home for a limited period to treat acute psychiatric symptoms that would otherwise require inpatient admission" (British Columbia Ministry of Health 2002e, 40). The need for such a service is based on the view that many persons presenting and being admitted to acute care hospitals could in fact be treated at home by mental health clinicians and that if available this less intrusive intervention would have benefits with respect to both cost effectiveness and client satisfaction. It is suggested that this approach would work best with "previously admitted patients with known patterns of decompensation" (42) – that is, that one would not normally use home-based care as the first response to a crisis involving an unknown client. While this type of intervention appears similar in some respects to assertive community treatment, the latter is intended to be a long-term service, whereas home care might typically last only three to six weeks.

Acute home treatment is still relatively uncommon in Canadian and American settings – one provincial report, for example, refers to it as "experimental" (British Columbia Ministry of Health 2002e, 40) – which may in part be related to a tradition in North America of psychiatrists rarely making home visits, unlike the practice of their British and European counterparts (Clarke Institute of Psychiatry 1997). Although not widely implemented, acute home treatment is referred to in the "Romanow Report" as one of the "two types of home care services that should be available for people with mental health problems" (Commission on the Future of Health Care in Canada 2002, 179) (the other is case management, although the report authors would appear to be referring to assertive community treatment).

Wasylenki and colleagues (1997) describe an acute home treatment service, the Home Treatment Program for Acute Psychosis, established in Toronto. In this program services were provided by nurses, homemakers, and social workers, with a psychiatrist available for back-up support. In urgent cases services started immediately; otherwise, intensive support was initiated within forty-eight hours. Once the client was stabilized, he or she was referred back to the regular case manager at the Clarke Institute. The project was evaluated over an eighteen-month study period during which there were thirty-four episodes of home treatment averaging twenty-eight days in duration. It was found that there was a reduction in client symptoms, a reduction in the burden of family members, and that clients were satisfied with home treatment and preferred it to hospitalization. Home treatment was also found to be significantly less expensive than inpatient care at the Clarke Institute: $139.78 vs. $637.00 per diem.

A more common method of psychiatric crisis response in Canada is the **mobile crisis team**, which generally is a seven-day-a-week service with some after-hours capacity that provides brief crisis intervention through telephone contact or home visits. The staffing complement is made up of nurses or other clinicians with psychiatric experience and on-call physicians. These programs may be specialized by the age of the target group – that is, adults, older adults, and children and adolescents. Concerning the nature of the intervention, a manual on emergency mental health suggests that "the orientation of psychiatric emergency services should develop from an emphasis on triage to incorporate crisis resolution, based on thorough assessment of available patient coping resources and of environmental supports" (Mental Health Evaluation and Community Consultation Unit 2000, 16).

Examples of mobile crisis teams include Vancouver's Mental Health Emergency Services, which offers a crisis line that clients and other citizens may access and which can provide home visits with a nurse, sometimes with a plainclothes police officer as back-up; the police officer provides more security for evening calls in higher-crime areas and can also invoke a provision of the *Mental Health Act* whereby persons can be taken to hospital for an assessment. In some cases a psychiatrist will be called in to assess the person on-site. A survey of Canadian programs notes that crisis response systems – mobile crisis teams and free-standing crisis centres – have been particularly well developed in the province of Manitoba (Goering, Wasylenki, and Durbin, 2000, 349).

Early Intervention Programs
It has been consistently observed that persons experiencing mental health problems for the first time will avoid or delay seeking treatment (Scholten et al. 2003). There are several reasons for this: (1) lack of knowledge of resources and/or problems with accessing the mental health system, (2) stigma, (3) social isolation – which is more common among persons with mental disorders – and hence a lack of concerned others who could contact treatment resources, (4) family members and care providers who lack knowledge concerning psychiatric disorders, (5) a perception by the individual and others that there *is* no problem – that the person's experiences are within the realm of normality – or an attribution to other causes such as recreational drug use, and (6) that in some cases the onset of the disorder is insidious and hence more difficult to identify (Lines 2000).

Another factor contributing to treatment delay has been program mandates: until relatively recently, community treatment services have taken a "downstream" approach to mental health problems, with early detection and prevention not being high on the agenda.

Using untreated psychotic disorders as an example, one can identify a number of harmful outcomes that may result from treatment delays following the first onset of symptoms:

- *Greater disruption of domestic relationships, parenting roles, schooling, employment, and career planning* given that the onset of psychotic disorders is typically in early adulthood. That early social functioning is the best predictor of social functioning later in life points to the "importance of preserving or recovering social functioning capacity at the earliest possible point" (Lines 2000, 5; see also Birchwood, Todd, and Jackson 1998).
- *Risk of suicide.* Suicide rates for persons with schizophrenia are significantly higher than for the general population in any case, but with respect to early intervention, it may be noted that the risk is even greater within the few years immediately following the first presentation and for young males with higher IQs (Lines 2000).
- *Poorer long-term clinical outcomes.* A number of studies have examined the association between duration of untreated psychosis (DUP) and clinical outcomes, and while there are inconsistencies and "unresolved methodological differences" (Scholten et al. 2003, 561), the preponderance of evidence appears to support a relationship between these two variables – that is, that "long durations of untreated psychosis have been associated with slower and less complete recovery, more biological abnormalities, more relapses, and poorer long-term outcomes" (Mental Health Evaluation and Community Consultation Unit 2002, 4; see also Malla and Norman 2002; Marshall et al. 2004). Subsequent relapses, in turn, are associated with "more social impairment, higher levels of secondary morbidity, and more residual symptomatology" (Mental Health Evaluation and Community Consultation Unit 2002, 16). Lines (2000, 5) notes the "growing evidence that untreated psychosis is 'toxic' – that left untreated, neurological damage progresses."

With concerns being expressed among stakeholders about mental health problems going unrecognized and untreated in the general population, health authorities are increasingly being forced to address the issues of prevention and health promotion, areas where these bodies have not historically been prominent. In Canada, a Mental Health Awareness Week was launched in 1992, with the stated aims of destigmatizing mental illness, providing education, promoting public discussion and informed treatment decision making, and improving access to mental health services (Steiner and Amir 2003). This initiative has continued annually under the umbrella of the Canadian Alliance on Mental Illness and Mental Health and in many locations includes a depression screening day, which is held in venues such as shopping malls and community centres. In reporting on the depression screening day held in Montreal in 2002, Steiner and Amir (2003, 15) note that 5,639 citizens participated at twenty-seven sites and that of those completing the screening instrument (the Harvard National Depression Screen) roughly half (442/879) had a score "consistent with a 95 percent sensitivity ... for a diagnosis of major depressive episode."

In another area, **early psychosis intervention** (EPI) programs have been initiated in a number of Canadian centres (e.g., Tee and Hanson 2004). As reviewed by Lines (2000, 1), EPI "refers to current approaches to the treatment of psychosis that emphasize the importance of both the timing and types of intervention provided to persons experiencing a first episode of psychosis," with "early" being defined as "early as possible following the onset of psychotic symptoms." The aim of these programs is to "improve outcomes by promoting as full a recovery as possible, thereby reducing the long term disability and costs," with this being achieved by strategies "designed to limit the duration of the psychosis – prior to and during treatment – and prevent relapse" (2).

EPI programs contain elements that distinguish them from other psychiatric treatment programs. Lines (2000, 7) notes that treatment approaches targeting young persons need to be *stage sensitive*: "This population not only represents a unique developmental stage, but is naïve in terms of neuroleptic [medication] use and system exposure, and appears highly sensitive to the impacts of both."

Concerning medication use, treatment guidelines emphasize the need to start with lower doses that are increased only gradually because of the greater sensitivity of young persons to the effects of antipsychotic medication (Mental Health Evaluation and Community Consultation Unit 2002). Younger persons are now always started on newer-generation, "atypical" antipsychotic drugs, which, compared to older products, produce fewer side effects in the form of movement disorders and offer some benefits with respect to cognitive functioning. There is often great ambivalence on the part of young clients about being on medication and consequently a dilemma for the clinician as to whether pharmacological treatment should be "intermittent" (discontinued once symptoms disappear) or continuous (lasting one to two years after a "first break"). While published practice guidelines emphasize the importance of medication and favour the use of longer-term maintenance regimens, there is the acknowledgment that "development of the therapeutic relationship may take precedence over treatment initiation in order to increase the probability of long-term success" (7).

Concerning "system exposure," receiving a diagnosis and being processed by the mental health system for the first time can be extremely traumatic for a young person, who has no frame of reference for this experience. Often times an initial hospitalization is precipitated by a crisis in the family home, necessitating in some cases the involvement of the police and resulting in involuntary treatment and detention in a psychiatric ward. The experience is also traumatic because of the longer-term implications: what does this diagnosis/intervention mean for the individual's life and career plans?

The potentially traumatic experience of hospitalization speaks to the importance of early identification and treatment of psychotic disorders, thus – in theory – obviating the need for involuntary institutional care. Whether this can be achieved, however, is complicated by a number of factors. One is that, as noted, the individuals in question, as well as their significant others, may engage in denial and rationalization when presented with a mental health explanation for problem behaviours – which is, in many respects, an understandable response.

There is also the simple fact that psychiatric disorders, in their early stages, are not easily identified (Helling, Ohman, and Hultman 2003; Yung et al. 2003). Changes may not be abrupt; rather, there is typically a **prodromal** phase, wherein are manifested the signs and symptoms seen *before* the development of a full-blown psychosis, symptoms that are often nonspecific. Indeed, according to a document on EPI practice guidelines, the "prodrome" is by convention diagnosed retrospectively, only *after* the development of florid features of psychosis (Mental Health Evaluation and Community Consultation Unit 2002). While attempts have been made to better identify incipient psychosis at the prodromal stage (McGlashan and Johannessen 1996; Murray 1999), there is still, as noted by Lines (2000, 8), "lack of a sufficiently concise operational definition of the prodrome that will avoid the accumulation of false positives." As well, the ethical dilemmas inherent in treating persons at the prodromal stage – such as the effects of "labelling" and using antipsychotic medication before the presence of a disorder is clearly established – remain unresolved (Ehmann, Yager, and Hanson 2004). On this point, authors with the Mental Health Evaluation and Community Consultation Unit (2002, 18) at the University of British Columbia conclude that "it is not possible to accurately predict if a person displaying features of a prodrome will make the transition to psychosis. For these reasons, and because little is known about how to prevent the onset of psychosis,

psychosis-specific treatments (e.g., antipsychotic medications and education about psychosis) should not be implemented until a psychosis is definitely present." Rather, these authors recommend that clinicians address the presenting problems (e.g., depression, anxiety, insomnia), maintain a therapeutic alliance, monitor closely, and work on skills training to help the client deal with stressful events. (Concerning the maintenance of a therapeutic connection, the separation of mental health programs into age divisions – child, adolescent, adult, and older adult – may in some instances be a barrier to care: some "childhood" mental health concerns may represent the prodromal phase of an adult mental disorder, pointing to the importance of integrated care and linkages to avoid the gap between termination of one program and initiation of another.) Early identification, while a difficult task, is enhanced by public education programs, which would involve family doctors and other health care providers and, in particular, would include liaison with the school system.

Once a young person has been engaged in treatment, it is recommended that there be frequent reassessment, at least initially, because of the issue of diagnostic uncertainty and consequently the risk of applying inappropriate treatments and providing inaccurate information. Practice guidelines also emphasize the importance of professional involvement that is "ongoing and intensive" (Mental Health Evaluation and Community Consultation Unit 2002, 7).

Family involvement and education are key components of EPI. With the family being part of the therapeutic system, it is important that family members be given the resources, skills, and risk reduction strategies to better support their loved one. Similarly, for the young client, education and skills training are crucial and will probably require the involvement of occupational therapists and other rehabilitation staff. While stigma and demoralization are important issues for psychiatric clients of any age, it is particularly important that they be addressed in programs for persons who have had a "first break."

In summary, as reviewed by Lines (2000), emerging best practices with respect to early psychosis intervention include:

- reduction of periods of untreated psychosis through public education
- building a therapeutic alliance, which is so crucial at this first entry point into the mental health system
- family engagement and support
- comprehensive, phase-specific, individualized treatment, including low-dose medication, education, and psychosocial rehabilitation
- prolonged engagement to sustain gains.

In Canada clinical/research programs in EPI have been developed in a number of centres, including Calgary, Halifax, Toronto, Hamilton, Kingston, and London. London's Prevention and Early Intervention Program for Psychoses (PEPP), described on its website (http://www.pepp.ca), utilizes an assertive case management model wherein a case manager "walks the client through the mental health system, though whenever possible, relying on generic community services to reintegrate the young adult to his/her full potential over a two-year follow-up period." In a published description of the program, the authors note the importance of a flexible intake policy and quick response to referrals (twenty-four to forty-eight hours) in attempting to reduce treatment delays (Scholten et al. 2003). Concerning barriers to treatment, a mobile, home-based intervention program for early psychosis was introduced at the Centre for Addiction and Mental Health in Toronto in 2001 in an attempt to deal with the stigma that is attached to receiving treatment from a psychiatric clinic or hospital.

Programs for Persons with Co-occurring Disorders

As noted earlier, persons suffering from mental disorders have much higher rates of co-occurring substance use disorders than the general population. (The term "co-occurring," referring to mental disorder and substance abuse/dependency, has been used interchangeably in the literature with "concurrent disorders" and "dual diagnoses," although readers should be aware that the latter term has also been used to describe persons with mental disorders and intellectual handicaps.)[4] Individuals diagnosed with schizophrenia or bipolar disorder seem particularly vulnerable, with surveys suggesting that roughly one-half of this population may have a substance use disorder (British Columbia Partners for Mental Health and Addictions Information 2003a; Ziedonis and Trudeau 1997). The use of street drugs by a person with a condition such as schizophrenia is associated with a number of negative outcomes, such as an exacerbation of psychotic symptoms, greater risk of violence – with respect both to commission and victimization (Steadman et al. 1998) – increased risk of infectious disease (Davis 1998), criminal involvement, high service utilization, and homelessness (Davis 1987b).

Despite their numbers and care needs, persons with co-occurring disorders have not typically been well served by the health care system or, in particular, by mental health practitioners. Several potential barriers to service can be identified.

First, staff working in community mental health have not traditionally been trained in the assessment and treatment of persons with addictions, which has been seen as a separate specialty, with services being delivered in a separate location.

Second, there is the unfortunate fact that "helping professionals" can be quite judgmental when it comes to persons with drug addictions. This may have to do with the perception that drug addiction – unlike, for example, the manic state of a person with bipolar disorder – is a volitional condition, meaning that the individual is responsible for his or her own demise and is in some sense less deserving than other clients (Committee on Addictions of the Group for the Advancement of Psychiatry 2002). On this point, researchers who conducted focus group interviews with clients in three provinces as part of a Health Canada (2001a, 72) report on co-occurring disorders found that "the strongest theme that emerged was the *additional and severe stigma* associated with having both substance use and mental health problems. The stigma expressed itself in various forms, including repeated and chronic self-harm experiences, self-deprecation, the fear of being judged, and the hurtful experience of judgmental attitudes" (emphasis in the original).

A third barrier to service is the reality that co-occurring disorders may still be underrecognized. This can happen in different ways:

- Despite all the clinical and empirical evidence, some clinicians may still not appreciate the magnitude of the problem with respect to co-morbidity. While practitioners may be disappointed with the fact that a client has more than one set of challenges, they should not be surprised; indeed, as one authority states, "dual diagnosis should be *expected* rather than considered an exception" (Minkoff 2001a, 597, emphasis added).
- Clinicians may not adequately screen for substance use disorders among their mental health clients. Health Canada (2001a) describes several "Level 1" screening procedures, so-called because they require little time and effort on the part of the clinician. These include (1) asking a few questions (although it is noted that clients may not be forthcoming about drug use before a trusting relationship has been developed); (2) case manager judgment, based on knowledge of the signs and symptoms of intoxication and withdrawal and associated emotional and behavioural indicators; (3) similarly, use of an **index of suspicion**, which is a checklist of indicators that include housing instability, difficulty budgeting, prostitution, sudden unexplained mood shifts, employment problems, suicidal behaviour, hygiene problems, weight loss (especially with stimulant use), and legal difficulties; and (4) a brief screening instrument, such as the CAGE-AID (Brown 1992). "Level 2" procedures include four instruments, validated with persons with mental health disorders, that take somewhat more time to incorporate into practice: the Dartmouth Assessment of Lifestyle Instrument (DALI), the Michigan Alcoholism Screening Test (MAST), the Drug Abuse

Screening Test (DAST), and the Alcohol Use Disorders Identification Test (AUDIT) – all of which are in the public domain.

- Mental health practitioners may see only the drug addiction and miss the accompanying/underlying mental disorder – which can result in misdiagnoses and persons being turned away from psychiatric treatment. This can happen at "entry points," such as intake by a mental health team or attempted admission to a general hospital psychiatric unit, where incoming clients are commonly deflected or given short shrift if there is any sense that the psychotic symptoms seen are related to drug use (Johnson 2004).

A fourth barrier has to do with psychiatric traditions that do not account for the reality of co-morbidity. An example here is the concept of the **primary diagnosis**, which is usually defined as the condition that is the main focus of attention or treatment, a definition that is not particularly helpful when considering persons with two equally challenging sets of problems, each affected by the other.

A fifth barrier has to do with the lack of integration of services, at either the governance or the program level. At the governance level, addiction and mental health programs have often been placed in different government ministries or departments, which usually did not communicate with one another. At the program level, these two services have not only operated in different physical locations, but are also influenced by different philosophical traditions, resulting at times in poorly coordinated treatment. Examples of these competing perspectives include:

- Differences in the educational backgrounds of mental health and addictions practitioners: the self-help emphasis and practice of hiring former addicts in some addictions programs may be contrasted with the "professional" model seen in mental health programs.
- Differences in the client's role. As noted by Minkoff (2001b), some addictions services, such as traditional twelve-step programs, emphasize individual responsibility rather than disability and use confrontational methods in group meetings (generally considered inappropriate for persons with serious, persistent mental disorders), which may be contrasted with mental health case management approaches, where care – versus confrontation – is emphasized and more is done *for* the client.
- Different views about medication, with some addictions and residential treatment programs having low tolerance for the use of prescribed psychotropic drugs by clients (particularly anti-anxiety agents).

- Different views about abstinence. Some programs mandate abstinence from the drug of abuse as a precondition to participation. Critics have suggested that this approach discourages or prevents engagement in treatment (Minkoff 2001b) and that abstinence should be considered a *goal* rather than a prerequisite. **Harm reduction** approaches – where ongoing substance use by the client is tolerated – have the potential of better maintaining a therapeutic relationship but in some cases have produced discomfort among practitioners.

By contrast, in an integrated approach to treating persons with co-occurring disorders, efforts should be made "to ensure that the individual receives a consistent explanation of illness/problems and a coherent prescription for treatment rather than a contradictory set of messages from different providers" (Health Canada 2001a, vii).

In addressing the lack of integration in the provision of services to persons with co-occurring disorders, American psychiatrist and addictions expert Ken Minkoff (2001b, 598) suggests "[the] adoption of a consensus mission statement incorporating a coherent set of principles on which system design will be based, embodying an integrated philosophy that is acceptable to both mental health care and substance use treatment providers." Minkoff outlines the principles as follows:

- Co-morbidity is an expectation, not an exception, necessitating a service delivery system that is welcoming and accessible.
- Admission criteria should be designed to promote acceptance of clients at all levels of motivation rather than preventing persons from receiving services.
- *Both* psychiatric and substance use disorders should be regarded as "primary," with each requiring specific and appropriate treatment.
- Both co-occurring disorders should be considered persistent, relapsing conditions, conceptualized by using a disease and recovery model, with parallel phases of treatment or recovery.
- Treatment should be phase-specific, corresponding to the stage that clients are in with respect to recovery from both conditions.
- Whenever possible, treatment should be provided by individuals, teams, or programs with expertise in both mental health and addictions.
- The system should promote a longitudinal perspective on the treatment of persons with co-occurring disorders, with service providers being available for the long term.

- The system should include interventions to engage the most detached or marginalized persons – for example, by providing outreach to the homeless.

Canadian jurisdictions are gradually seeing greater integration of mental health and addiction services. In British Columbia, for example, after years of "bureaucratic drift," Addiction Services was finally located administratively alongside other health and mental health programs with the creation of the regional health authorities in 2001 (prior to this it had been within the Ministry for Children and Families, a department whose mandate was child protection and services for the mentally handicapped).

Health Canada (2001a) reviews a number of strategies to support integration at the program level, including the co-location of mental health and addictions treatment services, centralized intake and referral, shared data systems, shared training and education of staff, adding substance abuse specialists to mental health services (or vice versa), and creating "blended" teams. At the systems level, integration may be facilitated by the creation of interagency planning committees and networks, partnerships that could "go beyond joint planning exercises to the level of service agreements or potentially merged organizations" (85). Concerning the dissemination and transfer of knowledge, the creation at the national level of a concurrent disorders resource centre and website has been proposed (Health Canada 2001a).

Bearing in mind that local contingencies – attitudinal, fiscal, and bureaucratic – will influence how, or if, integration occurs at the level of individuals as opposed to teams or units of service, one can note that a number of different scenarios are possible. One approach is to broaden the skills of workers in existing programs: as noted above, one version of case management is a "generalist" model, where all mental health case managers are trained in techniques relevant to the treatment of addictive disorders; an example is the technique of **motivational interviewing,** an approach used in the field of addictions but not traditionally taught to mental health specialists (see Chapter 11). Clearly, notwithstanding traditions and individual preferences, it is hard to support a status quo where mental health practitioners do not have at least a basic understanding of epidemiology and techniques in the area of co-occurring disorders.

Another approach to integrated treatment is the inclusion of substance abuse specialists on mental health teams. This strategy has been most clearly developed in assertive community treatment program guidelines; for example, one overview of "indicators of high fidelity" in Assertive Community Treatment (ACT) programs stipulates that there should be two or more full-time equivalent (FTE) staff with substance abuse training in each ACT program (Phillips et al. 2001, 774).

A different strategy from integrating treatment is to co-locate addictions and mental health programs. In the Vancouver, British Columbia, health region, "one stop shopping" arrangements were under discussion at the time of writing – that is, the creation of facilities where primary care, mental health, addictions, and other specialized services are offered under one roof (Carrigg 2004). The core addiction services to be offered at each of these facilities are to be counselling, home detox, needle exchange, opiate replacement (methadone) therapy, and school prevention programs. The beginning stages of implementation – with mental health and primary care being housed together – has produced mixed results and some doubt as to whether integration is really being achieved, underlining the importance of establishing protocols with respect to information sharing and interagency cooperation.

Another strategy has been the development of programs specifically focusing on the treatment of persons with co-occurring disorders. As reviewed by Health Canada (2001b), a number of these specialized programs have been developed in Canada, although there is variation with respect to the range of services offered, with some focusing more on treatment (narrowly defined) and others also offering case management and outreach. Specialized co-occurring disorder programs represent an attempt to provide a more coherent approach to treatment and are a valuable resource not just for clients, but also with respect to consultation and training of staff in other units of service. At the same time, there may be some danger of this model working against the goal of integrated services at the "macro" level: these stand-alone programs may become ghettoized within the larger system, with case managers on mental health teams routinely relegating clients with addictions to this other service without attempting to incorporate addictions treatment strategies in their own practice. It is almost certainly the case that no single stand-alone program can cope with the huge numbers of persons with co-occurring disorders (Carrigg 2002).

Acknowledging the historical attitudinal and bureaucratic barriers, Health Canada (2001a, 82) notes that achieving service integration in the field of co-occurring disorders is a difficult, "slow, evolutionary" process dependent on the leadership of individuals championing the cause and on the participation of stakeholders such as service users and family members.

Telepsychiatry

Canada is a vast country with many sparsely populated regions, and persons residing in more remote areas have had for the most part limited access to health care resources in general and to specialized mental health care in particular. Earlier attempts to address this problem included "travelling clinics," where psychiatrists were periodically flown into rural locales to provide assessments and consultation. Now, with advances in a number of technologies, **telepsychiatry** has become a more common method of providing support to persons in remote areas, with Canada indeed being "at the forefront" of this movement (O'Reilly et al. 2003, 18). Telepsychiatry is defined as "the use of electronic communication and information technologies to provide or support clinical psychiatric care at a distance" (American Psychiatric Association 1998, 2). While this may refer to various modes of communication, telepsychiatry commonly involves the use of video conferencing, which is a real-time, usually two-way transmission of video images. Telepsychiatry can be seen as a branch of "telehealth" or "telemedicine," the applications of which now include "hospice care, cancer support groups, substance abuse and depression screening, teleconsultation to ... the military, remote consultation to obviate language or cultural barriers at the local site, and telepsychiatric care of deaf mentally ill via ... sign language" (1). Telepsychiatry is designed to supplement, not replace, local treatment initiatives: a group with the University of Toronto Psychiatric Outreach Program (2002) notes that for legal and practical reasons *consultation* should be the primary model for telepsychiatry – that is, the local clinician should retain responsibility for ongoing care. Telepsychiatry can involve disciplines other than medicine, notably nursing (Hunkeler et al. 2000).

While most episodes of telepsychiatry involve assessment, diagnostic clarification, and treatment recommendations, it is noted that applications are "theoretically limitless" (Hilty et al. 2003, 11) and can include case conferencing, psychological testing, student supervision, and continuing education. The University of British Columbia's Department of Psychiatry, for example, now uses video conferencing to deliver education modules to mental health staff in outlying areas.

There has been some discussion about the use of telepsychiatry in emergency assessments, which might form the basis for involuntary hospitalization. Although video conferencing for the purposes of certifying clients under relevant mental health statutes has been sanctioned in Australia and New Zealand, as of 2003 the Canadian Psychiatric Association had no published position on this issue, and a survey of Canadian provincial mental health acts found that "all acts [were] either silent on whether assessments [had to] be conducted face to face, or their interpretations [were] ambiguous" (O'Reilly et al. 2003, 18).

Concerns have been expressed about the ramifications of "virtual" interviewing – for example, how this affects rapport and whether the assessor can detect nonverbal cues, particularly when there are problems with the video transmission (Hilty et al. 2003). Calgary psychiatrist Doug Urness (2003, 21) notes that clients approaching video conferencing for the first time may have different comfort levels, may wonder whether they will experience the "social presence" of the other person, and may ask themselves if they will be "treated as human beings or as depersonalized images on a television screen." It is thus noteworthy that a review of published evaluations of telepsychiatry found, notwithstanding expectations, generally high rates of client satisfaction with the process, concomitant with increased access to care (Hilty et al. 2003). In particular, reduced travel time, less absence from work, reduced waiting time, and more client choice and control were noted in the studies reviewed. Urness (2003, 25) suggests, with respect to concerns about new technologies, that therapist qualities are still more influential than the medium used (apologies to Marshall McLuhan) and that "the success of a telepsychiatry interview is more a function of traditional communication processes than of technology."

There have been some evaluations of the cost effectiveness of telepsychiatry. A study in rural Australia, for example, determined that over $100,000 per year was saved due to a reduction in employee travel costs and patient transfer costs, although equipment maintenance and (future) upgrade costs were not factored in (Trott and Blignault 1998). An American study in Maryland, which concluded that remote treatment of depression had comparable outcomes to in-person sessions, found a cost advantage for remote delivery, provided the distance from the medical centre was greater than twenty-two miles (Ruskin et al. 2004). Similarly, other studies indicate that because of the costs of maintaining the program, there needs to be a minimum number of consultations – approximately seven per week – for a telepsychiatry service to break even (Hilty et al. 2003) and that it may be premature to assume that this new technology is cost effective (Whitten, Kingsley, and Grigsby 2000).

The Nonprofit Sector
The treatment programs referred to so far are generally provided under the auspices of provincial governments or health authorities. Complementing these programs are a number of services offered by nongovernmental, not-for-profit agencies. These are sometimes referred to as "support" programs, which, depending how this term is interpreted, sells them short since their many services – which may include respite, advocacy, housing, education, and employment – are for many clients and care providers the ones that really "make a difference." Indeed, the evolution of these programs, a number of which were started by family members or clients themselves, was at

least in part a result of the deficiencies or limited scope of existing government services, deficiencies propagated by service providers who were "often reluctant to recognize these additional services ... as equals" (Health Canada 2002c, 4).

While it is impossible to list all the various nonprofit organizations, two will be mentioned here because of their prominence and because they have both national and regional representation. One is the Canadian Mental Health Association (CMHA), founded in 1918, which has chapters in all provinces and territories. The CMHA provides direct services to clients, such as drop-ins and social/recreational programming, and also plays a major role in combating the stigma of mental disorders through systemic advocacy and public education. To this end, the CMHA sponsors workshops, seminars, and research projects, and issues pamphlets and newsletters. The CMHA has produced position papers for governments and bodies such as the Romanow Commission, and has published influential policy documents – a number of them used as references for this book – such as *A New Framework for Support for People with Serious Mental Health Problems* (Trainor, Pomeroy, and Pape 1993), which highlights the importance of services and supports that have traditionally been outside the formal mental health service delivery system (Health Canada 2002c).

The other organization that has become an important voice for advocacy and public education is the Schizophrenia Society of Canada (SSC). While representing the interests of both clients and significant others, the SSC is especially known for its support groups and education programs for family members. In 1994, through prize money donated by a Canadian Nobel laureate whose son had schizophrenia, the Schizophrenia Society of Canada Foundation was established, the main focus of which is to fund fellowships for research in the areas of genetics and biochemistry (Schizophrenia Society of Canada 2002-03).

Notes

1 By the year 2000 there were an estimated 11,000 beds in provincial psychiatric hospitals and about 10,000 beds in general hospital psychiatric units in Canada (Goering, Wasylenki, and Durbin 2000).

2 For example, entering the phrase "case management" in the Internet search engine *Google* in December 2005 returned approximately 23.8 million "hits."

3 Even in programs serving persons with serious, persistent disorders, most clients will not be hospitalized in any given year. For instance, a 1999 survey of Vancouver, British Columbia, mental health teams found that only about 30 percent of clients had used "intensive clinical services" in the previous year, this term being defined as hospitalization, admission to a subacute facility, or contact with the mental health emergency service (Peters and Hay 1999).

4 Other terms have also been used, which, as reviewed by Health Canada (2001a), include "CAMI" (chemically abusing – mentally ill), "MICA" (mentally ill – chemically abusing), and "SAMI" (substance abusing – mentally ill).

Other Resources

- The Evidence-Based Practice Project at Dartmouth University has a website with downloadable documents on assertive community treatment, family education, supported employment, and other topics (see http://www.mentalhealthpractices.org/fam.html).
- The *Emergency Mental Health Education Manual,* published by the Mental Health Evaluation and Community Consultation Unit at the University of British Columbia, is available online at http://www.mheccu.ubc.ca/publications/emh-manual/emh-manual.pdf.
- The website for Shared Mental Health in Canada is http://www.shared-care.ca.
- The website of the Canadian Centre on Substance Abuse (http://www.ccsa.ca) has a number of downloadable documents on issues such as epidemiology, treatment, prevention, and harm reduction.

Housing

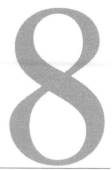

In the last chapter a number of treatment programs were reviewed. While these are clearly vital, no discussion of a comprehensive mental health system and the ultimate goal of long-term client recovery is complete without addressing the issue of housing.

Housing is one of the key determinants of health (Dunn 2003; Health Canada 2002a, 2004b). As one author (Thomas 2000, 5) puts it, there is a "critical link between mental health and housing. A lack of safe, secure, affordable and appropriate housing is shown to have negative effects on both physical and mental health, resulting in increased need for and use of emergency, treatment, and support services. Research also points out that adequate, appropriate housing is often the essential ingredient needed to help people with mental illness move forward toward recovery. Having housing helps people better manage their illness, reduces the need for treatment and support services, increases stability, and generally improves quality of life."

Further, it can be argued that housing is a fundamental right, one enshrined in the United Nations' *Declaration of Human Rights*.[1] Unfortunately, for many mental health clients, the reality is that appropriate accommodation has been either unaffordable (in the case of independent market housing) or limited in range (in the case of assisted/supervised housing), with a "custodial" approach predominating. This chapter looks at the increasingly inaccessible rental market in Canada and the link between mental disorder and homelessness as well as at developments in assisted housing for clients that – on a more positive note – have led to better outcomes with respect to choice, satisfaction, and mental health.

Homelessness

"Homelessness" may be defined narrowly, referring to the *absolute* homeless – persons "living rough" or in emergency shelters – or in *relative* terms, referring to people "who pay too much of their income for rent, or are residing in

inadequate housing, or lack security of tenure" (Eberle 2001c, 22). A definition of adequate housing provided by the United Nations includes five standards: (1) protection from the elements, (2) access to safe water and
sanitation, (3) secure tenure and personal safety, (4) access to employment,
education, and health care, and (5) affordability (Bryant 2003).

Because of the different methods and definitions used, estimates of
homelessness may vary widely; one author observes that "this is not surprising, given that homeless persons are often difficult to locate, the condition
of homelessness tends to be episodic, and homelessness is an ideologically
saturated concept with powerful political connotations" (Allen 2000, 16).

Concerning absolute homelessness, there is evidence that this is a significant and growing problem in Canada. A report published by the National
Housing and Homelessness Network (2001) gave the following "snapshots"
of homelessness in Canada:

- In Edmonton, on a single night in 1999, a municipal count found 836
  homeless persons – 523 in shelters and 313 on the streets. Occupancy rate
  for the 511 beds in the hostel system was 102 percent. That night 113 people
  were turned away from shelters. In addition, 32 people were discharged
  that day by hospitals or prisons onto the streets, with no place to live.
- In Toronto 30,000 persons stayed in hostels in 1999, a figure that per
  capita is higher than that for New York City. The biggest increase was among
  two-parent families. It was further noted that "many shelters do not meet
  the basic United Nations standards for refugee camps" (13).
- In Vancouver 600 people sleep outside every night. The number of people
  at one shelter sleeping on mats on the floor (because of no beds) tripled
  from 1995 to 1998.
- A number of cities showed an increase in shelter use over time. In
  Peterborough, Ontario, bed-nights increased 98 percent from 1994 to 1998,
  and in Barrie, Ontario, the increase was a staggering 1,235 percent over
  this same period.

Are the figures for homelessness increasing? The Toronto Mayor's Task
Force on Homelessness has noted a "continuous rise," with 2,000 more staying in hostels in 2002 than was the case three years earlier (see above) (Irwin
2004). In Vancouver, notwithstanding critiques of methodology, a report
from the city's housing office concluded that the numbers sleeping outside
on the streets had doubled from 2001 to 2004 (Deveau 2004; Howell 2005).

Concerning relative homelessness, the Federation of Canadian Municipalities estimated that across Canada 834,000 tenant households (representing over 2.25 million people) were spending more than half of their

pretax income on rent, meaning that they were potentially "one rent cheque away from being homeless" (Davies 2000, 37). In Calgary, Edmonton, Regina, and Kitchener one in five households spend more than half their monthly income on rent, with this figure rising to one in four for Montreal, St. John's, and Vancouver (National Housing and Homelessness Network 2001). In Greater Vancouver the proportion of this at-risk population grew between 1991 and 1996 by 65 percent for individuals and 50 percent for households (Laird 2004).

Researchers also distinguish between episodic and "chronic" homelessness, the latter term describing persons whose status may persist for several years before stable housing materializes. It is estimated that the chronically homeless represent 15 to 25 percent of the cross-section of all homeless persons (Bula 2004).

Allen (2000) notes that the ranks of the "old" homeless – older, working-class males who resided in areas close to transient labour opportunities – have been swelled by the "new" homeless, who include women, young persons, and families. For example, in Toronto in 1998 shelter users aged fifteen to twenty-four comprised 21 percent of all persons using shelters that year, well above the 12 percent proportion of youth in the general population in Toronto (Canadian Housing and Renewal Association 2002).[2] In its 2003 annual report, the Toronto Mayor's Task Force on Homelessness found that of nearly 32,000 persons staying in the city's hostels in 2002, 4,779 were children. There is also now the phenomenon of the "working homeless," with studies in Calgary finding that as many as half of its shelter population already have jobs (Laird 2004).

What about persons with mental disorders? Estimating rates of homelessness among this population is complicated by the definitions used, with some studies referring to diagnosis – with a varying range of included categories – and some to symptom profiles, based on prospective assessments of study subjects. In any event, it seems clear that a large proportion of the homeless population have mental health problems. Speaking of the American scene, one author concludes that about 35 percent of the homeless population have a "severe mental illness," referring mainly to persons with psychotic disorders, bipolar disorder, and major depression; he adds that this figure increases to 75 percent if one includes alcohol and drug addictions as mental disorders (Torrey 1997).

In Canada surveys have arrived at similar numbers, with two reviewers concluding that about one-third of the homeless are persons with mental disorders, although individual survey results vary (Allen 2000; Eberle 2001a). Examples include: (1) a study of emergency shelter users in Vancouver by Acorn (1993), which found that one in five met the criteria for schizophrenia, bipolar disorder, or major depression listed in the American Psychiatric Association's *Diagnostic and Statistical Manual (DSM)*; (2) a 1999 Toronto survey determining that 30 percent of that city's homeless population had a mental disorder (Golden et al. 1999); (3) a study of shelter users in Calgary involving the assessment of persons for symptoms of depression, anxiety, and psychosis, which found that one-third had a "significant mental health problem" (Stuart and Arboleda-Florez 2000, 55). There is also evidence that rates of mental disorder among the homeless may be higher for women (Eberle 2001a; Stuart and Arboleda-Florez 2000): a study of female street youth in Toronto found that more than one-half had attempted suicide and suffered from clinical depression (Hagan and McCarthy 1998). Regarding reported rates of homelessness among persons with mental disorders, these figures may be considerably higher if one is looking specifically at *chronic* homelessness (Todd 2004).

The effects of homelessness on the health of individuals and on the health care system itself are substantial. A Toronto task force on homelessness concluded in their report that "homeless people are at much higher risk for infectious disease, premature death, acute illness and chronic health problems than the rest of the population" (Golden et al. 1999, 103; see also Ambrosia et al. 1992; Toneguzzi 2005). As reviewed by Eberle (2001a, 6-7), several factors negatively affect the health of homeless persons:

- Homelessness increases a person's exposure to infectious and communicable diseases, such as tuberculosis.
- Homelessness is a severely stressful experience, and severe stress can trigger genetic predispositions to diseases, such as hypertension.
- Long periods of malnutrition can cause chronic conditions such as anemia and degenerative bone disease.
- There is a higher likelihood of experiencing violence or trauma on the street or in a shelter.
- Difficult living conditions also result in poor hygiene, inadequate diets, exposure to the elements, lack of sleep, and physical injuries.

For persons who are homeless *and* have a mental disorder the situation, if anything, is worse, with one psychiatrist stating bluntly: "this kind of life is often a living hell" (Torrey 1997, 19). In the Calgary study by Stuart and Arboleda-Florez (2000) the authors found that homeless persons with mental disorders experienced more hardships on the streets, took greater public health risks, more often abused substances, were more often victimized, suffered greater negative economic and interpersonal life events, experienced greater dissatisfaction, and suffered more stress. Persons with mental disorders are particularly vulnerable to financial and sexual exploitation while on the streets, with a number of studies documenting an alarmingly high incidence of rape among female clients in this population (Torrey 1997).

Homeless persons also tend to use health care services in an inefficient and ineffective manner. A survey of homeless persons in Toronto found that half did not have a family doctor, with most using hospital emergencies for routine care – half having gone to an emergency room in the past year (Golden et al. 1999). Similarly, data from an inner-city hospital in Vancouver showed that the number of patients with no fixed address seen at the hospital increased by about 300 percent from 1995 to 1999, while total admissions actually declined in this period (Eberle 2001b).

Causes

Numerous factors contribute to homelessness, although discussions about the significance of these have produced some sharp divisions of opinion (Allen 2000; Torrey 1997). Barak and Bohm (1989) provide a framework by suggesting that homelessness may be caused by (1) individual characteristics, (2) family disruption, (3) institutional policies, and (4) market forces. Concerning family disruption, a Toronto study found that 70 percent of young persons leaving home for the streets did so because of physical and/or sexual abuse (Eberle 2001a), and a report on homelessness among young women in Canada concludes that "the predominant reason for homelessness among young women is family breakdown in all its manifestations" (Canadian Housing and Renewal Association 2002, 53).

A study by this author (Davis 1987b) involving mental health clients shows in microcosm these different forces – individual, familial, systemic – at work: it involved a survey over three years of 232 persons with mental disorders residing in Vancouver emergency shelters, with one question being "how did you arrive here?" The results were:

- In 30 percent of cases persons had been evicted from their previous residence, 24 percent from a psychiatric boarding home and 6 percent from private accommodation. In most cases this was because of substance misuse and/or "problem behaviours."
- In 19 percent of cases – almost one in five – persons had just been discharged from a hospital psychiatric ward with no fixed address. While in some of these cases hospital staff and the client would agree about the need for supported housing, the waiting lists for this type of accommodation were too long to allow the client to continue taking up a bed in the hospital.
- In 17 percent of cases persons had just arrived from out of town with no money and no contacts.

- In 11 percent of cases persons had voluntarily left the previous residence because of a perceived need for greater support or because of troubling psychiatric symptoms (which were dealt with by constantly moving).
- In 10 percent of cases clients had left, or were forced out of, the previous residence because of a fight or argument with friends or relatives (often parents).
- In 8 percent of cases persons had just come from jail, and in 3 percent of cases they had come from detox.

While the link between homelessness and mental disorder seems clearly established, there continues to be debate about the interpretation and policy implications of this association. Some have argued that this unfortunate situation is indirectly a result of deinstitutionalization and directly a result of the disorder itself – that is, an inability among this population to recognize the need for treatment, or to have "insight" – in turn supporting the necessity of more coercive approaches to service provision, such as community treatment orders (Torrey 1997). On the other hand, there is the argument that homelessness is a problem of poverty and resource distribution and that focusing on individual factors, such as mental disorder, in effect blames and further stigmatizes the victim for government policies and cutbacks beyond his or her control. In an article entitled "How psychiatric status contributes to homelessness policy," one author suggests that a preoccupation with individual characteristics "removes from the level of discourse any indication of the macro-level changes that create and affect the day-to-day situation of homeless persons" (Lovell 1992, 256). Allen (2000, 18) points out that mental disorder or substance misuse can be a *result* of homelessness as well as a cause, noting that "the poorer an individual is, the more likely individual problems will precipitate homelessness, and it is arguable which is cause and which is effect."

In looking at structural factors leading to homelessness, a number of researchers point to unemployment and the increasing unaffordability of rental housing (Bula 2004). A five-year study of homeless persons in New York found that the strongest predictor of homelessness was the lack of affordable housing, rather than individual traits or characteristics, and that "subsidized housing succeeds in curing homelessness among families, regardless of behavioral disorders and other conditions" (Shinn et al. 1998, 1651; see also Shinn 1997). In an interview on this subject, University of Toronto urban economics professor William Strange concludes as follows: "Some observers argue – often based on personal observation – that because many of the homeless are substance abusers or are mentally ill, that homelessness is not a housing problem ... while it is no doubt true that homelessness has some of its roots outside the operation of housing markets, it is demonstrably false to claim that homelessness arises independently from the housing market ... although the deinstitutionalization of the mentally ill occurred simultaneously in many places, the rise in homelessness did not. Instead, increases in homelessness accompanied increases in income inequality" (quoted in Bula and Skelton 2004, A4). Interviewed for the same report, David Hulchanski, a University of Toronto professor and authority on housing, notes the impact of government programs for housing and income assistance: "There are so many people on the edge, it just takes small cuts to any of those [programs] to push people over the edge" (quoted in Bula 2004, B3).

In Canada one can note a number of social and economic factors that contributed to the rise of homelessness in the 1990s. At the federal level, the national housing program, mandated to fund social housing projects, was eliminated in 1993. At the provincial level, social programs were cut and more restrictive welfare policies implemented in a number of jurisdictions (Deveau 2004). A number of neighbourhoods underwent "gentrification," whereby rental units were renovated or demolished to make way for office buildings and condominiums. In some cases cheap single-room occupancy (SRO) hotels were converted to daily rental units or "backpacker hostels" (student dormitories) (Carrigg 2003a). All this, combined with high rents and low vacancy rates – around 1 percent in most of the larger cities – has made life difficult for low-income renters in Canada. Using Ontario as an example:

- Rental housing starts declined significantly in the 1990s, falling from 27 percent of all housing starts in 1993 to only 2 percent in 1998 (Eberle 2001c).
- Vacancy rates in Toronto and Ottawa have hovered at or below 1 percent since the late 1990s (National Housing and Homelessness Network 2001).
- The average rent for a two-bedroom apartment in Toronto broke the $1,000 ceiling in the late 1990s (National Housing and Homelessness Network 2001).
- Tenant incomes actually declined overall in Ontario from 1990 to 1995 (Eberle 2001c).
- In 1995 the newly elected Conservative government ended the period of unilaterally funded social housing programs in Ontario.
- Legislation regulating the demolition and conversion of rental buildings was weakened with the repeal of the *Rental Housing Protection Act* in 1998 (Eberle 2001c).

- Eligibility for welfare was made more restrictive – for example, with the advent of the Ontario Works Program in 1998 – while income assistance benefits were reduced in 1995 (Eberle 2001c).
- A number of social agencies that provided support to homeless or "precariously housed" persons had their budgets cut in the 1990s, forcing many to close (29).

Libby Davies, member of Parliament and New Democratic Party spokesperson for Social Policy and Housing, argues that the housing crisis is a direct result of these federal and provincial government cutbacks; she writes: "The [federal government] solution is to institutionalize shelters, and that is no solution at all. What they should be doing is admitting that the federal decision to retreat from social housing was not only shortsighted, it was shameful ... We need the government to commit to a national housing strategy, a strategy that calls for ... a federal investment of an additional one percent of overall spending on housing, or two billion dollars annually; and an approach that is national in scope and in vision" (Davies 2000, 38).

The National Housing and Homelessness Network (2001) suggests that federal and provincial investment in housing would produce a number of other social and economic benefits, including direct and spin-off employment, income tax revenues, neighbourhood stability, and empowerment. In fact, there is increasing evidence that providing affordable rental housing to marginalized persons is not only more humane, but also fiscally defensible. For example, a report authored by David Hulchanski at the University of Toronto found that it cost $40,000 annually to provide shelter as well as social, criminal justice, and health services for a homeless person, compared to $28,000 if that individual was given permanent housing (cited in Irwin 2004). On the question of cost benefit, a study of homelessness in British Columbia reached the following conclusion: "Homeless individuals tended to use more costly emergency type services than the housed individuals. Of the homeless individuals in this study, the cost of service use exclusive of housing was 33 percent higher than the housed individuals for the one year time period. When the costs of housing are included, the data showed that providing adequate supportive housing for these homeless individuals saved the government money" (Eberle 2001b, 40). A large-scale study of homeless mentally disordered persons in New York similarly found that provision of supportive housing was a cost-effective solution. Researchers collected service utilization data from 1989 to 1997 on 4,679 persons placed in supportive housing as well as from a matched group of control subjects who were not placed in housing. The study concluded that decreased costs of shelter use, hospitalizations, and jail time for the group in supported housing compensated for the per-unit cost of the housing – that is, apart from improving the clients' quality of life, stable housing paid for itself (Culhane, Metraux, and Hadley 2002).

At this point, we move to a discussion of just what "supported housing" for persons with mental disorders looks like.

Assisted and Supervised Housing

Depending on their needs and abilities, mental health clients will require different models of housing. Indeed, the availability of a *range* of options is an important aspect of a best practices housing program. Many clients will manage quite well in independent housing, although given that a large number of clients are on income assistance, the cost of appropriate market accommodation – as noted – may be prohibitive. Another obstacle is that some clients lack the skills to live independently, skills that in many cases can be taught and developed. As a result, there is the need for housing where assistance and support can be provided, either on-site or on an outreach basis. Assisted housing, broadly speaking, can be categorized as follows:

- *Residential* housing, defined as housing services that are provided "to enable individuals who cannot live independently at this time and/or who choose to acquire skills and confidence in a group setting to maximize their independence" (British Columbia Ministry of Health 2002d, 22).
- *Supported* housing, which refers to dwellings that offer greater independence and privacy (through self-contained suites) and where support services are offered on an "as-needed" basis (9).
- *Emergency* housing, which is provided for clients "who have no other housing or who require intensive stabilization (but not hospitalization) to return to adequate housing" (31). In some cases this will be in the form of specialized mental health facilities, but in many other cases this (unfortunately) will be in the form of shelters or hostels. As noted earlier in this chapter, emergency shelters have become a necessary evil in Canada partly due to deficiencies in other areas of the social service and health care systems.

These three categories of housing – residential, supported, and emergency – are discussed in more detail below.

Residential Housing

Group homes and boarding homes represent one of the earliest approaches to mental health housing; indeed, this type of accommodation predominated in Canada for a number of years following the initial wave of psychiatric hospital downsizing. These facilities were usually large, older buildings with shared bedrooms that were run for profit by private operators. Parkinson, Nelson, and Horgan (1999) note that the approach tended to be *custodial*: client autonomy was limited, there was an emphasis on rules (regarding smoking, drinking, visitors, curfews, set meal times, etc.), and residents had little or no decision-making input. Older-style residential homes may have provided the basic necessities, but they tended to foster dependency by not involving clients in activities, chores, or rehabilitation and by "focusing on deficits, rather than strengths" (147; see also Browne and Courtney 2004; Segal and Kotler 1993). While it could be argued that the most severely disabled clients required this degree of structure and supervision, a problem for practitioners working in the 1960s and 1970s was that there did not appear to be any alternatives for clients to this "one size fits all" approach. (Self-described psychiatric survivor Pat Capponi gives a moving account of life in a custodial boarding home in Toronto – which housed as many as seventy other people – in her biography *Upstairs in the Crazy House* [1992].) On the question of independence, a survey by this author (Davis 1987b) of clients referred to residential housing found that, of the 41 percent of persons who refused placement, most did so because of a wish for independence and an unwillingness to accommodate the rules and regulations of residential housing – even though at the time of referral they were homeless and residing in emergency shelters.

An early example of residential housing that aimed for tenant empowerment – and, not surprisingly, that came out of the self-help sector – was (and is) the group home program of Vancouver's Mental Patients Association, founded in 1972. In these homes the expectation is that residents will clean their own rooms, make their own meals, and look after their own health care and medications: "The aim of this program is to provide individuals with communal supportive housing while they are developing the skills and support contacts needed to live independently in the community. This is accomplished through the use of a self-help empowerment model used in a democratic environment" (Mental Patients Association 2001b, 1). This was one of very few programs that allowed residents some say in who their housemates would be by requiring that prospective tenants be "ratified" by the other members.

Currently, best-practice guidelines stipulate that residential facilities should be small and homelike, offer more privacy, have more of a rehabilitation focus, and be run by nonprofit societies (Mosher 1999; Nelson, Hall, and Walsh-Bowers 1997; Parkinson, Nelson, and Horgan 1999). On this last point, a government document gives the example of a housing society where the land is owned by the province but services are contracted with care providers on the basis of proposal calls; with services separated from property ownership, residents do not lose their housing if contractors change (either voluntarily or as a result of not meeting standards) (British Columbia Ministry of Health 2002d). Concerning privacy, this same document recommends that, either by policy or regulation, a standard of one person per room be established in licensed facilities.

Types of housing within this model include (1) fully staffed, licensed facilities that offer twenty-four-hour support; (2) partially staffed, unlicensed facilities; (3) family care homes, which are unlicensed facilities housing one or two individuals; and (4) "step-down" facilities, which provide short-term, supported housing for persons leaving hospital (British Columbia Ministry of Health 2002b). With the exception of step-down programs, client tenure in these facilities may be short- or long-term.

Residential housing is "segregated" in the sense that all tenants of a particular facility are mental health clients. Critics and researchers have argued that this approach promotes stigmatization and social isolation while "creat[ing] environments that foster deviant behavior" (Ridgeway and Zipple 1990; see also Aubrey and Myner 1996). To overcome these drawbacks, different authors have suggested that these facilities should be located within easy access to services and amenities and be indistinguishable from other houses in the neighbourhood, and that residents should be encouraged and empowered to develop networks for peer support, family contact, and social support (Carling 1993; Dixon et al. 1998; Hall and Nelson 1996).

There are several potential systemic barriers with respect to developing residential housing that meets best-practice standards and that is accessible to clients who need it. One, unfortunately, is lack of community acceptance, more commonly known as the "not in my back yard" (NIMBY) syndrome. Fears expressed by neighbours about having group homes located in their neighbourhoods are often based on myths and ignorance about mental disorder, which again speaks to the importance of public education. A concern sometimes voiced is that social housing will lower the property values in the area, although research conducted on the issue contradicts this claim (Hamid 2000b). Local opponents of residential housing may not appreciate that mental health clients will be living among them in any case – the days of the asylum are long gone, after all – but (potentially) as marginalized, unsupported citizens, a situation that benefits neither the clients themselves nor the other residents of the area. In attempting to overcome the NIMBY problem, a general strategy is to enhance public education about mental disorder. Particular projects may also require that project leaders make contacts with local officials: in describing the opposition to a group home in a small town in British Columbia, author Sarah Hamid (2000b, 28) describes how the mayor, city council, and police chief were invited for dinners where clients attended and made presentations; these officials were "surprised to see people ... that they knew from other contexts ... [and] by the time the mayor and council left ... were in full support of this project."

Another barrier to residential placement concerns client access to income and adequate support funding. In some jurisdictions a client's income assistance is suspended when that person goes into a residential facility, with the facility then receiving direct payment from government sources and the client getting a small amount of money for personal expenses. In British Columbia, at the time of writing, the "comfort allowance" given to clients was about $80.00 per month. While practitioners can attempt to persuade the client that he or she is getting a good deal in some respects – housing, meals, and other services are being provided – the small amount left over as "cash in hand" can make it a very tough sell when discussing residential placement. A recommendation here, in keeping with principles of client autonomy, is that clients receive income assistance directly and pay shelter and food costs out of this (British Columbia Ministry of Health 2002d).

Another barrier concerns restricted access to housing across health region boundaries, an issue that has come up with the move in many jurisdictions to region-based funding of mental health programs. This policy may restrict the ability of clients to make choices about where they wish to live and may effectively block access to specialized programs that are only available in other regions. The recommendation is that "health authorities be required to establish policies and procedures that will maintain and support consumer choice in housing across boundaries" (British Columbia Ministry of Health 2002d, 30).

Supported Housing

The move to supported housing in mental health reflects an increased emphasis on the principles of recovery and empowerment and in particular the importance of client choice. As reviewed by Browne and Courtney (2004, 37), more recent surveys "indicate that, for people with a mental illness, boarding homes are the least desirable type of community accommodation and that living in their own homes is the most desirable." A survey of 300 mental health clients in London, Ontario, for example, found that almost 80 percent stated a preference for living in their own apartment or house (Nelson, Hall, and Forchuk 2003).

Supported housing also represents a move toward greater physical integration – that is, dwellings that are "located in ordinary residential areas and widely dispersed in the community, rather than segregated" (British

Columbia Ministry of Health 2002d, 15; see also Parkinson, Nelson, and Horgan 1999). Supported housing can take different forms, such as block apartments with self-contained suites, supported hotels, and satellite apartments, which are subsidized units in regular apartment buildings. In this model, particularly in the case of satellite apartments, the aim is to "delink" services from the building, with clients then utilizing outreach support and/or office-based programs in the community.

Historically, there has been a tendency to see more independent, supported housing programs as something clients could "work toward" after successfully completing a placement in residential housing. The thinking on this has shifted, however, to the view that placement in supported housing should be the *first consideration*, to be ruled out only if the degree of client disability and potential risk are so high as to necessitate using other options (such as licensed facility care). This view is based on the finding that supported housing is associated with increased client satisfaction, greater community integration, and increased residential stability as well as with favourable outcomes in clinical domains such as hospitalization rates and symptom reduction (Boydell and Everett 1992; Brown et al. 1991; Canadian Housing and Renewal Association 2002; Champney and Dzurec 1992; Dixon et al. 1994; Hurlburt, Wood, and Hough 1996).

It is acknowledged that, compared to residential housing, there can be a greater risk of social isolation in supported housing. Different approaches to addressing this problem include the provision of outreach support as well as communal kitchens and shared activity groups in the block apartments. Another potential problem area concerns medication assistance: supported housing models do not normally make provision for supervising clients' medication, consistent with principles of autonomy and self-determination. In the worst-case scenario, this can lead to rehospitalization and loss of housing. Client independence with respect to health care would normally be assessed prior to placement; additionally, options such as injectable forms of medication, medication delivery, outreach support, coaching, and use of blister packs and dosette containers may be considered to assist clients.

Major barriers to client access to supported housing include the supply and affordability of these units. In Vancouver, for example, a 2003 publication estimated that waiting lists for supported mental health housing averaged four years in length, although, at the time of writing, the waiting lists were in fact substantially longer (British Columbia Partners for Mental Health and Addictions Information 2003b). Lack of timely access to housing may mean that persons are held longer than necessary in hospital beds awaiting placement, or that persons must spend extended periods in more costly housing, or that eventual transitions to supported housing are more difficult due to persons becoming acclimatized to supervised residential settings. A best-practices document recommends that provincial governments and health authorities should "aim to provide housing services for a minimum of 30 percent of persons identified as having a serious and persistent mental illness" (British Columbia Ministry of Health 2002d, 20).[3] Access to apartment-style housing is also limited by high rents and inadequate income assistance for mental health clients. The result of this is that clients may be forced into inadequate, unsafe housing, a stressor that in turn may lead to greater clinical instability and greater use of hospitals and crisis shelters (Niles 2000). One author observes that "a person's home may root them to a point in the landscape that exposes them to things that are unhealthy such as pollution, crime, vandalism, violence, discrimination, exclusion, social isolation, and a lack of services. In this way, people can easily become 'prisoners of space,' especially if they are poor and cannot afford to move and live elsewhere" (Dunn 2000, 4). It is consequently recommended that supported housing programs come with rent subsidies, which would be portable should the individual wish to relocate to another health region.

Emergency Housing

The discussion here considers two types of emergency housing: shelter/hostel accommodations and short-stay crisis units. Concerning the need for emergency shelters, it is noted that, "while emergency housing programs must exist to provide services to the homeless and must engage in best practices, they are clearly a stop-gap solution. Emergency shelters should be viewed as symptomatic of the lack of affordable, appropriate, safe and secure housing and as a reflection of an inadequate and inappropriate response to housing needs" (British Columbia Ministry of Health 2002d, 34).

Housing mental health clients in shelters or hostels is problematic in a number of respects. Shelters usually provide services to a wide range of individuals, with the potential that mentally disordered clients may be marginalized within the shelter setting or exploited by others. Shelters are often located in inner-city or skid-row areas, meaning a greater probability that vulnerable mentally disordered persons will be exposed to unsafe situations and activities, such as drug use (Davis 1998). Clients may be fearful enough to simply refuse placement; as a former shelter worker notes, "Large shelters tend to be dangerous places, especially for those who lack the social skills of getting by and surviving in a desperate milieu" (Allen 2000, 25). Shelters also tend to get clients with the greatest needs or who are the hardest to house – for example, persons with multiple diagnoses, such as mental disorder, intellectual impairment, and substance misuse – despite having limited resources to assist these people. Operating with minimal funding and staffing makes it difficult for shelters to intervene effectively in the lives of clients prior to discharge. Mental health clients face additional challenges with respect to emergency housing: transition houses for battered women may not take persons with mental illness even if they have been battered (MacPhee 2002), and older-style "men only" shelters (sometimes run under religious auspices) may force clients out of the building during the day even though the individual may be fragile and in need of respite. Daly (1996, 157) describes these older shelters: "These practices [of the shelter] include placing a large number of residents in a dormitory-like setting; inappropriate short-term limitations on length of stay (which tend to induce transience); night use only (residents are forced to leave early in the morning); minimal staff-to-resident ratios (which makes it difficult to provide a secure environment); staff members who adopt a controlling or punitive approach to residents; limited resident involvement in the planning of the shelter or its operations; and only tenuous connections to supportive community."

A document produced by Canada Mortgage and Housing Corporation (1999) makes several recommendations concerning emergency shelters: (1) that staff have a nonjudgmental manner, offer support respectfully, and empower and encourage clients to accomplish the goals they have set for themselves; (2) that safety and security be emphasized; and (3) that services be provided flexibly, particularly that length of stay be negotiable and based on client needs with a view to longer-term stability. Some shelter organizations have ancillary services, such as an outreach program whose workers help clients to locate housing and make other linkages that support long-term tenancy. In Toronto, the Shared Care Hostel Outreach Program, an initiative of the Centre for Addiction and Mental Health, provides outreach workers, nurses, and part-time physicians to five city hostels so that clients in need of health care services can be identified, given immediate assistance, and linked up with a doctor (Lechky 1999).

Crisis units are programs for persons who need short-term stabilization but not hospitalization (ideally, a stay in such a program will obviate the need for hospital care). These facilities offer a safe environment with twenty-four hour staffing, although they vary in terms of staff composition and the treatment model applied. In some cases the approach is medically focused, with the staff consisting of nurses and sessional doctors; in other cases a nonmedical, self-help model is used, an example being Toronto's Gerstein Centre, whose target group is persons aged sixteen and over "who are experiencing an acute crisis and severe or persistent mental health problems" (Bhullar 2000, 16). The Gerstein Centre offers telephone crisis intervention and a mobile crisis team, in addition to the centre itself, where the average length of stay is three days. A program that uses a peer-support model is

Seneca House in Winnipeg, which provides crisis support for persons "18 years of age or older with mental health problems" and where the length of stay is seven days at a time (16). Peer counsellors help clients to make linkages, assist them with problem solving and goal setting, and endeavour to have people become "empowered in their own recovery process" (16).

In settings where twenty-four-hour assertive community treatment is offered, crises may be managed in the client's own residence, a "least restrictive" alternative that some clients may prefer (Owen et al. 1996; Reding and Raphelson 1995). Alternately, some clients may prefer the safety and security of a staffed facility. Unfortunately, particularly in more remote settings, neither option may be available.

The best-practices guidelines for crisis housing are similar to those for residential housing (see above). In particular, it is recommended that these facilities be small and homelike, be indistinguishable from other houses in the neighbourhood, be located within easy access of services and amenities, and offer single-occupancy bedrooms (British Columbia Ministry of Health 2002d; Rakfeldt et al. 1997).

There are several systemic problems with respect to the effective operation of emergency housing resources. As with residential housing, there is the question of community acceptance, with residents of suburban areas not uncommonly objecting to emergency shelters being built in their neighbourhoods. While these objections should be considered, citizens and practitioners must be aware of the problems associated with locating shelters only in inner-city areas, particularly the vulnerability of mentally disordered persons to drug use, assault, and financial and sexual exploitation.

Emergency housing resources also face the problem of increasing acuity in the cases presented to them, which is related to diminishing resources in other areas, particularly the relative unavailability of hospital beds. Because clients refused admission to a hospital emergency department are in many cases sent to a shelter, these facilities become de facto hospital wards (Torrey 1997). Some of these clients may be elderly or medically compromised, in addition to having mental health problems.

Finally, staff at emergency facilities may find it difficult – practically, clinically, and ethically speaking – to discharge persons due to a "lack of safe, affordable, secure and appropriate resources" (British Columbia Ministry of Health 2002d, 40). This author recalls the situation of a demented man being placed in a subacute facility because he was at risk living in his own apartment; the facility, which normally housed people for only about a week, had to hold onto this individual for two months while staff scrambled to arrange priority placement in a nursing home. Having persons wait a long time in a shelter or crisis unit decreases access to the resources by other persons, who may also be in dire need, while discharging persons into unsuitable housing may only fuel the cycle of transience, instability, and shelter use. That shelter costs in many cases are higher than the costs of supported housing again speaks to the need for better housing options for mental health clients.

A form of temporary housing that exists in some centres is *respite* accommodation. Respite is primarily for clients who are living with or receiving care from a friend, partner, or family member who may be away, ill, or temporarily unable to provide care. In some cases respite is provided to clients who are living independently but who need a brief reprieve in a setting where some support and meals are provided.[4] Respite options have been established for some time for persons looking after an older relative with a dementing illness such as Alzheimer's, but are relatively new in the case of younger adults with other mental disorders. In Canada family support groups such as the Schizophrenia Society have been instrumental in organizing respite services.

Notes

1 See Section 25 of this document at http://www.un.org/overview/rights.html.
2 This author was told by the director of a Vancouver emergency shelter that the average age of shelter users there changed from fifty-seven in 1971 to thirty-two in 1985 (Davis 1987b).
3 It was estimated that the waiting list in British Columbia in 2000 for all forms of mental health housing (residential and supported) was close to 3,000 persons (Hall 2000).
4 In this author's experience, clients living in skid-row hotel rooms would negotiate brief stays in emergency shelters as respite; despite some of the negative features of these shelters, they were still seen as an escape from the noise, drug activity, or bleak surroundings associated with life in SRO hotels.

Other Resources

- The website of Toronto's Gerstein Centre (http://www.gersteincentre.org) describes the different services of this client-run program, which include a residential crisis intervention centre.
- The website of Vancouver's Lookout Emergency Aid Society (http://www.lookoutsociety.bc.ca) describes the programs of this agency, which runs several shelters and longer-stay residences.
- The National Homelessness Initiative, a federal government program, is described on the website of Human Resources and Development Canada (http://www.homelessness.gc.ca/home/index_e.asp).
- The Ladybug Foundation is a charitable Canadian organization supporting the homeless (see http://www.ladybugfoundation.ca).

The Interface with the Criminal Justice System

This chapter addresses the unfortunate fact that persons with serious mental disorders are overrepresented in the criminal courts and corrections systems. Hypotheses are advanced concerning what some have termed a "criminalization" process, and in particular the role of the police and the courts are examined. The chapter concludes by looking at a specialized branch of the mental health system: forensic psychiatry.

Criminalization

Apart from the mental health system, another large, publicly funded institution provides for the care and containment of persons with mental disorders: the criminal justice system. This assertion is supported by the large numbers of studies showing that the prevalence of serious, persistent mental disorder in remand/pretrial centres and prison populations far exceeds that seen in the general population (Davis 1992; Lamb and Weinberger 1998). For example, a study by University of Montreal researchers Sheilagh Hodgins and Gilles Cote (1990) found the prevalence of schizophrenia, bipolar disorder, and major depression among Quebec penitentiary inmates to be, respectively, 7.5, 4.8, and 16.9 percent, each figure being several times higher than the corresponding rate seen in the general public. This study found strikingly high rates of other, "less serious" disorders, notably dysthymia and anxiety disorders, especially post-traumatic stress disorder (PTSD). A secondary finding from the survey was how few inmates received psychiatric help: of 112 persons identified as having a serious, persistent mental disorder, only 40 had discussed their symptoms with a professional, and only 24 had been transferred to psychiatric care.

High rates of mental disorder have also been seen among remand populations: studies conducted at the Pre-Trial Centre in Vancouver, British Columbia, by Gingell (1991), who reviewed 313 consecutive admissions, and Hart and Hemphill (1989), who reviewed 576, determined that 8 percent of the groups studied met the diagnostic criteria for schizophrenia and that 7 percent were actively psychotic at the time of admission. In her 2001 annual report, the mental health advocate of British Columbia noted that approximately 15 percent of persons in the BC corrections system had a serious, persistent mental disorder and that the recidivism rate of these individuals (the number who reoffend) was about 62 percent (Hall 2001).

The situation in the United States is apparently even worse, especially considering the huge number of persons incarcerated, the lack of treatment resources, and the "pressure cooker" atmosphere of the institutions in question. A report from the organization Human Rights Watch (2003) determined that about 16 percent of American inmates had a serious, persistent mental disorder and that correctional facilities had become the nation's largest de facto psychiatric inpatient facilities, an example being the Los Angeles County jail, which houses approximately 3,400 mentally disordered prisoners. According to the report, American prisons now contain three times as many persons with mental disorders as do units in general and psychiatric hospitals.

Life in prison is not easy for anyone but is especially difficult for those with a psychiatric diagnosis. Such individuals, referred to as "bugs" in prison jargon, are low down on the inmate hierarchy and are often victimized and physically or sexually exploited by others. The Human Rights Watch (2003, 2) report describes prisoners "who, because of their illness, rant and rave, babble incoherently, or huddle silently in their cells. They talk to invisible companions, living in worlds constructed of hallucinations. They lash out without provocation, beat their heads against cell walls, cover themselves with feces, mutilate themselves until their bodies are covered with scars, and attempt suicide."

Not surprisingly, mentally disordered inmates are often considered a management problem by corrections staff (Hart and Hemphill 1989), who may have little training in mental health. These inmates are sometimes punished for symptoms of the disorder itself, such as being noisy, disruptive, refusing orders, or even self-mutilation. A common response is to put such persons in isolation, which can actually have the effect of exacerbating psychotic symptoms. In examining this response, Hodgins and Cote (1991, 181) surveyed inmates of Quebec penitentiaries who had been transferred either to "special handling units" or to "long term segregation units," finding persons with schizophrenia and bipolar disorder to be overrepresented relative to the total inmate population in both of these special units; the same did not apply to those suffering from depression, leading the investigators to conclude that "withdrawn mentally disordered inmates are left within the general penitentiary population, while the troublesome ones are sent to isolation."

In considering the plight of mental health clients who, in disproportionate numbers, are ending up in criminal justice settings, the remaining questions are "how did this come about?" and "what – if anything – can be done about it?"

With respect to the first question, this state of affairs has usually been seen as another failure of deinsitutionalization. Like homelessness, the incarceration of the mentally disordered has been linked to the larger numbers of these persons now present in the community because of psychiatric hospital downsizing and to the fact that community treatment and support services are insufficient and/or unresponsive (Davis 1992). The phenomenon has in fact been given a name, **"criminalization,"** which refers to the hypothesis that troublesome behaviour by mentally disordered persons that would have presumably been dealt with previously by the mental health system – usually by hospital detention – is now being dealt with by the criminal justice system in the post-deinstitutionalization era. These "troublesome behaviours" could be the result of a disorder – for example, an extremely paranoid person committing a minor assault – or in some cases the result of volition, necessitated by poverty and a lack of resources, such as a "dine and dash" at a restaurant, or seeking arrest in order to get room and board (Abramson 1972). Apart from the large numbers of mentally disordered persons seen in correctional settings, the criminalization hypothesis is also supported by "the observations of both clinicians and researchers that a high proportion of mentally ill persons found today in the criminal justice system resemble in most respects the persons who used to be patients in long-term ... hospitals" (Lamb 2001, 13).

An alternative explanation for the numbers of mentally disordered seen in jails and prisons is that the stress of these environments *precipitated* the disorders being manifested. This seems unlikely, however, given what we know about the etiology of conditions such as schizophrenia and bipolar disorder, and is contradicted by Hodgins and Cote's (1991) findings from Quebec, which determined that the vast majority of subjects found to have a serious, persistent mental disorder had this diagnosis before entry to the penitentiary. At the same time, it must be conceded that long-term incarceration would have a damaging effect on anyone's mental state.

Interestingly, "criminalization" is not a new concept. In 1939 a British researcher named Penrose published a paper based on a survey of service utilization data from eighteen European countries, which proposed that the size of psychiatric hospital populations was inversely proportional to prison populations and that a dynamic relationship existed between the two. In other words, depending on the zeitgeist, care and containment of the mentally disordered was apparently being passed back and forth between these two systems, a proposition that is supported by the observation that in earlier periods in Canada, before there were asylums, "insane persons were ... placed routinely in local jails" (Rochefort 1992, 1084). However, determining the extent to which the prevalence of mentally disordered persons in correctional settings in Canada has changed over time is made difficult by the lack of reliable archival material, not to mention the changes seen in diagnostic systems. It has been suggested that the number of mentally disordered persons in jail and prison populations has in fact always been high but previously underidentified (Davis 1994b). The process of shifting the care and containment of individuals with mental disorders from one institution to another has been referred to by some authors as "**transinstitutionalization**" (e.g., Bradley 1991; Dickinson 2002).

To better understand the problems and dilemmas that arise when mental health clients encounter the criminal justice system, it is necessary to take a closer look at the components of this system as they are encountered, sequentially, by the client.

The Role of the Police

In evaluating the criminalization hypothesis, a considerable amount of attention has been given to the role of the police since they represent the key "entry point" to the criminal justice system and since they can exercise a fair degree of discretion in how they respond to community disturbances involving persons who are apparently mentally disordered (Teplin and Pruett 1992). As to the frequency with which this happens, a Canadian study estimated that over 30 percent of mental health clients had contact with the police while making, or attempting to make, their first contact with the mental health system (Canadian Mental Health Association, British Columbia Division, 2003).

Concerning police decision making, it can said that generally, depending on contingencies, police officers may take no action, may informally intervene (such as removing a person from the scene), may attempt to use another resource (such as taking a person on a voluntary basis to hospital or detox), or may invoke statutory powers, either under mental health legislation (which authorizes initiating involuntary hospitalization) or under the *Criminal Code*, whereby the person is arrested. Of course, police discretion is limited by the nature of the disturbance, with more serious incidents being more likely to lead to arrest. So how is police discretion used in the case of mentally disordered persons?

Going back to the 1960s – the early stages of post-deinstitutionalization – a number of American studies found that persons with mental disorders were being arrested at a higher rate than the general public (Mulvey,

Blumstein, and Cohen 1986) (no comparable studies were published in Canada). The interpretation of this, however, was unclear; did it mean, for example, that "dangerous" ex-hospital patients were now running amok in the community? To better examine the police decision-making process, American academics Linda Teplin and colleagues conducted a number of participant-observation studies in the 1980s, which involved "ride-alongs" with Chicago police officers (Teplin 1984; Teplin and Pruett 1992). Based on a large number of documented encounters with persons who were apparently mentally disordered, Teplin (1984, 794) concluded that these individuals were "indeed being criminalized" – that is, that all things being equal (the seriousness of the charges being constant) they were more likely to be arrested than the general public.

Why was this happening? Teplin found that the mentally disordered subjects were not committing more serious offences but that other factors were in operation. In some cases, the mental disorder was not recognized by the police. There was also the "visibility factor" – that is, the disturbance was public, or the persons in question lacked social skills and might have been disrespectful, or they were more easily caught, or the behaviours/symptoms were disconcerting to other citizens, resulting in demands (implicit or explicit) that the police officer "do something." (The publicness of these incidents is made more likely by the fact that mental health clients are disproportionately homeless.) Finally, and most significant, other options were blocked for bureaucratic reasons. For example, in the case of someone with a drug addiction and a mental disorder, police would find that a detox centre refused to admit the individual because of symptoms of psychosis. Hospital admission, which one might think would be the most appropriate intervention, was relatively unavailable because of a shortage of beds, because the involuntary admission criteria were (or were interpreted to be) very narrow, and in general because of the "red tape" and amount of time needed to attempt this intervention. Teplin (1984) found that the police officers were all too familiar with the statutory criteria for hospital admission. Thus persons ended up being arrested "by default."

In drawing inferences from this, one can see that a number of the same factors could apply to the Canadian scene, particularly the possibility that not all officers recognize the symptoms of mental disorder (which becomes a training issue), the reality of an unsympathetic public, and the lack of alternate resources due to, for example, hospital overcrowding. With respect to the police authority to take a mentally disordered person to hospital, which exists under provincial mental health legislation, readers should note (1) that *admission* to the facility still requires the consent of the receiving doctor and (2) that in many Canadian jurisdictions the statutory criteria for police apprehension are narrower – with references to "danger," for example – than those applying to physician certifications (Gray, Shone, and Liddle 2000; see also Chapter 13). Indeed, on this second point, this author has encountered situations involving the police and the possible transport of a client to hospital where the officers in question were nervous about overstepping their authority.

Another area of police involvement that has received considerable attention is the use of lethal force when dealing with apparently mentally disordered persons. For example, according to one published report, at least six mentally disordered persons (all with psychiatric histories, at least three with diagnoses of schizophrenia) were shot by Vancouver-area police from 1996 to 2000, four of them fatally (Wittek 2001). Another report identifies thirteen such incidents across Canada between 1992 and 2002 (Bryan 2004). In some of these cases police officers were faulted, with witnesses arguing that lethal force was unwarranted given the proximity of the parties to one another, the lack of imminent threat, and the availability of alternatives (such as mental health personnel, who were present but ordered to back off). On the other hand, police officers in such situations may feel they have little choice given the apparent unpredictability of the individual and especially if that person is wielding a weapon. There is in fact evidence that the victims in these situations may in some cases provoke the response, a phenomenon referred to as "suicide by cop." Support for this claim comes from research conducted by Richard Parent, a former Vancouver-area police officer who went back to university to complete a master's thesis (Parent 1996). Parent reviewed fifty-eight incidents, spanning the period 1980 to 1994, where British Columbia police officers were confronted by a "potentially lethal threat." Of the twenty-eight cases where officers shot and killed the persons confronting them, Parent concluded that roughly 50 percent could be considered "victim-precipitated homicide." Parent later expanded his research in a PhD dissertation, analyzing 409 police shootings across Canada between 1980 and 2002 and 434 others in the United States during this same period. He concluded that 273 of these incidents – roughly one-third – could be considered victim-precipitated (Bisetty 2004; Parent 2004).

Despite the difficult realities of police work, officers are not necessarily unsympathetic when it comes to attitudes about mentally disordered persons. A recent editorial in a client-run newsletter, for example, is entitled "Compassion by law enforcers more common than may be expected," with the author relating a critical early experience with a compassionate policeman (Sterle 2004, 14). On the issue of police compassion, Ontario psychologist Dorothy Cotton surveyed 150 officers in Ontario and British Columbia using a questionnaire that measured four attitudinal dimensions (authoritarian, socially benevolent, socially restrictive, and oriented toward community integration) as well as their perception of the role of police in working with mentally ill people (Dorrance 2003). When the results were compared with those from the same survey given to the general public, it was found that the police officers were relatively more benevolent and less authoritarian: 80 percent of respondents believed the mentally ill to be "far less dangerous than most people suppose," 94 percent believed society should adopt more tolerant attitudes, and 93 percent believed the mentally ill should not be denied their individual rights. The study's author noted that "most police officers in fact have a great deal of trouble arresting individuals with mental illnesses and are much more interested in linking them to appropriate services" (quoted in Dorrance 2003, 8). An American survey of 382 police officers found that persons diagnosed with schizophrenia, all things being equal, were considered to be "more dangerous" but that – similar to the Canadian study's findings – individuals with this diagnosis were "less responsible for their situation" and "more worthy of help" (Watson, Corrigan, and Ottati 2004, 49).

Fortunately, concern about the involvement of the police with mentally disordered persons in Canada has stimulated discussion, research, and some procedural changes and program developments. The Canadian Mental Health Association issued a report on this subject in 2003, wherein a number of potential barriers to effective interventions, in addition to those identified above, were outlined. These included: (1) inadequate advance information – that is, information on mental health concerns not being passed on by dispatchers; (2) inadequate information systems, which could potentially identify mental health clients in advance and provide information about successful prior interventions; and (3) lack of access to consultation from mental health workers at the scene (Canadian Mental Health Association, British Columbia Division, 2003).

Program developments include the following:

- *Changes in technology:* officers in Toronto, Victoria, the Vancouver area, and other centres may now use the "taser," a device that immobilizes suspects with a jolt of electricity and that has been brought in specifically as a nonlethal alternative for dealing with mentally unstable persons (Nuttall-Smith 2000).[1]
- *Increased emphasis on training* for working with the mentally disordered. Hall (2001, 16) notes that "the RCMP [Royal Canadian Mounted Police] ... are developing crisis intervention training programs as well as a new curriculum ... to give new recruits a better understanding of the needs of mentally disabled people in crisis."

- *Partnership programs,* such as the one between the Toronto Police Service and St. Michael's Hospital, piloted in 2000, where plainclothes police team up with mental health nurses to respond to emergency calls involving mentally disordered persons. This program is designed to "better improve the police's response to dealing with people with emotional disturbances" and to "both reduce costly policing delays and move people with mental illness from the court system into the health care system" (Centre for Addiction and Mental Health 2001, 2). Similar programs exist in Hamilton, Vancouver, and Ottawa.
- *Establishment of a new national body, the Canadian National Committee for Police/Mental Health Liaison,* which held its first conference in 2002. Composed of police officers and mental health professionals, this organization's "issues of concern" include: training police in the area of mental health and training mental health practitioners in the area of criminal justice; effective liaison and partnerships between criminal justice and mental health programs; research and data collection; and less lethal uses of force (Cotton 2002).

The Role of the Courts

Once a police officer makes the decision to charge and arrest an accused person, that person is taken into custody at a remand centre and subsequently appears before a judge, usually the following morning. Because many mentally disordered persons are poor, they are typically represented by legal-aid lawyers.

A key decision to be made early in this sequence is whether the individual, if mentally disordered, is *fit to stand trial* – that is, whether they can competently participate in an adversarial criminal proceeding. The accused's lawyer, for example, may point out to the judge that he or she is unable to communicate effectively with the client because that person is psychotic. The judge may then order a fitness assessment, which is usually carried out by a forensic psychiatrist, sometimes at the remand centre and sometimes following a transfer to a forensic facility (see more on the role of the forensic system below). To assist persons doing fitness assessments, clinicians have developed structured guidelines, such as, in Canada, the Fitness Interview Test (Viljoen, Roesch, and Zapf 2002). The available evidence suggests that most accused persons are found fit following the assessment (e.g., Davis 1995a; Ohayan et al. 1998), which may be the result of the courts applying a low standard of fitness since a finding of unfitness results in further delays and deprivation of the accused's liberty.[2] Some have observed that the fitness threshold may be too low and judicial decisions too idiosyncratic, despite the criteria available in the *Criminal Code*; for example, interviews conducted by this author as part of a research project on the fitness process turned up the following quotation from a forensic psychiatrist: "Different judges can have much broader, or narrower conceptualizations of fitness. I've been in court when the accused is so psychotic he doesn't even know where he is, let alone what the 'role of the prosecutor is,' and yet the judge will declare him fit" (Davis 1994b, 115).

Indeed, it is distinctly possible that an accused person's impaired mental state may be underestimated – or not recognized at all – during the remand process. One of the reasons for this is that the provincial courts in larger urban centres deal with a huge volume of cases, meaning that persons with serious mental disorders may simply get swept along with the mass of other unfortunates entering the criminal justice system – which speaks to the need for adequate screening for mental disorder at the point of remand (Roesch 1995).

Persons found fit are, in most cases, released with bail conditions, requiring them to report to a bail supervisor and to return for further court appearances. This can be a problem for some mentally disordered persons: disorganization and cognitive impairment caused by the disorder or substance misuse, and a lack of community supports, may mean that they fail to make these appointments, which may lead to further charges since "failure to appear" is itself an offence.

If convicted, persons may be sentenced to probation or time in custody. As noted earlier, serving time in a correctional facility is especially difficult for persons with a mental disorder, who may be abused by other inmates, considered a management problem by facility staff, and offered very limited treatment services. Persons on probation face other difficulties: as with persons on bail, cognitive impairment may mean that they fail to make appointments or have a more difficult time following conditions such as geographical restrictions.

Some persons given probation may be ordered to receive psychiatric treatment as a condition of their probation order, which in most cases means that they will be seen by the forensic psychiatric system. Nonforensic mental health services have historically been reluctant to accept these sorts of cases (1) because they are a "voluntary" service (although with the increasing use of community treatment orders, this is a debatable assertion) and (2) because of discomfort in dealing with clients who carry the "criminal" or "offender" label. As an editorial in the *Canadian Journal of Psychiatry* notes, "Most psychiatrists, like most physicians ... prefer not to deal with the often unpleasant characters with which forensic psychiatrists inevitably must deal" (Hucker 1998, 456). In this way mental health programs make a distinction between the "mad" and the "bad," with the latter group often being turned away, despite being diagnosed with serious mental disorders. One of the problems with this response is that it becomes a self-fulfilling prophecy: the denial of services to "mentally disordered offenders" (as they are referred to in the forensic literature) may mean further deterioration of their mental state, resulting in more charges and subsequent reinforcement of their "bad" label.

In Canada there has been a growing consensus, among a range of stakeholders, that rather than convicting and sentencing mentally disordered persons for minor offences, it is more appropriate, humane, and effective to *divert* these individuals from the criminal justice system. "**Diversion**" refers to the suspension of criminal charges with the understanding that the accused person will instead receive prompt treatment within the mental health system (in theory at least). While diversion can refer to an earlier point in the proceedings – for example, decisions made by a police officer before charges are laid – it is usually defined as a procedure that occurs postarrest and pretrial.

Diversion has gone on for some time on an informal basis. In British Columbia persons charged with minor offences, detained, and subsequently certified under the *Mental Health Act* were until the 1980s channelled directly from the pretrial centre to the provincial psychiatric hospital, all of which ended because of policy changes and, more specifically, the downsizing and closure of many of the wards at that facility. There are problems, however, when diversion occurs informally – that is, without explicit guidelines and protocols. For example, is the consent/nonconsent of the accused person taken into account? Another problem is that, without guidelines, diversion decisions may be idiosyncratic and biased. Evidence for this comes from a study of pretrial diversion in British Columbia, where it was found that 13.4 percent of persons (103/771) undergoing pretrial psychiatric assessment were diverted (Davis 1994c). In this study diversion decisions were related primarily to three factors: (1) charge seriousness (with less serious charges more likely to be suspended), (2) court jurisdiction, and (3) the discretion of the assessing psychiatrist. While the first factor seems reasonable and predictable, it was hard to rationalize the significance of the other two.

In the United States the issue of diversion has been handled by the creation in a number of centres of "mental health courts." As reviewed by Watson and colleagues (2001), the development of mental health courts was influenced by the earlier establishment of drug courts in the United States, a "therapeutic jurisprudence" model that identified substance misuse as a public health (not simply a criminal justice) problem and that emphasized immediate intervention, a nonadversarial process, a team approach, and having clear rules and goals. As of 2004 Canada had two drug courts, in Toronto and Vancouver, although in this same year the federal government asked for proposals to provide pilot funding for drug courts in other centres (Howell 2004).

The goal of the mental health court is to "prevent criminalization and recidivism by providing critical mental health services" (Watson et al. 2001, 477), with defendants having charges deferred if they agree to participate in mental health treatment programs. There are eligibility requirements around the nature of the criminal charge and the accused person's diagnosis, with most jurisdictions requiring a "serious, persistent" condition. The idea of a mental health court carries with it some legal and ethical complexities – for example, the question of the accused person's competency to surrender legal protections and to understand the consequences of his or her actions.

In Canada court diversion programs have been established and formalized in a number of cities. In Ontario, for example, a partnership was formed in 1994 between the Ministry of the Attorney General and the Canadian Mental Health Association (CMHA) to form the Mental Health Diversion Program. As described on a CMHA website, the program is "designed to give a more suitable response to mentally disordered offenders, both adults and young offenders, who find themselves in conflict with the criminal justice system because of their mental illness ... [and] to gain the necessary treatment and support they need to prevent future criminal activity" (Canadian Mental Health Association, Thunder Bay Branch, 2001). Diversion is decided by the judge on a case-by-case basis, with diverted persons being referred either to a hospital, to a mental health professional, or to the Canadian Mental Health Association to seek treatment.

Diversion programs, as noted, have eligibility criteria. An example comes from the Provincial Forensic Psychiatric Program in Alberta (Alberta Mental Health Board, n.d.), which stipulates that the target population consists of individuals who are:

- Adults (eighteen years of age or older).
- Suffering from a mental disorder, defined as a substantial disorder of thought, mood, perception, orientation, or memory that grossly impairs judgment, behaviour, capacity to recognize reality, or ability to meet the ordinary demands of life.
- Charged with a minor low-risk offence, such as assault (simple assault in a nondomestic context), theft, possession of stolen property, fraud, false pretense, and mischief (property related; causing a disturbance; transportation, lodging, and meal fraud; obstruction of a peace officer; or other minor charges on a case-by-case basis).

Further,

- Crown counsel must be satisfied that the charge has a reasonable likelihood of conviction.
- Diversion must not be contrary to the public interest, with the safety of the public being a paramount consideration.
- A prior criminal record or diversion under the program or other programs does not preclude diversion, although both factors are relevant considerations in the exercise of the Crown's discretion to divert.
- The accused must accept mental health diversion.
- To participate, it is not necessary for the accused to admit guilt.
- Substance abuse in addition to suffering from a mental disorder does not preclude eligibility for participation in the Calgary Diversion Project.

Does diversion work? While these programs are relatively new in Canada, an evaluation from Ontario offers some insights (Swaminath et al. 2002). Investigators studied diversion programs in Elgin County, a predominantly rural area, and Middlesex County, a more populous area that includes the city of London. The diversion team in Middlesex was made up of three psychiatric nurses, based at the courthouse, while the Elgin team had just one nursing position, based at the police station. In both cases the nurses provided assessment, linkages for the client, and consultation with Crown and defence lawyers, and also organized individualized support and supervision plans. The study appeared to show positive results, with recidivism – defined as a re-arrest for any charge within the year following the initiation of the diversion agreement – being low in both locales: 2 to 3 percent, which the authors note compares favourably to rates of comparison groups taken from the literature. At the same time, the study, and by extrapolation the diversion program itself, suffered from what is called *selection bias:* offenders could be ruled ineligible for diversion either (1) because of previous criminal convictions, (2) because the victim did not agree to diversion, or (3) "if a program of treatment and rehabilitation was unavailable or could not be monitored," with Middlesex County in particular suffering from a lack of coordinated services. While the courts have a right and a duty to screen out "high-risk" clients from diversion programs, application of overly restrictive eligibility criteria may at the same time result in the exclusion of the very persons that these sorts of programs were set up for in the first place. As well, the problem of appropriate treatment services not always being available speaks to the importance of community resources since diverted persons, after all, have to be diverted "to" somewhere.[3]

The Forensic System

Mental health clients entering the criminal court process may become involved with the **forensic psychiatric system,** which provides assessment and treatment that is mandated by the courts. Involvement with the forensic system can come about in several different ways:

- Pretrial assessment of an accused person can be requested to determine that person's fitness to stand trial, referring to his or her mental state while at court, or to determine criminal responsibility, referring to the mental state of the accused at the time of the offence and to whether mental disorder negated the *mens rea* (the "guilty mind," or criminal intent) required to secure a conviction. In most cases these assessments are undertaken by psychiatrists with a forensic specialty. Assessments may be done at a remand centre, at a secure forensic hospital, or on an outpatient basis.
- Persons who are found either unfit to stand trial or **not criminally responsible by reason of mental disorder (NCRMD)** may be detained in

The "Multisystem" Client

A Canadian author (Roesch 1995, 524) notes that a subset of mental health clients, referred to as "mentally disordered offenders," "cycles continuously through the health, mental health, forensic and criminal justice systems" and that "traditional methods ... have not been especially successful in dealing with these individuals."

Several factors contribute to the plight of the "multisystem" client. Many of these individuals have co-occurring substance-use disorders and criminal or forensic histories, both of which have been used as the basis for exclusion from traditional mental health programs. Diagnostically, these persons may not clearly fit the "serious, persistent" designation, suffering from conditions that include attention-deficit hyperactivity disorder, fetal alcohol syndrome, organic brain disorder, and intellectual impairment. These individuals may have a hard time connecting with an office-based service that requires close adherence to scheduled appointments. As well, because they will typically have been rebuffed, turned away, and barred from many programs, trust is hard to establish. And the different systems involved may have no history of or interest in cooperation or establishing linkages, resulting in the attitude that the client is always "someone else's problem." Roesch suggests that any adequate response "will require inter-ministerial, inter-agency, and community cooperation" (524).

In 1987 an attempt was made to address these barriers to care with the establishment in Vancouver, British Columbia, of the Inter-Ministerial Program, a partnership between three government agencies: provincial corrections, the forensic system, and mental health. Using an assertive case management model, the program targeted those individuals who cycled through the different health care and criminal justice systems and attempted to maintain continuity of care for the long-term regardless of where in the system the client was at any given time. Workers endeavoured to keep clients in treatment, to provide advocacy, to consult with court personnel, including defence and Crown counsel, to assist with and teach skills concerning activities of daily living, and through frequent contact and knowledge of clients, to anticipate and head off any crises (Davis, Eaves, and Wilson 1999).

The program was evaluated to see if, in particular, there was any impact on recidivism, defined as "jail days" (Wilson, Tien, and Eaves 1995). Clients in the program were compared with a quasi-control group of clinically and demographically similar individuals over an eighteen-month baseline period and then over an eighteen-month in-treatment period. The results showed that the group followed by the Inter-Ministerial Program spent substantially less time in jail: a mean of 80.4 days at eighteen months compared to a mean of 213.6 days for the comparison group. An earlier evaluation of the same program (Bradley 1991) also found an association between program involvement and "decriminalization" – that is, less time spent in jail – but uncovered the additional interesting result that clients of the program saw something of an *increase* (not reaching statistical significance) in their use of beds in the hospital system. In explaining this, the author notes that advocacy works in opposite directions in the corrections and mental health system: "In the corrections system, advocacy is likely to produce more lenient sentences or probation or bail in lieu of incarceration, while in the mental health system it is likely to encourage doctors, nurses and other mental health professionals to give multi-problem clients greater access to treatment" (63).

Given the current emphasis in the best-practices literature on reduced numbers of hospital admissions as an indicator of "success," the increase in bed days seen here might be counted as a negative outcome. This, however, views resource use, and "success," in a narrow fashion and does not account for the flow of clients between the different systems. As well, it would seem to be uncontroversial that persons with mental health problems are more appropriately cared for in a mental health, rather than a criminal justice, setting.[4]

custody or given a conditional discharge, as determined by a board of review (or in some cases by the court itself). In these cases ongoing treatment and supervision of the review board order is provided by forensic practitioners, either in secure hospitals or in outpatient clinics in cases of conditional discharge. Persons found NCRMD and initially held in custody will in most cases graduate to conditional and then absolute discharge status. Persons found unfit to stand trial will return to court once they have been found fit. The conditions attached to conditional discharges are in some respects similar to probation conditions, with references, for example, to abstention from alcohol, having no contact with certain individuals, and "no-gos" to certain areas, in addition to the requirement that the accused take treatment as directed. Applications for discharge are made at review board hearings, when there are submissions from both the accused's representatives and forensic clinical staff. Historically, persons found "not guilty by reason of insanity" could expect to be detained in custody for lengthy periods, so in Canada defence lawyers tended to avoid this plea, except for in the case of very serious charges (often murder). This has all changed; following a series of court decisions and *Criminal Code* amendments, there is now an onus on review boards to come up with "least restrictive" dispositions and for persons found NCRMD to be granted absolute discharges unless there is evidence that the individual is a "significant threat" to public safety (Verdun-Jones 2000).

- In some cases persons may be required to report for psychiatric treatment as a condition of bail or probation, which is usually provided at a forensic psychiatric outpatient clinic. This can be recommended when an individual has been unwilling to see a mental health team voluntarily and if there is evidence that when unwell the person gets into conflict with the law. Enforcement of these orders can be a cumbersome process: if a client "breaches" an order by not showing up for treatment, no immediate action is necessarily taken; rather, the individual may be required to make another court appearance at some future date.

- Forensic clinicians may also become involved in the criminal process at the point of sentencing. After a defendant is convicted, the court may ask for a pre-sentence report, wherein material is gathered and opinions offered on the likelihood of reoffending – in particular under what conditions – and on the question of treatability. This typically happens in cases where there has been repetitive violent behaviour and in particular sexual offending.[5] (It should be pointed out that while conditions such as pedophilia are included in the American Psychiatric Association's *Diagnostic and Statistical Manual [DSM]*, sexual deviations are not usually included in the "serious, persistent" category of mental disorders, and there is considerable debate among practitioners as to whether they should be considered mental disorders at all.) Whether mental health practitioners should be in the business of predicting future violence is a very controversial issue, with opponents arguing that accurate prediction is impossible and that attempting to do it is therefore unethical (Rogers and Mitchell 1991). A counterargument is that, like it or not, practitioners on a routine basis are forced to make risk assessments and that in the forensic context this process can be improved by the application of structured guidelines that incorporate clinical, actuarial, and environmental factors (Borum 1996).

- Treatment for sex offenders is provided by forensic clinicians, either at correctional facilities or on an outpatient basis. A range of therapeutic approaches may be tried, including (1) drugs that reduce testosterone levels; (2) behavioural techniques such as aversion therapy, covert sensitization, and masturbatory satiation; (3) cognitive techniques that look at the rationalizations that support deviant behaviour; (4) social skills training; and (5) relapse prevention, a process that attempts to interrupt the "crime cycle" by identifying behavioural precursors to sexual offending (Glackman 1991).

Some built-in limitations arise with court-ordered treatment. To begin with, there is the fact that the client-practitioner relationship in this situation is by definition involuntary and may be perceived as more adversarial given that the "control agent" function is emphasized and that clinicians report to the courts, probation officers, and review boards. Of course, nonforensic practitioners may also have an involuntary relationship with clients, and in either case there is the potential for a skillful, compassionate clinician to make therapeutic gains. Court-ordered treatment is also time-limited, meaning that investment and commitment, on the part of either client or practitioner, can be compromised. As well, court orders are a clumsy, cumbersome means of enforcing treatment given the postponements and delays endemic to the court system and the unfamiliarity of court officers with mental health issues. Finally, because of mandate, philosophy, or fiscal restraint, forensic psychiatric services tend to be more narrowly focused and may not have the important ancillary and rehabilitation services offered in other mental health programs.

While forensic psychiatric programs have historically been separate from other mental health services with respect to location, governance, and organizational culture, the move to regionalization in Canada means that forensic programs are coming under the umbrella of local health authorities, although not yet in all jurisdictions. It is difficult to talk about "integration" of forensic and nonforensic programs given that there are different legal mandates, with forensic staff dealing with orders from the courts and review boards that operate under the *Criminal Code* (however, see box on p. 185). At the same time, there is room for improvement with respect to linkages between forensic and nonforensic programs, particularly concerning how, or if, clients leaving forensic treatment are received by the other system. There has been, as noted, a tendency to distinguish the "bad" from the "mad" – that is, for nonforensic practitioners to consider clients tainted by the forensic label as somehow different and not appropriate for regular mental health follow-up. This is arguably a misperception; as we have seen from the research on "criminalization," which system a client winds up in at any given time depends to a large extent on resources, environmental contingencies, and happenstance. Nonforensic clinicians may also assume, incorrectly, that forensic staff have some special techniques for working with clients who get into conflict with the law. The methods, both pharmacological and counselling, are much the same, and it may be that comfort level is the main characteristic that distinguishes staff from the two programs.

Notes

1 Although, concerning "nonlethality," see O'Brian (2004a).
2 The fitness standard may be lower than the certification standard: this author has encountered cases where a client has been certified after arrest but still found to be fit for court.
3 A further implementation problem noted by the study authors was that diversion had to be initiated by defence lawyers, who were often unaware of the diversion option or, if aware, had the view that the process was overly cumbersome.
4 Despite having received these positive evaluations, the Inter-Ministerial Program folded in 2002 due to funding cuts.
5 The Canadian *Criminal Code* contains "dangerous offender" provisions, referring to persons who have committed a "serious personal injury offence" – in practice, usually a sexual offence. The application of these provisions must be supported by psychiatric testimony, and convicted persons given this special status may be detained in custody indefinitely.

Other Resources

■ The website of the Canadian National Committee for Police/Mental Health Liaison is at http://www.pmhl.ca.
■ The Canadian Mental Health Association's report on police encounters with mentally disordered persons, "A Study in Blue and Grey," is available online at http://www.crpnbc.ca/policereport.pdf.
■ Simcoe County, Ontario, sponsors a Mental Health and Addictions Foundation website (http://www.mhcva.on.ca), whose forensics page provides useful information on mental disorder and the criminal justice system.

Assessment and
Medical Management

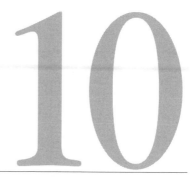

Assessment and medical management are the basic, "core" functions performed by practitioners working in most public mental health treatment programs in Canada. "Medical management" is used here to refer to a process, led by a psychiatrist or physician, that involves the diagnosis and subsequent treatment and stabilization of acute psychiatric symptoms, primarily with the use of medications. Nonpharmacological approaches to treatment – education, skills training, and psychotherapy – are described in the next chapter. The separation of pharmacological and nonpharmacological treatments is an artifact of this book's construction: in reality, clients of mental health teams may simultaneously receive services from a prescribing physician *and* a practitioner using psychological approaches such as cognitive-behavioural therapy. That being said, the fact remains that in some cases mental health clients do not receive more than "medical management," despite their own wishes and despite evidence that other types of treatment and education are effective. There are three main reasons for this. One is ideological, reflecting the dominant position of biological approaches in North American psychiatry. The second has to do with resource allocation: family physicians and practitioners on mental health teams generally have large caseloads, with clients being booked at short intervals, so brief assessments and medication renewals may be favoured over longer counselling sessions. The third has to do with training: not all practitioners have been exposed to, for example, cognitive-behavioural approaches.

This chapter provides a description of the assessment process and of the most commonly used psychotropic medications as well as some brief comment on the use of electroconvulsive therapy (ECT) and hospitalization. Discussing the use and effects of medication is fraught with difficulty because of the speed with which new products are developed and because our understanding of the benefits and costs associated with their use is constantly changing. As a result, the reader is strongly advised to consider other sources of information, such as the *Compendium of Pharmaceuticals and Specialties*, published annually by the Canadian Pharmacists Association; the *Clinical Handbook of Psychotropic Drugs*, published in revised editions by Hogrefe and Huber Publishers; *Psychotropic Agents*, published in revised editions by IGR publications; the Health Canada website (http://www.hc-sc.gc.ca); or, of course, a physician.

Assessment

The clinical assessment is an ongoing process, one that involves interviews, gathering collateral information, using psychometric instruments, and in some cases laboratory tests as well as scanning and imaging techniques. While sometimes seen as separate parts of the therapeutic endeavour, assessment and treatment can in fact inform each other and be conceptualized as one process (Mental Health Evaluation and Community Consultation Unit 2002). In particular, since the early phase of any intervention often involves the client describing and setting goals, the assessment is an opportunity to engage the individual and motivate him or her to participate in the recovery process (Kopelowicz and Liberman 2003).

What follows is an overview of components of the assessment process, namely the mental status examination, medical tests sometimes used, risk assessment and in particular suicide assessment, structured rating scales, and assessment of psychosocial functioning. Readers should note that while the assessment is a structured process, it is, to use the old cliché, an art as well as a science – not simply a mechanical recitation – one that is dependent on the assessor's ability to conduct an interview skillfully and in particular to be empathetic and to engender trust.

History and Mental Status Examination

The initial assessment usually begins with the "chief complaint," or presenting problem (e.g., "So, what brings you here?"). Even if the client's version of events does not coincide with other sources, the practitioner should be respectful and serious in considering this information. Indeed, the treatment team must to some extent accept where the client "is at" for engagement to be successful. Following this step there is an attempt to get a history of the present illness and previous encounters with the psychiatric system as well as a personal and family history (not always possible in one session and usually involving collateral material from elsewhere). Assessors need to be alert to the possibility of histories of physical/sexual/emotional abuse or neglect and also of substance misuse; while these are both sensitive issues, they are known to be present at high rates among mental health clients and to have considerable significance for treatment planning. An initial assessment may occur at a time of crisis for the client, so assessors must be tuned in to the possibility of suicidal thoughts or intentions.

The **mental status examination (MSE)** involves a consideration of:

- *Appearance and behaviour*, including hygiene, grooming, attitude toward the interviewer, signs of excessive energy, or psychomotor retardation.
- *Speech*: is speech *pressured* (characteristic of mania) or is there poverty of speech?
- *Emotional state*: is the person elated, sad, tearful, or labile (changes mood suddenly), and is affect normal, restricted, or blunted? "Euthymic" refers to an emotional state that is not excessively high or low. A crude test used by practitioners is to ask persons in each session to rate their mood from zero to ten as a way of tracking changes over time. Assessors commonly ask about the "vegetative signs" that are often associated with mood disturbances, such as changes in appetite, energy, and sleep patterns.
- *Thought form*: this refers to disturbances in expression of speech or in the continuity of ideas. There are a number of examples of these, such as a flight of ideas, circumstantiality (taking a long time and many detours before getting to the point), tangentiality (moving away from, and never getting to, the point), echolalia (repetition of other people's words or phrases), loosening of associations (no logical connection between parts of speech), thought blocking, and neologisms (creation of new words).
- *Thought content*: this refers to evidence of delusions, obsessions/compulsions, phobias, and suicidal or homicidal intentions. Delusions may take many forms, including beliefs about persecution, beliefs in special signs or omens, beliefs that the individual is being controlled by external forces, grandiosity, and nihilistic delusions (e.g., that your internal organs are rotting). Beliefs that do not apparently reach the threshold of delusion may be referred to as *overvalued* ideas.
- *Perceptions*: this refers to hallucinations, which may be auditory, visual, or olfactory, and to other disturbances, such as heightened perception and depersonalization (e.g., feeling as if one is in a dream).
- *Cognition and orientation*: clients are typically rated on their orientation to time (what year, month, day is it?), place, and person (usually referring to individuals in the immediate proximity, such as family members). There may be assessment of memory, both short-term (e.g., by having the client repeat three words given earlier in the interview) and long-term (by seeing if recollection of childhood events is consistent with other sources of information). Concentration may be assessed by asking the person to subtract serial 7s from 100. Proverb interpretation is sometimes used to assess whether the person can think in the abstract by referring to

metaphorical meaning, as apposed to a concrete or literal interpretation (although answers here may be influenced by culture, education, and age). A pencil-and-paper test commonly used to assess cognitive ability is the Mini-Mental Status Exam (see below). While all parts of the assessment need to be done with sensitivity, tests of cognition and orientation in particular need to be approached tactfully.

■ *Insight:* the client's awareness of his or her disorder or situation. A common way of testing this is to ask: "Why were you brought to the hospital?" (referring to a psychiatric unit). Sometimes the response will be incongruous or a non sequitur, such as "my back was bothering me." Responses may also be along the lines of "I wasn't bothering anyone, when the police picked me up" – a version of events that needs to be corroborated.

Medical Tests

Medical or laboratory tests – such as computerized tomography (CT) scans – may sometimes be performed in an attempt to clarify diagnosis, particularly to rule out organic causes of psychiatric symptoms. These causes can include toxicity (drug-induced effects), trauma (e.g., concussion or subdural bleeding), infection (e.g., meningitis or syphilis), brain tumours, epilepsy, endocrine dysfunction (e.g., hyperthyroidism), and electrolyte imbalance. However, a care guide published by the University of British Columbia's Department of Psychiatry notes that while CT scans "may reassure patients and families ... the lack of specificity of abnormal findings associated with psychoses suggests that neuroimaging is not necessarily indicated if the neurological exam and history are normal" (Mental Health Evaluation and Community Consultation Unit 2002, 6).

Other lab tests relate to the use of psychotropic medication: for instance, liver and heart function may need to be assessed to make sure that a medication can be metabolized safely. Once started, serum concentrations of some drugs, such as lithium, need to be regularly monitored to ensure that they do not reach toxic levels.

Risk Assessment

Mental health examinations are in part assessments of *risk*, particularly risk of self-harm because of, for example, suicidal thoughts, reckless actions, or neglect of personal care to the point of physical deterioration. Practitioners may have an ethical if not legal duty to intervene in these cases, mandated by provincial mental health and guardianship acts that permit the involuntary hospitalization of persons with mental disorders who are apparently likely to bring harm to themselves. Practitioners may also intervene when there is the potential of harm to others, an example being dangerous driving as the result of a manic episode, which could involve a request to the motor vehicle branch that the individual's driver's licence be temporarily suspended or that the person in question be retested.

Risk factors can be categorized in different ways. On the one hand, there are demographic or actuarial risk factors (used, incidentally, by life insurance companies to calculate client premiums), such as youth, male gender, and First Nations status in the case of suicide risk (Kirmayer, Boothroyd, and Hodgins 1998). The limitations in this case are that risk is assessed in an aggregate-statistical, rather than idiographic, sense and that the factors are "static" – that is, fixed and not amenable to intervention. *Individual* risk factors can be historical – past suicide attempts being a strong predictor of future similar behaviour (Moscicki 1995) – or current, referring to the person's mental state as well as to environmental contingencies that either raise the risk of suicide (such as alcohol use) or are protective (such as a supportive family).

Assessment of risk may be unstructured, based on clinical impression, but may also involve the use of structured clinical guidelines. Examples from the field of forensic psychiatry, where violence to others may be a concern, include the Risk for Sexual Violence Protocol (RSVP), developed by the British Columbia Institute Against Family Violence (Hart, Kropp, and Laws 2003), and the HCR-20, used with persons suffering from serious mental disorders and also developed by Canadian clinicians (Douglas, Ogloff, and Hart 2003; Webster et al. 1997). The HCR-20 addresses twenty factors known to predict violence, Historical (past), Clinical (present), and Risk management (future). To enhance accountability, it is important in any risk assessment process that practitioners consult with colleagues wherever possible, document their actions, and in particular articulate how the assessment conclusion was reached.

Suicide Assessment
As noted previously, persons with mental disorders, particularly depression, bipolar disorder, and schizophrenia, are at higher risk for committing suicide, with one estimate being that 90 percent of all completed suicides are associated with mental or addictive disorders (Moscicki 1995). A study of a large Canadian community mental health program found that the forty-three documented completed suicides over a three-year period by clients of the program represented a rate twenty-five times higher than that seen in the general public (Davis 2000). There is thus a clear indication that mental health practitioners need to regularly consider clients' thoughts and intentions concerning suicide, a process that involves assessment, documentation, and consultation with colleagues and supervisors.

Risk factors for suicide completion can be categorized as follows[1] (American Psychiatric Association 2003; Davis 2000):

(1) Vulnerable populations:
  - includes males, persons with a mental illness, youth, First Nations, the elderly, widowers, and those suffering from a painful, chronic, or terminal physical illness or condition.
(2) Historical factors:
  - previous attempts, history of suicide in the family or among friends, history of abuse or trauma, history of impulsivity, and the proximity of anniversaries of significant events, such as the birthday of a child who was taken away.
(3) Current risk factors:
  - current symptoms of mental illness, such as "command" hallucinations or delusions that support suicide
  - loss of a job, social standing, or relationship (or anticipation of same)
  - living alone or in isolation
  - recent death by suicide of another significant person
  - rigid, "black-and-white" thinking
  - perfectionism
  - recent discharge following a hospitalization for psychiatric reasons[2]
  - use of substances that are depressive or disinhibiting (such as alcohol).
(4) Current thinking:
  - a sense of hopelessness
  - thoughts of suicide that are frequent, persistent, and specific
  - having a plan and the means to carry it out.

A number of psychological and social factors are known to be *protective*, including a positive therapeutic relationship, coping and problem-solving skills, religiosity, sense of humour, having social support, a sense of belonging, and having others to care for, such as children or pets (American Psychiatric Association 2003). There is some debate among mental health practitioners as to whether persons who make a number of (apparently) less serious suicidal attempts or gestures – sometimes referred to as *parasuicidal* behaviour – can be seen as a qualitatively different group. On this question, the evidence suggests that the likelihood of suicide completion increases with each parasuicidal event (Sakinofsky 1994) and that suicide attempters constitute "a distinct but overlapping population with those who die by suicide" (American Psychiatric Association 2003, 21).

In assessing risk of self-harm, it is recommended that the practitioner speak directly and openly about suicide: "Although some fear that raising the topic of suicide will 'plant' the issue in the patient's mind, this is not the case. In fact, broaching the issue of suicidal ideation may be a relief for the suicidal patient by opening an avenue of discussion and giving him or her an opportunity to feel understood" (American Psychiatric Association 2003, 9). There should be a supportive stance and a validation of the pain that the person is going through. The assessor explores current stressors, the history of previous acts and efforts at self-rescue, urgency (is there a plan – e.g., medication stockpile – or a date?), persistence of thoughts of self-harm, and resources (e.g., coping skills and social supports). Where it is clear that there is an imminent risk, hospitalization may need to be arranged. Short of this, the client should be provided with a plan that includes contacts and phone numbers with twenty-four-hour access (such as crisis lines) and contingency measures if contacts are not available. Means of committing suicide, such as pills, should be removed (and future prescriptions for psychotropic medications may need to be for short intervals). In some cases the client is asked to sign a "contract" stipulating that he or she will not attempt suicide within a certain period of time, although there is some debate about the effectiveness of this tactic and whether it creates a sense of false security.

With respect to longer-term case management, the following are important for recovery (Michel et al. 2002):

- a steady therapeutic relationship with (at least initially) frequent contact
- a treatment approach that "works the ambivalence" of the client
- an approach that puts behaviour in historical and biographical context
- the development of coping and problem-solving skills
- the building of a supportive network outside of the mental health program.

Structured Rating Scales

A practice guidelines document notes that during assessments "semi-structured interviews and the use of standardized clinical rating scales are recommended, since they increase diagnostic reliability, ensure consistent coverage, quantify symptom severity, permit later comparisons, and are useful for program evaluation" (Mental Health Evaluation and Community Consultation Unit 2002, 6). A large number of risk assessment and psychometric instruments have in fact been developed that can be applied in community mental health settings, and the interested reader may refer to published compendiums of these rating scales (e.g., Ehmann and Hanson 2004a; Fischer and Corcoran 1994b; Impara and Plake 1998; Murphy, Conoley, and Impara 1994; O'Donovan 2004).

In considering the use of these instruments, the following should be noted: (1) Scales are created for different purposes and are not necessarily used for assessment or clinical applications. Some, such as the Brief Psychiatric Rating Scale, are more commonly used in research, where reliability and comparability of results is the foremost concern (Woerner, Mannuzza, and Kane 1988). An example of a scale used for diagnostic purposes is the Structured Clinical Interview for Axis I DSM-IV Disorders (SCID) (see First, Spitzer, and Gibbon 1995). (2) Some scales have been thoroughly evaluated for validity and reliability, while others have not. (3) Some scales are in the public domain, while use of others may require permission of the copyright holder. (4) Some scales require trained raters, some do not, and some are self-reports. In the case of depression, a commonly used *self*-rating scale is the Beck Depression Inventory (BDI),[3] while the Hamilton Depression Rating Scale (HDRS) is a widely used and accepted *clinician*-rated instrument (O'Donovan 2004).

Rating scales are often used by practitioners working with older clients to test and track cognitive impairment and dementia over time (for a review, see Lorentz, Scanlan, and Borson 2002). One test commonly used with clients where dementia is suspected is the Mini-Mental Status Exam, scored out of 30, which provides a quick assessment of orientation, attention, recall, and use of language. A longer version of this test is the Modified Mini-Mental Status Exam (3MS), which is scored out of 100. While some practitioners may be reluctant to use rating scales, it is advisable in the case of assessing dementia and cognitive impairment since quick, subjective impressions can often be at variance with the client's actual functional ability.

Rating scales are commonly used in the field of addictions to help determine the seriousness of drug and alcohol misuse among clients. Given the high rates of concurrent disorders seen in mental health practice – clients having an addiction as well as a mental disorder – these scales may see greater application by mental health practitioners, who have not traditionally been regarded as addictions experts (for a review, see Health Canada 2001a).

Psychosocial Assessment
More narrowly focused psychiatric assessments may also include, or be supplemented with, assessments of social functioning. A practice guidelines document on interventions with clients experiencing a first psychotic break notes that a psychosocial assessment should obtain information on the following (Mental Health Evaluation and Community Consultation Unit 2002):

- the status of social relationships, including school, work, and recreation
- activities of daily living, including money management, self-care, and domestic roles
- strengths and intact functions to support self-efficacy

- the rate of change of these functions
- cognitive and intellectual status
- stressors, coping abilities, and beliefs about illness
- developmental, academic, occupational, and social histories.

There may be inconsistencies between settings and practitioners as to when (or if) and by whom these psychosocial assessments are performed. While social functioning may be addressed, at least in part, in the initial assessment, often times in multidisciplinary programs, psychosocial assessments are carried out by an occupational therapist (although this may require a referral from a case manager, leading to the potential danger that this important component may be overlooked). Occupational therapists may refer to structured instruments or rating scales for this purpose. It is unfortunately the case that psychosocial assessments and interventions are sometimes regarded as belonging to the area of rehabilitation and thus as "nonclinical," which may diminish their importance; Kopelowicz and Liberman (2003, 1491) point out that such reasoning is fallacious in that "there are no conceptual or operational differences between 'treatment' and 'rehabilitation'" (see also the next chapter).

Special Considerations
Practitioners need to be sensitive about the age, literacy, and cultural background of clients they are assessing. A number of assessment instruments have been developed specifically for children (for a review, see Rapoport and Ismond 1996). Concerning clients from different cultural backgrounds, practitioners may need to make arrangements for translation services and, more generally, should be aware that Western psychiatric terms and concepts may not be easily translated into the idiom of another culture. This in turn speaks to the need for resources – training, consultation, specialized liaison workers – that may assist practitioners in understanding the use of metaphor and imagery particular to the group of people with whom they are working (Bose 1997; see also Chapter 14).

Psychotropic Medication
The medications used in psychiatry are referred to as "psychotropic," which is defined (not very helpfully) as "having an effect on the mind" (Andrews et al. 2000, 110). Since the 1950s the number and type of medications used in psychiatry have increased dramatically, and currently in Canada they form the cornerstone of the treatment offered to persons with serious, persistent mental disorders. To quote the editor of the *Canadian Journal of Psychiatry*, "while many areas have made significant contributions [to psychiatric prac-

tice], the area of psychopharmacology has been in the forefront since the introduction of chlorpromazine for schizophrenia" (Rae-Grant 2002, 513). Critics argue that there is an overreliance on drug therapy, particularly in psychiatry and more generally in medicine (e.g., Smoyak 2004). The counterargument is that until acute symptoms such as psychosis and mania are stabilized, which usually requires the use of medication, the individual will be unable in any case to avail him or herself of other, complementary treatments. Even specialists in psychosocial approaches to rehabilitation concede that "psychosocial services are of little value unless the client is adhering to maintenance antipsychotic, mood stabilizer, and antidepressant regimens" (Kopelowicz and Liberman 2003, 1492). The use of medication as the *sole* treatment is more difficult to defend, especially when one is talking about nonpsychotic and nonmanic disorders.

Before considering the separate categories of medication, it is necessary to speak, more generally, about the mechanisms, effects, and side effects of the drugs used in psychiatry.

To begin with, it is understood that psychotropic drugs affect the activity of **neurotransmitters,** which are chemicals that transmit nerve impulses across the synapse (gap) between nerve cells by attaching to receptor sites (receiving cells) on the neighbouring cell. A number of different neurotransmitters are believed to play a role in psychiatric disorders, including dopamine, serotonin, acetylcholine, norepinephrine, and gamma aminobutyric acid (GABA). How exactly the regulation or dysregulation of these compounds affects the manifestation of psychiatric disorders is not yet clearly understood, although it is known, for example, that dopamine dysregulation plays a role in schizophrenia and that serotonin helps regulate mood and is implicated in depressive disorders.

Psychotropic drugs modify natural physiological events in several ways: (1) they may alter presynaptic activity to prompt neurotransmitter release; (2) they may alter postsynaptic activity by affecting the binding at the receptor site; (3) they may interfere with normal neurotransmitter reuptake processes; and (4) they may alter the manufacture of the receptor cells. These medications can be classified as *agonists*, which means that they increase neurotransmitter effects, or as *antagonists*, which means that they decrease neurotransmitter effects.

One important distinction between different drugs has to do with a drug's *half-life*, which refers to how quickly it is metabolized and clears the system. Injectable antipsychotic drugs, for example, stay in the system for a long time (they may be injected as infrequently as every four weeks), which has advantages with respect to administration but which is a concern if the drug is producing an adverse reaction. Other drugs have short half-lives:

the anti-anxiety agent lorazepam (Ativan) has a shorter half-life than other drugs in its class, which means less daytime sedation and decreased risk of psychomotor impairment but, at the same time, more pronounced withdrawal symptoms and greater likelihood of rebound anxiety (Andrews et al. 2000).

Psychotropic drugs, like all medications, have side effects. While these may diminish with time, it is unfortunately the case that some side effects are persistent and unpleasant enough to deter clients from taking the medication. When this happens, the practitioner must consider alternatives, such as reducing the dose, switching to a different agent, or adding another medication to deal with the side effects. The practitioner is often struggling with a cost-benefit situation while attempting, through trial and error, to arrive at a medication regimen that is the least complicated and that provides maximum therapeutic benefit with minimum side effects. One great difficulty concerns the fact that medication response is very idiosyncratic, meaning that, despite double-blind drug trials, product monographs, and clinical experience, a practitioner can never be certain that any two individuals with the same diagnosis will respond to a medication in the same way (for a discussion of the difficulties of applying "global evidence" from drug trials – "average effects" – to individual cases, see Kravitz, Duan, and Braslow 2004). Some differences in metabolism between individuals, and consequently differences in drug response, are more predictable, being based, for example, on the age or ethnicity of the client; however, some are less predictable, an example being the roughly 8 percent of the Caucasian population that, because of "less efficient" liver enzymes, do not metabolize the antidepressant Paxil as well (Kirkey 2004). While newer medications, such as the "atypical" antipsychotics (see below), have been marketed with the promise of a reduced side-effect profile, it is almost certainly the case that dealing with side effects will be a preoccupation of clients, practitioners, and family members for the foreseeable future.

Particular medication side effects come about because of activity at particular neural receptor sites (for an overview, see Ehmann and Hanson 2004b). Movement disorders associated with the use of antipsychotic drugs (see below), for example, are a side effect of dopamine blockade occurring at the D2 receptor.[4]

Some of the most commonly encountered side effects seen with the use of psychotropic medications include:

- **Extrapyramidal symptoms (EPS),** often seen with the use of older antipsychotic drugs. EPS refers generally to movement disorders, which can include akathisia (a feeling of restlessness in the legs), dystonia (a muscular spasm that can affect the neck, jaws, back, or eyes – the latter referred to as an "oculogyric crisis"), Parkinsonism (stiffness, tremor, loss of facial expression, drooling, or stooped posture), and **tardive dyskinesia** (enduring involuntary movements, usually in the facial muscles, such as the lips and tongue). "Tardive" by definition refers to a late onset; thus a tardive dystonia, for example, is one appearing after sixty days, whereas an acute dystonia is one that manifests right away.

- Anticholinergic effects, which can include dry mouth, blurred vision, and constipation. These are seen particularly with older antipsychotic and antidepressant medications.
- Gastrointestinal effects, including constipation, diarrhea, and nausea. These are seen with a wide range of drugs, including mood stabilizers and antidepressants, although effects are transient in many cases.
- Weight gain, seen particularly with the use of lithium (a mood stabilizer) and antipsychotic drugs such as olanzapine and clozapine.
- Sedation, seen with a range of different medications (response can be idiosyncratic).
- Diminished sex drive and performance, seen with antidepressant drugs such as the selective serotonin reuptake inhibitors (SSRIs) (see below).
- Anxiety and insomnia, seen sometimes with the use of antidepressant medications.
- Rarer, but potentially serious, conditions such as (1) neuroleptic malignant syndrome, which is seen with the use of older antispychotics and which can lead to muscle rigidity, fever, and in some cases death; (2) agranulocytosis, which refers to the diminishing of white blood cells, and consequently of the body's ability to fight infection, and which is a particular concern with the use of the newer antipsychotic clozapine.

Helping a client to talk about and manage side effects, a crucial role for practitioners, is addressed later in this chapter.

In the following description of different drug categories, the reader is reminded that medications have both a generic and a trade name, an example being the antidepressant fluoxetine, which is better known by the trade name Prozac. (Drug companies may manufacture generic forms of a drug originally produced by another company once the patent protection has expired.) In most cases the references here will be to the generic name.

Antipsychotics

Currently, antipsychotic medications (also known as neuroleptics) are classified as either first generation ("typical") or second generation ("**atypical**"). The first generation commenced with the discovery by French researchers in the early 1950s of the antipsychotic properties of chlorpromazine, a drug that is still in use today. Building from this discovery, other agents were developed, including thioridazine, fluphenazine, haloperidol, and loxapine, all of which are now available in generic form. These medications have been found to be effective treatments for the positive symptoms of psychosis – delusions, hallucinations, and thought disorder – although it is estimated that about 30 percent of clients will show only a partial response or no response (Kane 1996). In the jargon of psychiatry, persons who don't respond are said to be **refractory** to a particular type of treatment.

Concerning the mechanism of these agents, it has been found that stimulating the activity of the neurotransmitter dopamine increases symptoms of psychosis and that antagonist medications such as chlorpromazine work against this by blocking dopamine at neural receptor sites. Unfortunately, by doing so, these first-generation medications interfere with motor function and in up to 75 percent of cases produce extrapyramidal side effects (see above) (Blin 1999). Further, in about 5 percent of cases a year, clients may develop tardive dyskinesia, a movement disorder that may be irreversible even after the discontinuation of the medication (Tollefson et al. 1997). To address this problem, most mental health settings now require physicians to assess persons on antipsychotic medication regularly with tests for involuntary movement, an example being the Abnormal Involuntary Movement Scale (AIMS). Other problems associated with using first-generation antipsychotics include oversedation, particularly with "low potency" drugs such as chlorpromazine and thioridazine, as well as hormonal effects (Andrews et al. 2000). Finally, while beneficial for positive symptoms, the first-generation antipsychotics have been found to have little or no impact on the negative symptoms of schizophrenia – such as apathy, blunted affect, and lack of spontaneous speech (Kane and Mayerhoff 1989).

More recently, a number of "atypical" antipsychotics have been developed, including clozapine, risperidone, olanzapine, quetiapine, ziprasidone, amisulpride, and aripiprazole. It has been found that these agents block not just dopamine but other transmitters, such as serotonin, and that they achieve a therapeutic effect at a lower level of dopamine blockade than is the case with the first-generation antipsychotics, one result being that the newer medications are less likely to produce extrapyramidal side effects and tardive dyskinesia (Bailey 2004; Correll, Leucht, and Kane 2004; Ehmann and Hanson 2004).[5] There is also evidence that the newer-generation drugs, by more selectively blocking different receptors, have a beneficial effect on some negative and neurocognitive symptoms, such as working memory and verbal fluency (Blin 1999; Green, Marshall, and Wirshing 1997; Keefe, Arnold, and Bayen 1999; Meltzer and McGurk 1999). A meta-analysis of studies of relapse prevention in schizophrenia with atypical antipsychotics, published in the *American Journal of Psychiatry*, found that "rates of relapse and overall treatment failure were modestly but significantly lower with the newer drugs" (Leucht et al. 2003, 1209) but that "the number of treatment failures was high in both the atypical and conventional drugs groups" (1219) (treatment failure refers to poor medication response and/or non-adherence to treatment, the latter often a result of intolerable side effects). In another study, 1,493 persons diagnosed with schizophrenia were followed for eighteen months after being randomly assigned to treatment with either an older-generation antipsychotic or one of four "atypical" drugs; the overall treatment dropout rate was 74 percent, and it is notable that three of the four atypicals had a higher dropout rate than the older medication (Lieberman et al., 2005).

While the atypical antipsychotics produce fewer extrapyramidal symptoms, they are not without side effects (for a review, see Andrews et al. 2000). One significant problem associated with the use of these newer drugs is weight gain and higher cholesterol levels, which in turn have other medical consequences (Abidi and Bhaskara 2003; Marder et al. 2004; Saari et al. 2004). Data from the Canadian National Outcomes Measurement Study in Schizophrenia found weight gain – defined as over 7 percent of baseline – in 56 percent of persons using quetiapine, 24 percent of those using olanzapine, and 24 percent of those using risperidone (McIntyre et al. 2003).[6] While there is some controversy as to whether weight gain and effects on glucose and lipid metabolism are directly caused by medications, as opposed to an independent, co-existing "metabolic syndrome," schizophrenia treatment guidelines now stipulate that clients should have regular measures of body mass index as well as screening for lipid and glucose levels (Marder et al., 2004).

Another medication that has had its impact limited by side effects is clozapine, which when introduced as an antisychotic showed great promise in achieving a response in individuals who had been resistant to other medications. However, because of the risk of white blood cell suppression, persons using clozapine must get regular, indefinite blood tests (weekly, then biweekly) and be monitored for signs of infection, which has made the product less attractive and usually a treatment of last resort. In commenting on the difficulty of risk-benefit decisions in the use of clozapine, Abidi and Bhaskara (2003) note that the risk of death by suicide among persons with treatment-resistant schizophrenia (1/10) is still considerably higher than the risk of death from agranulocytosis caused by the drug (1/10,000).

Antipsychotic medication is available in oral form (pills and in some cases liquid) and in long-acting injectable ("depot") form. Injections are intramuscular, usually given in the buttock, and are administered at intervals of two to four weeks. The compounds reach a peak plasma level, depending on the product, in two to nine days and have single injection half-lives ranging from four to twenty-one days. The choice of injection over oral administration usually has to do with a client's history of poor compliance with the oral form and is also recommended for persons who are forgetful or disorganized. Currently, the manufacturer of Zyprexa (olanzapine) offers a pill in instant-dissolve ("Zydus") form, another method of dealing with compliance in institutional settings where there is the possibility of clients "cheeking" the medication (Chue et al. 2002). One of the main reasons that clients may still be using the older, typical antipsychotics, apart from the much greater cost of the new products, is that for some time the atypicals were not available in injectable form. This is changing, with, for example, risperidone and olanzapine now being made available as an injection (Wright et al. 2003).

Antidepressants
The majority of antidepressant medications achieve their effect by enhancing the action of neurotransmitters such as serotonin and noradrenaline. As with antipsychotics, antidepressants can be classified as older- and newer-generation. One class of older antidepressants is the monoamine oxidase inhibitors (MAOIs), which include phenelzine and tranylcypromine and which work by inhibiting enzymes that break down serotonin and noradrenaline. Problems with this class of drugs include their toxicity in overdose, which is always a concern when prescribing for depressed persons, and the potential for a hypertensive crisis, which, in rare cases, can be fatal (Andrews et al. 2000). The risk of this reaction is partly managed by dietary restrictions. MAOIs can also be problematic with respect to drug interactions, so the use of other medications must be monitored closely by a physician. MAOIs are rarely prescribed now, although a newer class of antidepressant, *reversible* MAOIs, has been developed, which does not have the dietary restrictions and which is safer in overdose.

Another major class of older antidepressants is the tricyclics, which include amitriptyline (Elavil), clomipramine, and doxepin (all available as generics) and which work by blocking the reuptake of neurotransmitters that include noradrenaline and serotonin. The most common side effects are anticholinergic (see above), and this class is very toxic in overdose due to cardiac complications.

More recently (since the late 1980s), a number of new antidepressant agents have been developed that act more specifically on neurotransmitters, have fewer side effects, and are safer in overdose. One class that remains widely prescribed at the time of writing is the SSRIs, which include fluoxetine (Prozac), fluvoxamine (Luvox), paroxetine (Paxil), and sertraline (Zoloft). The longer-term side effects of this group include lethargy and, in 30 to 70 percent of cases, sexual dysfunction (Nurnberg et al. 2003). Bupropion (Wellbutrin), a newer agent of the class noradrenaline dopamine modulator (NDM), has fewer sexual side effects (this product is also marketed in Canada as a smoking cessation medication under the trade name Zyban).

Antidepressants, unlike some other classes of medication, can take some time to achieve a therapeutic effect, often several weeks, which can result in frustration and ending treatment early. While primarily used for the treatment of depression, the SSRIs may also be prescribed for other conditions, such as obsessive-compulsive disorder (OCD), panic disorder, and bulimia.

Through the 1990s, there was a considerable increase in the use of antidepressants in Canada; this finding does not apparently reflect an increase in the incidence of depression or a change in help-seeking behaviour but suggests "a change in practice patterns, which could be related to changes in the prescribing patterns of physicians or to greater public acceptance of these medications" (Patten and Beck 2004).

While there was initial enthusiasm about the newer-generation antidepressants (e.g., Kramer 1993), in more recent years the use and purported efficacy of these drugs have come under closer scrutiny. In 2002 a meta-analysis of data submitted to the United States Food and Drug Administration covering the years 1987 to 1999 found that approximately 80 percent of the response to SSRI medications was duplicated in placebo control groups, leading to the inference that the difference between the patient's response to medication and response to placebo was small enough to be considered clinically meaningless (Kirsch et al. 2002; see also Vedantam 2002).[7] The study authors qualified this by concluding that the effects of the medications were either very small or being missed by current effectiveness measurements due to how the drug trials were conducted.[8] (The issue of efficacy with respect to antidepressants is further complicated by the fact that they have been prescribed so widely, if not indiscriminately, that there may be some question as to whether users meet the diagnostic criteria for depression.) There have also been concerns expressed about an association between use of SSRIs and increased incidence of suicidal/parasuicidal behaviours (Fergusson et al. 2005). In 2003 concerns about adverse effects of SSRIs and about the lack of an evidence base to support their use in children with depression led to restrictions being placed on the use of most SSRIs with juveniles in the United Kingdom. Following the lead of the British, in February 2004 Health Canada issued an advisory on the use of SSRIs and serotonin noradrenaline reuptake inhibitors (SNRIs) by persons under eighteen, stating that these patients "should consult their treating physician to confirm that the benefits of the drugs still outweigh the risks in light of recent safety concerns," this referring to "an increased risk of suicide-related events in patients under 18" (Health Canada 2004a, 1).

Mood Stabilizers

Mood stabilizers are used for the acute treatment of mania and hypomania and for the ongoing management of bipolar disorder. They may be prescribed for other conditions where there is a mood component, such as schizoaffective disorder.

A trio of drugs has been used for some time as the main pharmacological treatments for bipolar disorder: lithium (in the form lithium carbonate) and two antiseizure agents, carbamazepine (Tegretol) and valproic acid. Lithium is a naturally occurring element that was found to have antimania properties by an Australian psychiatrist in 1949, although the physiological mechanism by which the therapeutic effects are achieved remains unclear (Sadock and Sadock 2003). Lithium, while clearly effective for mania, can become toxic at relatively low levels, which can, in some cases, lead to kidney damage, coma, and even death. As a result, blood levels need to be monitored regularly to ensure that the serum concentration is not below or above the therapeutic range. Apart from overdose, use of lithium may in the longer term produce a fine tremor and weight gain. Side effects associated with the other two medications include gastrointestinal problems and some less common but potentially serious effects, such as agranulocytosis in the case of carbamzepine (Andrews et al. 2000).

More recently, other antiseizure agents have been proposed as possible treatments for bipolar disorder, including gabapentin, lamotrigine, and topiramate. In a review article, Gorman (2003, 96) notes that evaluations of these newer agents as treatments for bipolar disorder have produced mixed results; gabapentin has not proven to be effective, although lamotrigine "demonstrated the most potent effect in treating the depressions suffered by bipolar patients."

Benzodiazepines

The benzodiazepines are the class of drugs most commonly used as antianxiety agents, although they may be prescribed for a number of other conditions, including insomnia and alcohol withdrawal, as a treatment for extrapyramidal side effects, and as an adjunctive treatment for schizophrenia, bipolar disorder, and other mood and anxiety disorders. Indeed, that they are *so* widely used has become a source of controversy, particularly the finding that, despite the recommended short duration of use, prescriptions often run for long periods of time (Valenstein et al. 2004; see also box on next page).

There are a large number of products in this class, examples being diazepam (Valium), lorazepam (Ativan), oxazepam (Serax), and clonazepam (Rivotril), all now available as generics. Physiologically, these agents cause more complete bonding of the neurotransmitter GABA to its receptor sites. The key difference between the various benzodiazepines has to do with their half-lives; longer half-life drugs such as clonazepam require less frequent doses, have more stable plasma concentrations, and have milder withdrawal symptoms but cause more daytime sedation, a greater accumulation of the drug in the body, and more psychomotor impairment (Andrews et al. 2000). Benzodiazepine use, in the long term, can lead to dependency and **tolerance**, which refers to the need to keep increasing the dose to achieve the same effect. Long-term use means that the body's natural benzodiazepine compounds diminish, so when the drug is withdrawn, particularly if this is done abruptly, a withdrawal syndrome can occur, symptoms of which include "rebound" insomnia, anxiety, restlessness, and irritability.

Stimulants

Stimulant medications are most often associated with the treatment of attention-deficit hyperactivity disorder (ADHD), although they may be prescribed for other conditions, such as depression and narcolepsy. Studies of the use of these drugs with schoolchildren have found that they improve concentration and academic performance (Sadock and Sadock 2003; Klassen et al. 1999), with one review concluding that "the effectiveness of stimulants for the short-term treatment of ADHD is well documented and constitutes the largest body of evidential literature in child psychiatry pharmacology" (McClellan and Werry 2003, 1392). The exact mechanism of action of these compounds is not clearly understood; one hypothesis is that stimulant drugs increase central nervous system activity in parts of the brain that are responsible for inhibition (Nathan, Gorman, and Salkind 1999). Examples of drugs in this category are methylphenidate (Ritalin), dextroamphetamine, and modafinil. Side effects, which can be seen as exaggerations of the main effects, include agitiation, tremor, and tachycardia. Other effects include weight loss (which is a desired effect when the drug is in the form of a diet pill), mood changes, and in some cases psychosis, with one Canadian study finding that in 6 percent of cases children with ADHD being prescribed stimulants developed psychotic symptoms (Cherland and Fitzpatrick 1999). Because of the potential for abuse and addiction, use of these medications must be monitored closely (medication orders require a triplicate prescription). Despite concerns about the use of these compounds,

Benzodiazepines: A Pill for Every Ill

Benzodiazepines are among the most widely used medications in Canada, with the number of prescriptions written increasing each year (Hermann 2002). In British Columbia alone, 1.585 million prescriptions (including refills) were written in 2001, an increase of 14.6 percent over four years (Hermann 2002). As noted, benzodiazepine use can be problematic because of the addictive properties of these drugs and because of withdrawal effects. Among the elderly – a group that is frequently prescribed benzodiazepines – using these drugs has also been blamed for falls and broken bones as well as incontinence (Landi et al. 2002; Hogan et al. 2003). A Vancouver woman, Joan Gadsby, went so far as to sue her doctor for allegedly turning her into a "benzo" addict, writing about her travails in the book *Addiction by Prescription* (2000).

Canadian writers who have interviewed physicians and specialists about prescribing benzodiazepines and other psychotropic drugs have found decision making to be driven by both good intentions and expedience (Branham 2003; Hermann 2002). A Vancouver psychiatrist sums up the "doctor's dilemma" as follows: "As physicians, we want to be helpful, but we often suffer individually and collectively from a pharmacological imperative: if we have a drug we feel compelled to prescribe it. We suffer from excessive therapeutic optimism" (quoted in Branham 2003, B3). Another psychiatrist notes simply that, for anxiety disorders, benzodiazepines "work" and more quickly than do antidepressants (Hermann 2002, A4). Other respondents suggest that family physicians, because of the fee structure, don't have the time to counsel patients or, for that matter, the interest or the skills necessary to deal with the patient's disclosures, finding it easier to write a prescription instead. Currently, provincial fee schedules result in physicians being paid the same "whether they do a 15 minute examination and prescribe a pill, or take twice as long to counsel patients and teach them strategies to cope with anxiety and depression" (Branham 2003, B3). While acknowledging that "'a pill for every ill' is still the dominant model," another physician speaks about the need for "moral integrity" among practitioners, which implies taking the time to establish a clear diagnosis and to explore approaches other than the use of tranquilizers (Hermann 2002, A4). Because of pressure from patient advocates, medical associations in Canada are now distributing manuals on benzodiazepine addiction and withdrawal to their members.

a survey of Alberta psychiatrists found that almost half – 47 percent – of respondents were prescribing stimulants to adult patients, a result that the authors concluded was "higher than expected" (Beck et al. 1999).

Cognitive Enhancers
These medications are for the symptomatic treatment of mild to moderate forms of Alzheimer's dementia and include donepezil and tacrine, both of which work by increasing the concentration of acetylcholine in the synaptic clefts. One review concludes that donepezil is "associated with a statistically significant but clinically modest improvement in cognitive function in a substantial minority of patients with mild to moderate Alzheimer's disease" (Flint and Reekum 1998, 689). Side effects of these compounds include gastrointestinal difficulties, drooling, and bradycardia.

Augmenting Agents
A number of different compounds, including lithium, tryptophan, thyroid hormone, and beta-blockers (Pindolol), have been found to enhance the activity of antidepressant medication.

Antiparkinsonians
These drugs are used to treat the side effects caused by antipsychotic medications, particularly extrapyramidal symptoms. There is some debate as to whether they should be used in an ongoing, prophylactic fashion or only when EPS has developed (Andrews et al. 2000). There are several different categories: anticholinergic agents (e.g., benztropine and procyclidine), antihistamines (e.g., diphenhydramine), beta-blockers (e.g., propranolol), dopamine agonists (e.g., amantadine), and benzodiazepines (e.g., lorazepam).

Special Considerations
How drugs are absorbed, metabolized, and excreted is affected by the age, gender, ethnicity, and physical health of the client, and these factors need to be taken into account when psychotropic medications are being considered. For example, it has been found that persons of Asian ancestry metabolize psychotropic medications more slowly and need to be given lower doses (Janicak et al. 2001). Metabolism also changes with age, meaning that elderly people are generally more sensitive to psychotropic agents, necessitating lower doses. Since older adults are also more likely to be on other types of medication, drug interactions may be a problem. A basic principle in prescribing for the elderly is "start low, go slow, and avoid multiple medications" (Andrews et al. 2000, 152).

Smoking can also affect how drugs are metabolized and can lower the blood levels of some antipsychotic medications by up to 50 percent (Mental Health Evaluation and Community Consultation Unit 2002).

Another area of concern is the client who is, or may be, pregnant. The approach in this situation is summarized by Andrews and colleagues (2000, 15): "In general, unnecessary use of medication is to be discouraged during pregnancy and, wherever possible, all medication is to be avoided during the first 12 weeks of pregnancy. However, in some cases medication is considered necessary and will be prescribed if the benefits ... outweigh all possible risks. For example, the risks associated with untreated psychosis or affective illness are generally higher than the risks of taking drugs." While not all drugs may be harmful, drugs that are associated with fetal malformation include lithium, carbamazepine, valproic acid, and clonazepam. Older antispychotics may increase the risk of fetal malformation if given in the first trimester of pregnancy, while at the time of writing there was insufficient information concerning the effect of atypical antipsychotics on the developing fetus (Patton et al. 2002; Seeman 2004).

Prescribing for young children carries with it a set of practical and ethical concerns, such as diagnostic uncertainty and the fact that the safety and efficacy of psychotropics with this age group has not been adequately tested in many cases (Jensen 1998: McClellan and Werry 2003). On this issue, a review article in the *Canadian Medical Association Journal* concludes that "because medications are less commonly tested in children, much of pediatric prescribing involves educated guesses about doses, safety and effectiveness. A lack of appreciation of the differences between children and adults often results in the inappropriate extrapolation of data derived from adults to the pediatric population. This situation is dangerous. It either deprives children of the benefits of drug therapy withheld because of lack of information, or exposes them to unknown side effects" (Matsui et al. 2003, 1033).

As noted above, in 2003 British regulators issued a directive stating that no new prescriptions for the SSRI class of antidepressants (fluoxetine being exempted) or for venlafaxine (an SNRI) should be written for persons under eighteen (this directive concerned clients diagnosed with depression, not anxiety disorders). These decisions were based on findings that the limited evidence of medication efficacy could not compensate for the fact that "adverse effects [were] at least as likely as any antidepressant effects" (Branham 2003, B2). Following this, in 2004 Health Canada issued a (more qualified) advisory concerning the use of SSRIs and SNRIs in persons under eighteen, requesting that young patients consult their physicians about the risk-to-benefit ratio of these drugs in light of reports of "an increased risk of suicide-related events" (Health Canada 2004a, 1).[9] The drugs in question included buproprion (Wellbutrin), citalopram (Celexa), fluvoxamone (Luvox), mirtazapine (Remeron), paroxetine (Paxil), sertraline (Zoloft), and venlafaxine (Effexor).[10] In the advisory it is noted that Health Canada had requested "a thorough review of worldwide safety data" from the drug manufacturers. The murky state of regulating drug use in children is reflected in the following disclaimer, contained in the advisory: "It is important to note that Health Canada has not approved these drugs for use in patients under 18 years. The prescribing of drugs is a physician's responsibility. Although SSRIs/SSNIs are not approved for use with children, doctors rely on their knowledge of patients to determine whether to prescribe them in a practice called off-label use" (1).

Despite not being approved for use in children, it was reported that in 2002 British Columbia physicians wrote 49,667 prescriptions of SSRIs for patients under eighteen, more than twice as many as five years previously, and that 45 of these prescriptions were written for children aged six or younger (Branham 2004).

The Issue of Medication Noncompliance

Not infrequently, practitioners and family members will have to wrestle with the issue of medication noncompliance, which may range from feelings of ambivalence to outright refusal on the part of the client to take psychotropic medication. Indeed, some methods of drug administration (e.g., injectable antipsychotics, instant-dissolve tablets) are specifically designed to get around the problem of noncompliance. It is estimated that over one-third of persons receiving oral antipsychotic medication will start varying from the prescribed regimen within the first month of treatment (Johnson 1990). Persons refusing medication may simply not believe that they have a condition requiring pharmacological treatment, and in these instances they may be characterized as "lacking in insight"; on this point, one author suggests that about 50 percent of persons with schizophrenia have "impaired awareness" of their condition (Levine 2004, 27). However, treatment refusal is a complex matter, and in many cases client concerns are eminently reasonable (Bentley and Walsh 2001; Valentine, Waring, and Giuffrida 1992). Further, developing an adversarial approach toward a client on this matter is usually fruitless since both practitioner and client need to be "on board" as collaborators for the relationship to work in the long run (Jeffries 1996).

To begin with, practitioners need to identify the client's concerns. While clinicians may feel sure that they know what the issues are, studies comparing clients' and physicians' responses to a "reasons for stopping medication" survey have found, in many instances, a low level of agreement between the two groups (Pope and Scott 2003).

One obvious area of concern is side effects, which can include movement disorders, weight gain, and diminished sex drive – matters no one should take lightly. As reviewed by Andrews and colleagues (2000), practitioners should closely monitor these effects and where necessary consider changing the medication, reducing the dose, prescribing divided doses, making sure medications are taken with appropriate food, or adding a medication to treat the side effects. Strategies can also be employed for particular side effects, concerning diet, exercise, and alcohol and caffeine intake, strategies that will be more or less onerous depending on the individual.

Another area of concern may be the complexity of the medication regimen, which may require taking a number of different pills at various times of the day and night. (Hospitals may initiate regimens to which adherence is difficult in community settings.) Administration orders should be streamlined as much as possible, and clients may be assisted by having medications put in blister packs or dosette containers.

Sometimes clients may not like the idea of having to take medications long term, particularly when troubling symptoms are no longer present. A common lay understanding is that medications are taken to deal with a particular problem, such as an infection, then stopped. However, in the case of mental disorders such as schizophrenia, psychiatric practice guidelines advocate longer-term, maintenance treatment even after symptoms have subsided – based partly on the concern that recovery from subsequent relapses, should they occur, will be increasingly difficult (Mental Health Evaluation and Community Consultation Unit 2002). Clients may be given the diabetes analogy – that is, that antipsychotic medications, like insulin, are given to manage symptoms but must be taken indefinitely and will not cure the illness.

Weighing up the costs and benefits of long-term medication use is not an easy matter. Practitioners may point to the danger of relapse and to the apparently degenerative effect of untreated schizophrenia. Nevertheless, because outcomes in schizophrenia are known to be variable, rational optimism and supporting the client's freedom to make mistakes are two psychologically important attitudes now being identified as core practitioner competencies in mental health (Coursey et al. 2000). Any decision about ending treatment must be balanced against the known likelihood and degree of risk if the client decompensates.

Sometimes clients will point out that it is their *right* to refuse medication, which is true in most instances (an exception is the case of persons certified for hospitalization and deemed incompetent with respect to treatment choices). In these situations practitioners should strive to keep communication channels open and maintain contact rather than shutting down the therapeutic relationship. The advantage here, apart from the ability to monitor the health and safety of the client when off medication, is that the client will hopefully see the worker as someone who will stick with him or her in good times and in bad.

A number of other factors underlie treatment nonadherence:

- Some persons may enjoy the effects of the disorder. For example, this author has been told by one individual that medication "prevents me from having a religious experience" and by another that the high he achieved when manic was "the greatest feeling in the world."
- Self-dosing and experimenting with tapering off medications may also speak to the sense of control that we all need and that is lost when we turn our lives over to drug regimens.
- Families and significant others may not support the view that medication is necessary.
- Medications may interfere with the ability to concentrate on various tasks.

In sum, a number of reasonable concerns underlie medication nonadherence, concerns that may reflect broader, existential struggles with which the client is dealing. Practitioners should work with clients to identify these concerns and to come up with strategies to deal with them, although this will not always be possible. To this end, nonphysician practitioners may need to advocate on behalf of clients with physicians or help clients to develop assertiveness skills so that they can negotiate with physicians themselves.

Other Physical Treatments

ECT
Electroconvulsive therapy (ECT) involves inducing a minor brain seizure by the application of a brief electric current to sites on the scalp. The procedure has been in use since the mid-1930s, when it was given to individuals with schizophrenia, this based on the observation that schizophrenic symptoms decreased after a seizure and on the (unfounded) belief that schizophrenia and epilepsy could not coexist in the same person (Sadock and Sadock 2003). A major problem with early versions of ECT was the discomfort that it produced and the fact that some seizures were severe enough to result in broken bones. With improvements in anesthesia and muscle relaxants, these severe consequences have largely been eliminated, and despite a negative public image, the technique is now considered safe and effective (Andrews et al. 2000; United Kingdom ECT Review Group 2003). The most common side effects are short-term headaches and muscle pain; while ECT has the

reputation of producing memory loss, the best evidence suggests that this is transient and that long-term impairment of memory is "minimal or absent" (Gray, Shone, and Liddle 2000, 92).

Nowadays ECT is primarily used for persons suffering from depression or bipolar disorder, particularly when other treatments (medication and psychotherapy) have failed or when there is an increased risk of self-neglect or suicide. ECT seems to be especially effective with forms of depression where somatic (melancholic) or psychotic symptoms are present. The exact mechanism by which this is achieved is still not fully understood. Treatments are usually given three times a week for one to five weeks. This is sometimes done on an outpatient basis, but usually the patient is hospitalized.

RTMS

A relatively new treatment for depression, which has some parallels with ECT, is repetitive transcranial magnetic stimulation (RTMS). This technique, developed in the mid-1980s, was only an experimental procedure in North America until recent years (Kozel and George 2002). It involves a handheld electrical coil, which is positioned on the scalp and which creates a magnetic pulse that passes through the brain. An advantage of RTMS is that it is noninvasive, does not require a general anesthetic, and does not produce seizures, possibly giving it some advantages for very frail patients (Haynes 2002). While there is some evidence that RTMS is as effective as ECT for persons suffering from depression (Dannon et al. 2002), at the time of writing, the procedure was not widely known by practitioners, and those treatments that were offered were through private-pay clinics.[11]

Psychosurgery

The practice of psychosurgery, vividly depicted in movies like *One Flew Over the Cuckoo's Nest*, "has gone down in history as one of modern medicine's most barbaric practices" (Simmie and Nunes 2001, 238). Introduced by a Portuguese doctor in the mid-1930s, the *lobotomy* involved severing white matter in the frontal lobes of the brain and had become a relatively common procedure for treating psychosis by the late 1940s (Sadock and Sadock 2003). These surgeries in some cases produced a calming effect but also altered personality and cognitive functioning. While lobotomies are no longer performed, a procedure called limbic surgery is currently used – in rare circumstances – as a treatment of last resort for persons with severe forms of obsessive-compulsive disorder and depression. Limbic surgery involves fixing the patient's head in a metal frame, bilaterally drilling small holes in the skull, then using a heated instrument to produce a small lesion (about the size of a pea) in the brain tissue. In a description of a program operated at the University of British Columbia, it is noted that persons accepted for surgery must have been suffering from severe incapacitation for at least five years (which often means chronic suicidality) and have tried and failed with every other available treatment (Haynes 2002).

Hospitalization

Hospitalization is primarily used when there are concerns about safety and security, although it may also be recommended for clarifying diagnosis or when procedures such as ECT or initiation of clozapine treatment are being undertaken. In a Canadian Psychiatric Association document on the guidelines for the treatment of depression, it is noted that indications for hospitalization include "concern for the safety of others or the patients themselves, crisis intervention, diagnostic evaluation (especially with comorbid medical or psychiatric conditions), poor response to outpatient treatment, rapid deterioration or marked severity of depression (including hopelessness, suicidal ideation, or psychotic features), inability to function at home, and breakdown of social supports" (Reesal and Lam 2001, 25S).

The duration of stay in Canadian general hospital psychiatric units declined from the 1980s through the 1990s: from 1987 to 1999 the mean length of stay fell by 20 percent for persons with major depression, by 27 percent for persons with bipolar disorder, and by 26 percent for persons with schizophrenia (Health Canada 2002b). While these findings can be seen as an indication that there are now better community supports in place, making longer hospitalization unnecessary in most cases, they are almost certainly also a reflection of increasingly scarce hospital resources and the consequent pressure to discharge patients as soon as possible (Reesal and Lam 2001). One result of this has been a perception on the part of community practitioners that clients are being discharged prematurely in many cases, based in part on the observation that clients may still be fragile in the period immediately after hospital discharge (Hirschfeld and Davidson 1988).[12] The perception that hospitals discharge clients prematurely may be based on a misunderstanding of what the hospital's role in the present era should be. A best-practices document describes the rationale behind hospitalization as follows: "The goal is to make 'sick' people less 'sick,' *not necessarily 'well.'* Once they can be managed in a less restrictive environment, they are discharged unless it can be demonstrated that remaining in hospital leads to a better clinical outcome" (British Columbia Ministry of Health 2002e, 17, emphasis added).

Pressure on inpatient resources may also (unfortunately) influence decisions about how, or whether, to hospitalize a client in the first place: while it can be argued that voluntary admission is preferable, the community physician may lean toward involuntary admission based on the fear that an individual presenting him or herself at hospital as a voluntary patient may not be taken as seriously (this is apart from the problem of persons having to wait for hours in emergency departments to see a doctor, getting fed up, and leaving). On the other hand, in decisions *not* to hospitalize the person, community practitioners may weigh the cost of certifying a client – in terms of damaged rapport with the individual – against the limited benefits that will be achieved, the assumption being, based on prior experience, that the client will be quickly discharged. However, practitioners need to be reflective and wary about this sort of cynicism in their decision making and should continue to advocate for the best care for their clients.

Following hospital admission, because the client is now dealing with (in most cases) a completely different treatment team, continuity and communication between the hospital and community become crucial. It is an obligation of both parties to transmit relevant documents so that, at point of admission, hospital staff have some history, background information, and a sense of the client's "baseline" functioning so that, at point of discharge, community staff get a review of what was done in hospital, whether there were changes in medication, and how the client responded. It is unfortunately the case that, because of the pressure on hospital beds and staff time, clients may be discharged with little or no warning to the community and with insufficient supports in place. (The BC Schizophrenia Society has created and posted on its website [http://www.bcss.org/information_centre/hospital_discharge_planning.html] a "discharge checklist" so that family members can see that issues such as medication, housing, and follow-up care have been addressed prior to discharge.) Hospital staff may in turn complain that they cannot get follow-up appointments from community programs in a timely fashion: for example, the mental health advocate of British Columbia noted in her 2001 annual report that only 20 percent of community mental health clients had contacts for follow-up care within thirty days of being discharged from hospital (Hall 2001).[13]

Hospital and community staff work with different pressures (as noted) and indeed different frames of reference. While a client readmission may be seen by the hospital – and by health authority evaluators – as a "failure," community practitioners may, paradoxically or not, see the same event as a "success" because it is seemingly so difficult to get clients into hospital or because at least now the individual about whom they have been worrying will have a roof over his or her head and three square meals a day. Disagreements may arise over the purpose and appropriateness of hospitalization, with the argument being made that long-term admissions are counterproductive – that one fairly quickly reaches a point of diminishing returns – or that with some clinical presentations, hospitalization should be ruled out altogether (see Dawson 1988). While these hospital-community tensions may not always be resolvable, face-to-face encounters between staff from the two areas are recommended, either in meetings, case conferences, ward rounds, or committees, as a way of understanding the vantage point of the "other." Having staff with cross-appointments – physicians who work both in hospital and community settings – can be helpful with respect to bridging the disconnection between the two perspectives.

Notes

1 The author is grateful for the assistance of Dr. Natalee Popadiuk with this section.
2 There are several hypotheses to account for this finding: (1) that patients are being discharged prematurely while still in a fragile state of mind; (2) that patients *successfully* treated can now see with some clarity how poor their career and relationship prospects really are; (3) that patients who were dependent on the care provided in hospital, and who had few resources in the community, became despondent when discharged (Davis 2000).
3 With the advent of the Internet, there are now "make your own diagnosis" websites, such as that of Canadian psychiatrist Dr. Phil Long (http://www.mentalhealth.com).
4 It has for some time been hypothesized that persons with schizophrenia have a predisposition for movement disorders *independent of* any medication side effects. Establishing this, however, is complicated by the difficulty in identifying "medication naive" subjects at the prodromal phase and by the limitations of retrospective research designs.
5 However, in commenting on the drug trial methodology, the authors of the second study cited note that "the doses of the haloperidol used in the comparator studies were relatively high" (414).
6 Interpreting these results is complicated by the hypothesis that persons with schizophrenia have a predisposition to becoming obese independent of any other contributing factors, such as medication effects (see Yager 2004).
7 The "placebo effect" has proven to be a complex phenomenon. While previously thought to be just a psychological process, research on Parkinson's disease conducted at the University of British Columbia discovered that placebo pills were able to achieve a biochemically based therapeutic effect, similar to that of a "real" therapeutic agent, by causing a release of the neurotransmitter dopamine, although the underlying mechanism remains unclear (Motluk 2001). Another author suggests that the benefit derived from taking a pill – whether that be a placebo or "active agent" – "may come from the care and concern shown to patients during a clinical trial" (Vedantam 2002, A01).
8 Statistically minded readers may note that the first of these refers to a "type I" error and the second to a "type II" error.
9 It is noteworthy that in the Canadian advisory, as opposed to the British directive, a clear onus is still placed on the consumer to monitor the safety of their own prescribed medications.
10 Concerning the association between suicidality and antidepressant use, a British review found that suicidal events were much more likely to occur in the first nine days after starting a prescription than they were to occur in the ninety days afterward, indicating a need for careful monitoring in the early stages of treatment (Jick, Kaye, and Jick 2004).
11 See the http://www.mindcarecentres.com.
12 In a study of suicide attempts by clients of a Vancouver, British Columbia, mental health program, it was found that, for those hospitalized within the year prior to the attempt, 40 percent (38/95) were discharged within *one month* of their subsequent suicide attempt (Davis 2000). It must be acknowledged, however, that the method used limits any conclusions about a causal relationship between hospital discharge and suicidal behaviour.

13 Unfortunately, it was not clear from the report whether this meant that clients were being referred and having to wait, whether referrals were not always being made, or whether appointments were given but clients did not show up.

Other Resources

■ A good resource for persons interested in assessing risk of violence is the webpage of Simon Fraser University (SFU) professor Stephen Hart (http://www.sfu.ca/psyc/faculty/hart), which links to "Violence Risk Assessment Resources" and SFU's Mental Health Law and Policy Institute.

■ The Canadian Association for Suicide Prevention has its website at http://www. suicideprevention.ca.

■ The Australian State of Victoria operates a website with information for consumers on psychotropic drugs (see http://www.health.vic.gov.au/mentalhealth/druginfo/index.htm).

Education, Skills Training, and Cognitive-Behavioural Approaches

11

Philosophies about psychiatric treatment have shifted considerably over the past half-century, from Freudian psychology and psychodynamic approaches – "talk therapy" – which still held sway in the 1950s, to biological psychiatry and pharmacotherapy, which were preeminent in the 1970s and 1980s, to present-day psychological treatments – particularly cognitive-behavioural therapies – which are once again a mainstream approach, even in cases of "serious, persistent mental illness." At the same time, and of equal if not greater significance, the *belief system* underlying our treatment approach has been challenged, particularly the ideas of the client as a dependent, passive recipient of professional wisdom and of the practitioner as a detached, expert/authority figure (Curtis and Hodge 1995).

In considering the growing emphasis on approaches to treatment and rehabilitation other than, or complementary to, pharmacotherapy, one can point out several contributing factors:

- *The limitations of medication.* Despite the advantages (actual and purported) of newer-generation products, the fact remains that, for a number of reasons, not all persons with mental disorders benefit from taking medications (Keller 2002). For example, it is estimated that 30 percent of persons with positive symptoms of schizophrenia experience only small gains with antipsychotics, while 7 percent do not respond at all (Johnstone and Sandler 1998). A large-scale study comparing the effects of cognitive-behavioural therapy with the effects of antidepressant medication found that 45 percent of subjects showed no clinically significant response to the medication (alone) after twelve weeks of treatment (Keller et al. 2000). On this point, it should be noted that conditions such as depression are often *multidetermined* by social and lifestyle factors as well as by biology; thus, as one treatment manual concludes, "Medication is seldom a *complete* treatment" (Paterson et al. 1996, 8, emphasis in the original). Even if effective in one domain, medications may not be effective in others: one rehabilitation specialist concludes that antipsychotic medication "does little if anything to improve individuals' social and instrumental role functioning" (Wallace 1998, 9).

- *Empirical support.* It can now be said that a number of nonpharmacological treatments and programs are evidence-based – that is, have been shown to be beneficial using systematic methods of evaluation.[1] In the United Kingdom, the National Health Service agreed in 2003 to publicly fund cognitive-behavioural treatments for persons with schizophrenia – a relatively new technique – on the basis of positive empirical support for the therapy (American Association for the Advancement of Science 2003).
- *Concerns of clients and advocacy groups.* For example, in a report from the mental health advocate for British Columbia, the author concluded that the government needed to "develop the workforce" – that is, improve the skill sets of mental health practitioners so that the system could move beyond a "custodial" approach to mental health care (Hall 2000, 31). In particular, the lack of staff training and service availability in the area of anxiety disorders – which are often responsive to behavioural treatments – came in for criticism. The mental health advocate noted that "the limited treatment strategies available through the regional system and fee for service medicine are not evidence-based and create dependencies" (14). The Anxiety Disorders Association of British Columbia (n.d.) similarly concluded that there were a "lack of available treatment avenues" and a "shortage of public funds." As another example, in an editorial entitled "Changing the paradigm," a self-described psychiatric user/survivor criticizes the system's preoccupation with pharmacotherapy and speaks about the need for "medical coverage for non-drug medical support," such as "counseling, 'talk therapy' ... and coping skills education" (Thor-Larsen 2002, 4).

This chapter gives an overview of the counselling approaches most commonly used in public mental health programs in Canada. Psychodynamic treatments, such as psychoanalysis, and approaches such as Gestalt therapy are not covered here for several reasons: (1) these interventions are used predominantly by private practitioners; (2) they are used mostly with individuals less disabled than those typically seen at public mental health centres[2] and, indeed, have been seen as contraindicated when the client suffers from a psychotic disorder (Fenton 2000; Gunderson et al. 1984; Norman and Townsend 1999); and (3) there is uncertainty about the evidence base and benefits of a treatment such as psychoanalysis (Paris 2005; Shorter 1997; Wood 1986).

In this chapter a number of divisions are made – for example, separating "education and skills training" from "cognitive-behavioural approaches." While perhaps convenient, this is a false dichotomy in that many cognitive-behavioural approaches explicitly *involve* skills training. Similarly – looking ahead to the next chapter – an awkward distinction is made in community mental health between "treatment" and "rehabilitation." Since the latter also involves skills training and has direct impacts on clients' mental health, it inevitably overlaps with the former. In commenting on what they see as the "mistaken belief that treatment and rehabilitation are different enterprises," Kopelowicz and Liberman (2003, 1491) note that "there are no conceptual or operational differences" between the two, with the main distinction being that interventions are applied at different points along the continuum of relapse and recovery; perpetuating the dichotomy, they argue, "can only have adverse effects on our efforts to ... provide continuous and comprehensive care to our clients."

It should be pointed out that many practitioners working in community mental health centres are eclectic in their use of psychological techniques. This stance has been supported by those who see the need for a range of approaches to address the diverse needs of mental health clients, as opposed to the rigid application of a single model (Maguire 2002). Using techniques drawn from different areas clearly has some advantages with respect to flexibility and pragmatism, although it must be acknowledged that this sort of eclecticism may also be driven by time restrictions and less than comprehensive knowledge of particular treatment models. Since some models require consistent application of a range of protocols, such as Linehan's (1993a, 1993b) program for working with persons diagnosed with borderline personality disorder, compromising this necessity may actually work against treatment gains. In the same vein, a commentator notes that persons who talk about having "failed" at cognitive-behavioural therapy (CBT) may in fact have been exposed to something "CBT-like" that fell short of a systematic application of the complete model (Lott 2001). Because eclecticism may result in "confusion instead of coherence" (Meyer 1983, 731), there is increasing recognition of the need to integrate the various components of treatment. For example, Andrews and colleagues (2000, 252-53) describe a management plan for persons with agoraphobia that includes medication, education, training in anxiety control strategies, and graded exposure to feared situations. Similarly, Hogarty (1995), working with persons diagnosed with schizophrenia, describes a "personal therapy" based on an individualized approach that pulls together various elements, such as medication, education, relaxation, and cognitive strategies.

With case managers now expected to know and put into practice a wider range of nonpharmacological approaches, there is some pressure on administrators to reexamine staff education as well as the mandates and service delivery models used in community mental health settings. Some comment on this issue is offered at the end of the chapter.

Education and Skills Training

Education and skills training have increasingly come to be recognized as crucial components in a comprehensive psychiatric rehabilitation plan. That this was not always the case is the result of several factors: (1) a model of "professional as authority/expert" that did not apparently include empowerment of clients; (2) during the mid-1900s, influential psychodynamic theories that placed the root of clients' psychiatric problems in the *unconscious* mind, meaning that self-help was by definition not possible; (3) clinical pessimism about the prognosis of disorders such as schizophrenia; and (4) evolution of a service delivery structure where there was an overreliance on pharmacotherapy to the neglect of other interventions.

Education and skills training for clients of the mental health system have more recently been referred to as elements of **self-management**, a term and set of concepts borrowed in part from the "chronic disease model," which has been applied to the treatment of persons suffering from, for example, asthma, diabetes, or arthritis (Bilsker 2003). In describing self-management, Canadian psychologist Dan Bilsker notes that this refers to "an active engagement of the health care consumer in dealing with his or her disorder, meaning that the person with the disorder is an active participant in care, rather than someone who simply follows recommendations and complies with the treatment plan developed by a health professional ... [clients are given] a central role in determining their care, one that fosters a sense of responsibility for their own health. Using a collaborative approach, providers and patients work together to define problems, set priorities, establish goals, create treatment plans and solve problems along the way" (4). Responding to the argument that persons with mental disorders are too uninsightful or cognitively impaired to "self-manage," Bilsker concludes that, notwithstanding transitory periods of incapacity, "individuals with mental disorders have a considerable and *largely untapped* capacity to engage in self-management practices" (5, emphasis added).

In considering the role of education, it can be said that knowledge, in and of itself, can provide benefits to clients. A manual on the treatment of depression notes that "simple awareness" of negative thinking may provide relief in that (1) when "you become aware of an automatic process, it becomes less efficient" and (2) when thoughts enter into your awareness, you can bring your critical mind to bear on them (Paterson et al. 1996, 19). Describing a personal experience with schizophrenia, Canadian author Pavlina Vagnerova (2003a, 19) describes her frustration concerning information that was not forthcoming from treating professionals:

> Another turning point was when I was finally provided information about schizophrenia: the first diagnosis my doctors gave me. I asked them repeatedly for it, but for some reason they were reluctant to give it to me until almost the end, when they deemed I was "ready." Once I held this information in my hands and was able to read academic text – just like I used to for my classes at university – I realized that all the delusions of grandeur, paranoias and hallucinations I experienced had also been shared by many others before me. I also realized that I was not as special as I thought I was, in the grand scheme of things, and that I would be able to lead the normal life I wished.

Self-described psychiatric survivor Pat Capponi (2003, xvi) summarizes the client perspective as follows: "The challenge for psychiatric survivors, then, is the same for anyone with a chronic illness: learn anything you can about what it is you're supposed to have; don't let it consume you; pay attention to triggers, learn what eases the pain; and understand how frustration and behavior can sometimes undermine you."

Practitioners can assist clients, and their friends and family, by imparting to them our best current understanding of a syndrome. To this end, often the most useful service is telling people what something is *not* since misconceptions about mental disorders continue to be widespread (Stuart and Arboleda-Florez 2001). Examples of these include the idea that depression is a sign of character weakness, that schizophrenia is a form of multiple personality, or that young persons in the early stages of a disorder are simply being willful and disobedient. There are a number of good sources of mental health information, such as the websites of organizations like Health Canada, the Canadian Mental Health Association, and the Schizophrenia Society as well as books written for clients, families, and nonspecialists, including some written by persons themselves recovering from psychiatric disability (some of these titles are included in the list of Other Resources at the end of this book). Some periodicals, such as the *Psychiatric Rehabilitation Journal*, will routinely publish clients' accounts of their own struggles with mental disorder and other, existential concerns.

Educational programs have achieved an evidence-based status (Torrey et al. 2001). For example, studies of programs that provide support, education, and skills training to family members have found outcomes such as stress reduction and enhanced efficacy among significant others, and reduced rates of relapse and hospitalization among the client group (Dixon et al. 2001; Jones 2005; Pitschel-Walz et al. 2001). A meta-analysis of fifteen controlled studies involving persons with schizophrenia found that the rate of "poor outcomes" (relapse, suicide, withdrawal from program) declined over a one-year period from 54 percent to 27 percent when family education was added to the standard treatment approach involving case management and education (Falloon, Coverdale, and Brooker 1996).

Education may be delivered in a number of formats, including by the practitioner (either one-on-one or in the presence of friends and family) and through groups led or co-led by a practitioner, staff from a partner agency, family members, or clients and peer-support workers. Presentations that include the insider perspective of a client are particularly powerful. Groups may be either less structured and more supportive or more structured and specialized, with sequences of "modules" covering particular topics. Of increasing concern in recent years has been the need to disseminate mental health information to the ethnic and immigrant community, preferably by persons familiar with the language and cultural values of this group.

Guidelines for practitioner-delivered education are given by Andrews and colleagues (2000) and summarized as follows:

- There should be the recognition that education is an important component of the treatment process that ultimately can provide the individual with a sense of greater control and wellbeing.
- Education should be made relevant to each individual and his or her circumstances.
- It is suggested that, when time is very limited, two sessions of "basic education" be given, one around the time of initial assessment and one about two months into treatment "when non-compliance often peaks" (176). When more time is available, sessions are best delivered during the early stages of recovery.
- Basic education will include information about the nature and prognosis of the disorder, treatment options, and issues such as side effects, duration and costs, and recognizing early warning signs (see "relapse prevention" below). A more detailed education session, or sessions, would include audiovisual material and/or handouts. Education should be seen as an ongoing process.
- Prior to the session there should be an assessment of the client's knowledge, beliefs, attitudes, and expectations about treatment.
- Information should be geared to the level of the audience, and in particular unnecessary scientific jargon should be avoided. If unable to answer a

particular question, the practitioner should consult with some other source or person and answer the question at the next session.

- The client and significant others should be encouraged to participate actively.
- Important points should be repeated, and the client can be asked to summarize what has been covered.

Education inevitably overlaps with **skills training**, which is defined here as techniques, either cognitive or behavioural, that assist an individual in coping with or managing the effects of a disorder. "Effects" refers both to particular symptoms and to social situations that may be made difficult or more stressful because of deficits created by the disorder or because of responses by others to the disorder. A more detailed rationale for social skills training is given as follows:

> Almost by definition and by diagnostic criteria, an individual with a mental disability is likely to demonstrate deficits in social skills and social adjustment. Sometimes this arises from never having learned social skills because the mental illness intervened early in adolescence or adulthood, before critical interpersonal and independent living skills could be acquired. Other deficits occur because of atrophy or disuse after many years of institutional life, intrusion of positive and negative symptoms of psychosis or depression, current lack of environmental stimulation and learning opportunities, and cognitive impairments. With social functioning being a prime diagnostic indicator of long-term outcome of mental disorders, it becomes incumbent upon practitioners to teach social skills to the severely mentally ill. (Liberman 1998, 5)

As with education, skills training can be delivered in a number of formats. In some cases prepackaged modules have been produced along with manuals for the practitioner, each focusing on a particular skill area. A well-known example of this is the work of Robert Liberman and associates at the University of California at Los Angeles, who have produced modules, for example, on "medication management," "symptom management," "recreation for leisure," "basic conversation skills," and "interpersonal problem-solving" (Liberman 1998). The symptom management module, for instance, covers the topics of "identifying early warning signs of relapse," "developing a relapse prevention plan," "coping with persistent psychotic symptoms," and "avoiding alcohol and street drugs." Concerning medication management, Kopelowicz and Liberman (2003, 1492) observe that "pharmacotherapy will be of no avail if psychoeducational efforts are not used to inform clients and members of their families about the benefits and side effects of medication and to involve them as partners and active collaborators in the treatment effort."

In many instances persons with mental disorders will come up with their own coping strategies in an attempt to confront, reframe, or deflect intrusive symptoms. While some will resort to using drugs and alcohol, credit must be given to the clients who have arrived at constructive strategies and lifestyle choices without the intervention of mental health professionals. Indeed, it can be argued that what we call skills training is simply a somewhat more systematic application of principles that clients have already been using in many cases.

Below are overviews of five potential problem areas commonly encountered in mental health practice and corresponding strategies that clients may employ to deal with them: (1) relapse prevention, (2) dealing with insomnia, (3) dealing with anxiety, (4) being assertive, and (5) structured problem solving.

Relapse Prevention

"**Relapse prevention**" refers to a client's recognition of the *early warning signs* of a particular disorder, attention to *high-risk situations* that may exacerbate the disorder, and putting into action *early intervention strategies* that may head off potential problems. Signs that a client may be "slipping" are specific and unique to that person. Since the practitioner typically has more limited contact with the individual, he or she needs to rely on the client's self-report or, failing that, on the report of someone with intimate knowledge of the client, such as a spouse or parent. Self-detection of early signs is not always easy: in some cases the onset is so gradual that the client will not feel that anything is wrong or different. In other cases the "window of opportunity" is extremely small: a client with bipolar disorder told this author that she tripped over into mania so quickly that there was no chance to respond other than to "go along for the ride." One client, diagnosed with bipolar disorder, describes the early warning signs as follows:

> I began to see patterns to my illness. There were certain reliable early signs of relapse that I could identify. I learned that an early symptom of my pending mania would be increased excitement and decreased need for sleep. The immediate effect of this would be fatigue. The fatigue manifested itself in several ways: a cold sore, a facial tic, hand tremor and neck stiffness. As the mania progressed, I developed racing thoughts, pressured speech and severe insomnia. Gradually I would turn the night into day – staying up all night, and sleeping only during the day. My apartment and my car would be a mess, and I would stay up nights writing poetry. Friends would

comment that I didn't look myself, and that would embarrass or irritate me. (Winram 2002)

Once identified, the warning signs need to be articulated in some fashion, which may be done with a standardized form that lists the signs and the planned responses (Falloon et al. 1993); an example of a form is given on the next page.

High-risk situations are those that are known to be associated with a worsening of the disorder or some other negative outcome. The logic here is often applied to persons with addictions, who learn to recognize that certain individuals or locations may prompt a return to substance use. For persons with mental disorders, a number of situations may be significant, such as reminders of loss (e.g., anniversary dates, visits to a previous residence) or stressful events (e.g., family reunions). Where possible clients should keep a journal and note when, where, and under what circumstances symptoms appear to get worse (Maguire 2002).

Early intervention strategies are those that the client can put into place before, or without, having to seek assistance from the mental health system – which may not be immediately available. Again, these strategies will be specific to the individual and can be written down for future reference. The client with bipolar disorder, cited above, speaks about his "emergency kit":

At the onset of hypomania, my "emergency kit" consists of:

- Taking a few days off work.
- Taking a sleeping pill (extra sleep early in the mania is the key).
- Increasing my mood-stabilizing medication and my antipsychotic medication.[3]
- Phoning my psychiatrist to arrange for an emergency visit (but taking my increased medication immediately without waiting for the appointment).
- Reduce stress (it's not the time for me to contemplate romances or finances).
- Regular sleep, regular exercise, regular meals, reduced caffeine, no cigarettes or alcohol.
- Increased walking and listening to classical music to relax.
- I avoid the news or upsetting television.
- I stop driving my car (because of sedation from the medication or impulsively from the mania) (Winram 2002).

An example of a personal relapse prevention/crisis plan, adapted from a model created by Eric Macnaughton of the Canadian Mental Health

Association (British Columbia Partners for Mental Health and Addictions Information 2003c), is as follows:

Signs that suggest I am doing well:

_____

Events or situations that triggered relapses in the past:

_____

Early warning signs that I experienced in the past:

_____

Effective ways that I can cope if I experience early warning signs:

_____

What early warning signs indicate that I need help from others:

_____

Who I would like to assist me (names):

_____

What I would like them to do:

_____

If in crisis:

_____

Ways that I can manage stress, regain balance, or calm myself:

_____

People that I can call and their phone numbers:

_____

Resources that I can use (agencies, support groups):

_____

Things that I or other people can do that I find helpful:

_____

Medications that have helped in the past:

_____

Medications that have not helped or that have caused an adverse reaction:

_____

Medications that I am currently on:

_____

Sleep Hygiene

A surprisingly large number of clients will present with difficulties in sleeping. This can become a major preoccupation and worry, leading to increased use of prescription drugs as well as over-the-counter remedies such as

Sominex, Gravol, and antihistamines. Sleep disruption at night can be caused by daytime inactivity and napping – which speaks to the importance of employment and meaningful activity as part of a complete rehabilitation plan. It may also be caused by stress, anxiety, and depression, with the consequent insomnia making these problems worse. In other words, "sleep difficulties are a cause *and* an effect of mood problems" (Paterson et al. 1996, 14, emphasis in original). Sleep can be complicated by medication use; for example, while benzodiazepines may be used to help with sleep, tolerance – the need for higher dosages – and withdrawal can actually make sleep difficulties worse.

Suggestions for dealing with insomnia are as follows (Paterson et al. 1996):

(1) Avoid over-the-counter sleeping medication, alcohol, and caffeine. Alcohol use may produce an initial sedation but results in a less restful sleep and often leads to early morning waking. Similarly, over-the-counter remedies do not usually produce a refreshing sleep. Caffeine, in the form of coffee, tea, hot chocolate, and soft drinks, will affect sleep patterns, so beverages of this sort should be avoided after lunch.

(2) Set a standard bedtime and keep to it; in particular, don't go to bed too early.

(3) Set a standard rising time and avoid the urge to sleep in.

(4) Use the bedroom only for sleep, not for activities inconsistent with sleep, such as working, eating, watching television, and so on.

(5) Create a good sleep environment with respect to noise, light, and temperature.

(6) Avoid napping during the day (unless you are one of a minority that can achieve brief "power naps").

(7) Avoid strenuous physical activity, heavy meals, or mental stimulation for at least one hour before going to bed.

(8) Avoid lying in bed worrying. Strategies here include setting aside time for problem solving during the day or occupying oneself with activities that are distracting yet relaxing, such as listening to a relaxation tape. This may involve getting out of bed for short periods.

(9) Do not smoke for about ninety minutes before bedtime.

(10) Exercise during the day.

(11) Consider a light snack at bedtime, such as warm milk or a banana (both of which are high in the amino acid tryptophan, which plays a role in inducing and maintaining sleep).

Relaxation Training
Relaxation exercises are used to cope with symptoms such as panic attacks

and are also used within the context of cognitive-behavioural treatments such as systematic desensitization (see below), where the individual is deliberately exposed to anxiety-producing stimuli. One common technique for dealing with acute anxiety is to breathe into a paper bag, which helps steady the level of carbon dioxide in the blood. A preferred method is a slow breathing exercise, which is used at the first signs of panic and at other times during the day for practice. The exercise takes about five minutes and involves the following steps (Andrews et al. 2000): (1) Hold your breath and count to five. (2) At five, breathe out and say the word *relax*. (3) Breathe in for three seconds, and out for three, saying *relax* with each outward breath. (4) At the end of each minute (ten breaths) hold your breath for five seconds. (5) Continue until the anxiety subsides. This exercise may be used on its own or as the lead-in to progressive muscle relaxation, which takes about another fifteen minutes. This involves alternately tensing (for about ten seconds) then relaxing (for about ten seconds) in sequence: the hands, lower arms, upper arms, shoulders, neck, forehead and scalp, eyes, jaw, tongue, chest, stomach, back, buttocks, thighs, calves, and feet.

Assertiveness Skills   Skip
Clients may lack the ability to communicate opinions, needs, and feelings in an effective manner. In particular, communication styles may be overly passive or overly aggressive; in the former case, one runs the risk of being taken advantage of, and in the latter, there is the danger of antagonizing and alienating others. While communication may be a problem area for any of us, mental health clients may be more likely to have deficits for a number of reasons: (1) the onset of the disorder may have interrupted the normal course of developing relationship skills; (2) clients may come from chaotic family backgrounds where role models were either absent, negligent, or abusive; (3) clients may be estranged from family, socially isolated, and have no way to practise conversation skills; (4) clients disproportionately reside in inner-city, skid-row, and institutional settings, where "getting by" requires placing a premium on toughness; and (5) alternately, passive styles may be fostered in psychiatric hospital, residential, and treatment settings, where the professionals "call the shots."

In teaching assertiveness, the costs of staying with the present style of interaction need to be weighed against the benefits, with at some point – hopefully – the scales being tipped in favour of more effective communication. For example, the client may acknowledge that being passive is a way of avoiding conflict but with encouragement may see that this has a cost in terms of self-respect, respect from others, and independence.

Common myths about assertiveness can be described to clients (Andrews et al. 2000): (1) the myth of humility – "be humble at all costs" – which may lead to putting oneself down all the time and creating a poor self-image; (2) the myth of the good friend, which is the idea that companions should somehow know intuitively what you want, when, more often than not, open discussion is needed; (3) the myth of anxiety, referring to avoiding anxiety-producing situations – such as being assertive – at all costs, when in reality some degree of anxiety is normal; (4) the myth of obligation, which holds that you must always grant a favour to an associate when asked; and (5) the myth of sex roles – "it's not feminine (or masculine) to do that" – an example being the woman as "nagging wife" who stands up for herself. Andrews and colleagues (2000) list what they call "protective skills," to be used as a last resort in extreme situations when nothing seems to be working. These include:

- *"Broken record"*: repeating an answer over and over – without explanation – to someone who is not prepared to let you say "no" gracefully, such as a pushy salesman.
- *"Selective ignoring"*: not responding when someone continues to badger you about something despite a clear message that you no longer wish to discuss the topic.
- *"Disarming anger"*: stating that you will not respond until the person calms down.
- *"Separating issues"*: for example, "It's not that I don't care for you, it's just that I don't wish to lend you money."
- *"Dealing with guilt"*: don't let people guilt-trip you, and in particular don't use the phrase "I'm sorry" unless there are good reasons to apologize.

In assertiveness training, clients may be given scenarios where they role-play or describe what they would do before practising these in real-world situations, later getting feedback from the practitioner or group.

Structured Problem Solving

Structured problem solving is a process by which clients learn to identify for themselves problem areas and optimal solutions. While the concepts may seem straightforward, it must be emphasized that for some clients the ability to focus and prioritize will be impaired by symptoms that can include thought disorder, anxiety, depression, rumination, perseveration, and diminished concentration. The steps involved are as follows (Andrews et al. 2000):

- *Identifying problems or goals.* One rule here is that problems/goals should be considered one at a time; additional problems may be addressed on another occasion. Another guideline is that goals should be specific, realistic, and achievable and that the client – not the practitioner – should "own" the goal. If someone sets a goal at a high level and doesn't achieve it (for example, because he or she is depressed), this failure represents another setback that may further reduce morale and motivation. For this reason, where possible working toward an ultimate goal in small steps, "minigoals," is recommended (Paterson 1997).
- *Generating ideas through brainstorming.* The individual comes up with as many alternative solutions as possible without worrying at this point about how useful they may be.
- *Evaluating solutions.* What are the pros and cons of each? How feasible are they?
- *Choosing the best solution.* Often it is better to choose something that can be implemented sooner rather than later: even if the results are mixed, the individual may still learn something useful from the experience.
- *Planning.* What specifically needs to be done to put this into action?
- *Review.* What went right (or wrong)? What alternatives might now be tried? Here the practitioner should be encouraging, and outcomes should be framed as partial successes rather than as failures.

Motivational Interviewing
Experienced clinicians use a number of generic techniques, approaches that may be used in a wide range of situations. One such approach is *motivational interviewing,* first developed to assist clients struggling with addictions but now applied more broadly to help people to move forward and make changes in different areas of their lives (Miller and Rollnick 2002). It starts with the premise that most clients approach the relationship with the practitioner with *ambivalence* – indeed, while in some cases they may have sought help voluntarily, in others they may have been cajoled or coerced. This ambivalence is seen as a natural state of affairs in that people rarely want to give up control over their lives, but it is not necessarily an indication that the client is unwilling to change. In the case of someone misusing drugs or alcohol, the substances may not initially be perceived as a problem but as the *solution* to his or her problems. For example, a survey of untreated heavy drinkers published in the journal *Addiction Research and Theory* found that, despite what others might think, perceived benefits of drinking outweighed the drawbacks for the subjects themselves (a fact that the authors noted "challenges ... health promotion efforts") (Orford et al. 2002, 347). Not accounting for this ambivalence may be an obstacle to engaging or keeping a person in

treatment. It is recommended that the practitioner avoid being judgmental and lecturing the client about problem behaviours; instead, treatment goals should be mutually developed.

Motivational interviewing starts with determining a client's readiness to change based on a model suggested by Prochaska and DiClemente (1986) that sees people as being at one of five stages:

- *Precontemplation:* The client is not thinking of making a change.
- *Contemplation:* The client is thinking of making a change but is undecided.
- *Preparation:* The client is prepared to take action – for example, "within the next thirty days."
- *Action:* The client is doing things to change his or her behaviour.
- *Maintenance:* The client has made changes and is working to stay on track.

The client may move through these changes or may in fact relapse and fall back to an earlier stage. In each stage the practitioner's tasks are somewhat different, with motivational interviewing used more commonly in the first two stages to move the person toward action.[4] (1) With precontemplation the worker's task is to raise doubt and to increase the client's perception of the risks and problems associated with current behaviours. (2) With contemplation the worker is endeavouring to "tip the balance," evoke reasons to change and the risks of not changing, and support client self-efficacy. (3) With preparation the worker gives the client options and helps him or her to determine the best course of action to take in seeking change (see "structured problem solving" above). (4) With action the worker helps the individual to take these first steps. (5) With maintenance the worker helps the client to identify and use strategies to prevent relapse (see discussion on "relapse prevention" above). (6) With relapse the worker helps the client to renew the process and to address possible demoralization.

When engaged in motivational interviewing the practitioner should be guided by the following principles:

- *Express empathy:* The worker should be accepting rather than judgmental, use reflective listening, and recognize that ambivalence is normal.
- *Develop discrepancy:* The worker contrasts client goals and values with current behaviours, develops the discrepancy between where the client is and where he or she wants to be, makes the person aware of consequences, and allows the client to present arguments for change.
- *Avoid argumentation:* Arguments and confrontation breed defensiveness and denial; resistance may be a signal to change strategies.

- *Roll with resistance:* Opposing resistance may only reinforce it; instead, validate the client's perspective and use the individual as a resource for finding solutions.
- *Support self-efficacy:* The client is ultimately responsible for choosing and carrying out change strategies.

Cognitive-Behavioural Therapies Skip

First developed in the 1950s, cognitive-behavioural therapy (CBT) is increasingly being used to address a wide range of mental health problems and, arguably, has become the predominant nonpharmacological approach to treating and managing mental disorders in North American settings. For example, one author (Stern 1993, 3) suggests that "if psychiatrists are not trained in behavioural-cognitive psychotherapy it leaves them *therapeutically impotent,* and therefore less able to lead a multidisciplinary team" (emphasis added). Historically, this area of practice has been associated more with clinical psychology and specialized clinics; however, in recent years the logic and techniques of CBT (or at least, elements of it) have been taught and utilized in "generic" public mental health programs. It should be said that "cognitive-behavioural therapy" is potentially a misleading term in that not one but a variety of techniques are used under this rubric. Further, some treatment models tend to be more "cognitive," others more "behavioural," and others a combination of the two.

Behavioural Techniques

Behavioural techniques are based on principles of conditioning and social learning first articulated by psychology pioneers such as John Watson, B.F. Skinner, and Albert Bandura. These techniques have traditionally been used with persons with anxiety disorders, behavioural problems, and sexual disorders such as pedophilia. A key underlying principle here is that the consequences of a client's behaviour will be either reinforcing or not; based on this, a clinician can design contingencies to diminish unwanted responses, such as severe anxiety in anticipation of being in a public place.

Using the treatment of phobias as an example, the approach used will usually involve either *systematic desensitization* – exposure to a graduated hierarchy of situations that the client finds anxiety-provoking – or prolonged exposure ("flooding") until there is a recognition that no harm will come to the person. An example of the latter would be a person extremely fearful of germs being asked to continue touching a "contaminated" object until the anxiety dissipated; an example of the former would be gradually – over a period of weeks – increasing the distance travelled from home for someone suffering from agoraphobia. To help manage the anxiety, clients are taught techniques such as slow breathing or muscle relaxation, used at the beginning of the session to try to ensure that the individual is calm, and used during the session if anxiety rises. Through conditioning – since the relaxation response is incompatible with anxiety – anxiety symptoms will hopefully be extinguished. For more detailed descriptions of these types of interventions see, for example, Andrews and colleagues (2000).

While behavioural treatments of anxiety disorders have traditionally been done *in vivo*, more recently virtual reality technologies have been used to create three-dimensional representations of anxiety-producing stimuli, with the results of these "virtual" exposure therapies apparently being generalizable to the real world (Beierle 1996; MacDonald 2002). This technique may be particularly beneficial in treating children.

Other behavioural techniques, referred to as "contingency management" (Nietzel, Bernstein, and Milich 1998, 284), involve systems of rewards and punishments designed to elicit positive and extinguish negative behaviours, an example being the (somewhat dated) concept of the "token economy." Such methods are usually only applied in institutional settings and with very disabled persons, such as children suffering from severe forms of autism.

Because behavioural treatments have been shown to be effective in diminishing distressing thoughts and behaviours, adherents have been able to argue that tracing a symptom back to its psychic origins, as per psychodynamic theory, is unnecessary. As one text concludes, "behavior therapies will have a secure and valued position in the history of psychology because they helped lay to rest the hallowed notion of *symptom substitution* ... as a result, the avenue was opened for the development of specific techniques for dealing with specific patient complaints" (Phares and Trull 1997, 399, emphasis in original).

CBT and Depression

Cognitive treatments consider the ways that distorted thinking – irrational, unrealistic, or self-defeating beliefs and interpretations – can impact on an individual's mental and emotional state. In other words, "how you feel and act depends more on what you *think* is going on than what really is happening" (Paterson et al. 1996, 1, emphasis in original). Pioneered by clinicians such as Aaron Beck (e.g., Beck et al. 1979) and Albert Ellis (e.g., Ellis and Dryden 1987) and originally designed for persons with mood and anxiety disorders (particularly depression), cognitive approaches have become increasingly influential and have been extended and modified for use with clients with personality and psychotic disorders.

As summarized by Nietzel, Bernstein, and Milich (1998), the strategies employed in Beck's model for the treatment of depression include: (1) helping the client recognize the connections between cognitions, affect, and behaviour; (2) monitoring occurrences of cognitive distortions; (3) examining the evidence for and against these distortions; (4) substituting more realistic interpretations; and (5) giving clients homework assignments focused on practising new thinking strategies and more effective problem solving. Examples of this approach are as follows (Paterson et al. 1996; Paterson and Bilsker 2002):

- Clients are asked to write about events that have been upsetting as well as about their *interpretations* of the events and their *responses*. A client might write about how a friend cancelled a lunch date, which was interpreted as "He doesn't like me; no one likes me; I'll always be alone" and which was responded to with "Stayed at home alone, felt sad." The practitioner works with the client to come up with alternative, more realistic interpretations.
- Clients are asked to write down "put-downs" – statements or thoughts such as "I'm so stupid" – each time they occur and to make note of how they affect their mood. They are asked to substitute a more realistic phrase, such as "I may not like this, but I'll get through it."
- Similarly, clients are asked to write down *automatic thoughts* – negative thoughts that seem to arise spontaneously – as well as problem beliefs, such as "everything I do must be absolutely perfect; otherwise, I am a failure." They may then be asked to identify the thought or belief that has had the biggest impact on them, describe the impact, then come up with ways to challenge the belief.
- Clients are asked to catch themselves using various forms of biased thinking, such as overgeneralizing ("It's always going to be like this"), disqualifying the positive ("Anyone can do what I just did"), mind-reading ("She thinks I'm stupid"), fortune-telling ("I'm sure to fail this course"), and catastrophizing (being stood up for a date means you'll spend your entire life alone). Clients are asked to come up with more reality-based ways of thinking and may be provided with axioms, such as "I need to pay attention to the whole picture."

Depending on the individual client, overcoming negative thinking can involve:

- *Awareness of the distorted thoughts* – so that they are no longer "automatic" and can instead be critically evaluated.
- *Thought-challenging:* For example, keeping a journal where the client writes about situations, automatic thoughts associated with the situation, and more realistic appraisals of the situation – which can then be read aloud or kept for future reference.

- *Thought-stopping*, which involves a routine where the client orders him or herself to stop ruminating by standing up, clapping his or her hands, and shouting "Stop!" Eventually, the sequence of three actions is reduced to one and then replaced by a mental image of a stop sign.
- *Worrying time:* The client writes down issues that are worrying but defers dealing with them until a set, limited time when he or she will not be distracted.
- *Worry inflation:* The logic here is for the client to exaggerate his or her fears until they become ridiculous and implausible so that the original problem shrinks in size.

While the psychological treatment of depression involves cognitive techniques, therapists specializing in this approach will often incorporate other components of recovery, including education about depression and stress, lifestyle choices (diet, sleep, physical activity, use of substances, recreation), assertiveness training, and building a supportive social network (Paterson et al. 1996).

CBT and Personality Disorder

As noted earlier, practitioners frequently approach clients who have been diagnosed with borderline personality disorder (BPD) with great apprehension and ambivalence. The belief that these persons are untreatable may become a self-fulfilling prophecy because of the clinician's strong response to the client's apparently manipulative and provocative actions. In her approach to working with persons diagnosed with BPD, psychologist Marsha Linehan (1993a, 1993b) takes this into account, noting that before anything can be accomplished, the clinician needs to accept some basic assumptions: (1) that the patient wants to change and, despite appearances, is trying to do his or her best; (2) that the behaviour is understandable given the person's background and life circumstances; (3) that, while the client may not be entirely to blame for the way things are, it is his or her responsibility to make them different; (4) that clients cannot fail in therapy; rather, if things are not improving it is the treatment that is failing; and (5) that the clinician must avoid thinking or talking about the client in pejorative terms since this will work against the therapeutic alliance and feed into problems that have led to the development of BPD in the first place. Linehan strongly cautions against using terms like "manipulative," which implies a degree of skill in managing other people or from which one can infer intentionality, both of which are likely incorrect conclusions.

Linehan's influential model for working with clients diagnosed with BPD, which is based on principles of cognitive-behavioural therapy, is described briefly here, although interested readers are advised to consult the original manuals (Linehan 1993a, 1993b) or other sources, such as Kiehn and Swale (1995). The approach is called dialectical behaviour therapy (DBT), the term "dialectical" referring to the tension (or balance) between *acceptance,* on the one hand (i.e., validation of the client) and *change,* on the other (i.e., achieving the goals of skill acquisition and learning more adaptive ways of dealing with problems). It is noted that *invalidating environments* are those where the client experiences rejection and in some cases punishment or where problems and solutions are oversimplified – responses not infrequently encountered in health care settings. A consequence of these sorts of system responses is that the client may be retraumatized (Harris and Fallot 2001) or that, because undesired behaviours are inconsistent and erratic, they may unintentionally be reinforced.

The two main modes of treatment in DBT are individual therapy with a clinician and skills training, which is done in a group format; the client is required to attend both. In the skills training component, four groups of skills are described: (1) "core mindfulness skills," which are "techniques to enable one to become more clearly aware of the contents of experience and to develop the ability to stay with that experience in the present moment" (Kiehn and Swale 1995, 7) (recall the discussion on BPD in Chapter 3, which refers to problems with *object constancy*); (2) "interpersonal effectiveness skills," which have some parallels with assertiveness skills and which aim to have the client maintain self-esteem in interactions with other people; (3) "emotion modulation skills," which are ways of changing distressing emotional states and which involve examining the *misinterpretation* of events (such as overgeneralizing and catastrophizing, similar to the logic seen in CBT with depressed persons); and (4) "distress tolerance skills," techniques for putting up with emotional states if they cannot be changed for the time being, this involving skills such as "distracting," "self-soothing," "improving the moment," and "thinking of pros and cons."

Individual treatment is approached in stages: stage one focuses on stabilizing suicidal and "therapy interfering" behaviours (which is necessary before advancing to later stages and could involve distress tolerance and other skills); stage two deals with problems related to post-traumatic stress; and stage three focuses on self-esteem and individual treatment goals. Clients are given homework, which includes recording targeted behaviours in journals. Core strategies in treatment are (1) validation of the client's behaviours as understandable in relation to his or her life situation and (2) problem solving, meaning the establishment of necessary skills. Treatment involves creating a crisis plan, using cognitive and graded exposure techniques (see above), and in some cases using medication. In the course of treatment, behaviour is examined through a "chain analysis," which looks at the sequence of events leading to unwanted behaviours while generating hypotheses about factors that may be controlling the behaviour. Subsequently, alternative ways of dealing with situations are considered before being put into place and compared. The clinician tries to promote self-efficacy rather than doing everything for the client (such as intervening with other care providers). Kiehn and Swale (1995, 9-10) conclude: "Particular note should be made of the pervading application of contingency management throughout the therapy, using the relationship with the therapist as the main reinforcer. In the session by session course of therapy care is taken to systematically reinforce targeted adaptive behaviors and to avoid reinforcing targeted maladaptive behaviors."

Linehan's own evaluation of DBT was a study that compared two groups of twenty-two clients, one group receiving DBT and the other "treatment as usual" (TAU) (which could constitute a variety of outpatient situations). The outcome measures were frequency of parasuicidal behaviours, number of hospital days, and attrition rate from therapy (a frequent problem for persons with BPD). Results showed that the group receiving DBT did better on all three indicators, having fewer suicidal behaviours, lower therapy attrition rates (16.7% vs. 50%), and fewer days spent in hospital (eight days per year compared to over thirty-eight for the TAU group) (Linehan et al. 1991). A subsequent meta-analysis of eleven studies of cognitive-behavioural treatment of personality disorder concluded that CBT was an "effective treatment" (Leichsenring and Leibing 2003).

It is noteworthy that Linehan's model has influenced the development of initiatives taught and led by clients who themselves were diagnosed with BPD, such as (in Canada) the Self-Abuse Finally Ends (SAFE) Program, described on two websites: http://www.safeincanada.ca and http://ca.geocities.com/safebc.

CBT and Psychosis

In recent years cognitive-behavioural techniques have been utilized in the treatment of persons with psychotic disorders such as schizophrenia and bipolar disorder (Buccheri et al. 2004; Fowler, Garety, and Kuipers 1995). This represents a major change in thinking given that these disorders were previously considered contraindications for CBT, having been relegated to the category of "biological" or "brain" conditions that were only appropriately managed with medications (Kingdon 1998; Lam et al. 2003). As a review article in the *Canadian Journal of Psychiatry* summarizes, for some time the prevailing view had been "that psychotic symptoms resulted from a core neurophysiological dysfunction or dysfunctions that [were] not amendable to a talking therapy" (Norman and Townsend 1999, 245), a view supported by findings that psychodynamic therapies were of little utility in the treatment of psychotic disorders (Fenton 2000). Case managers in mental health programs (such as this author) were often instructed not to challenge or even discuss the substance of a client's delusions or hallucinations (except to conduct risk assessments) since, so the reasoning went, the "beliefs [would only] be reinforced by such exploration" (Kingdon 1998, 177) or "talking about voices could only make them worse" (Row 2003, 27). Despite this, there has been increasing interest in the use of cognitive treatments for clients with psychotic disorders. The impetus for this comes from several directions (Norman and Townsend 1999): (1) evidence of the success of these techniques in other clinical domains, such as the treatment of depression; (2) the finding that a number of clients, on their own, had been developing coping strategies for dealing with psychotic symptoms (Vagnerova 2003a); (3) evidence of the importance of psychosocial factors in rehabilitation and the development of the stress-vulnerability model; (4) findings that a large proportion of clients on antipsychotic medications – 30 to 50 percent – were continuing to experience difficulties related to psychotic symptoms; and (5) recognition that psychological and pharmacological approaches could be viewed as complementary rather than incompatible.

Cognitive-behavioural therapy with persons diagnosed with psychotic disorders incorporates education, skills training, distraction techniques, and methods of belief-challenging. For example, Norman and Townsend (1999) identify several skills to be taught as part of the CBT approach, such as: (1) "reframing psychosis," which is explanation and reinforcement of the stress-vulnerability model so that clients will see "the possible role of their social and physical environment as triggers" (246); (2) "identifying triggers for psychosis," discussed under "relapse prevention" earlier in this chapter; (3) "reducing physiological arousal" by means of muscle relaxation and breathing techniques; and (4) "improving general coping skills," such as assertiveness, conflict resolution, and knowing when and how to withdraw from stressful situations. The more cognitive components of treatment include: "belief modification," where client and clinician examine the client's evidence for apparently false beliefs or perceptions, consider alternative explanations, and "empirically [test] their relative validity" (247); and "disrupting symptoms," where clients are encouraged to move their attention away from symptoms by means of other activities such as "listening to music, watching television, humming, and engaging in social interaction" (247). Using CBT with persons with psychotic disorders will not necessarily eliminate positive symptoms; rather, the rationale is that environmental stressors *leading* to increased symptomatology are alleviated through enhanced coping strategies and that the emotional *consequences* of psychotic symptoms are reduced (Haddock and Tarrier 1998).

A twenty-four-session module is described by Canadian clinicians Lecomte, Leclerc, and Wykes (2001). The first six sessions cover "ice-breaking," defining stress, personal reactions to stress, the stress-vulnerability model, protective factors (such as self-esteem), and subjective understanding of symptoms. The next six sessions involve identifying how beliefs affect behaviour, challenging beliefs, and looking for alternative explanations. Sessions thirteen through sixteen examine the role of drugs and alcohol, with the next two sessions addressing depression, suicidality, and how psychotic symptoms affect mood. The final six sessions have to do with coping skills, including relapse prevention and building social support networks. Each session has a small homework assignment. One can see here a number of similarities with the Beck model for treating depression – that is, looking at how cognitions affect mood and behaviour, monitoring the occurrence of distorted ideas, and evaluating the evidence for and against unrealistic beliefs.

Studies of the effect of CBT with clients suffering from psychosis have in a number of instances shown beneficial results – that is, improvement of positive symptoms among treated persons versus those in control groups (Grech 2002; Gumley et al. 2003; Morrison et al. 2004) – as well as improvements in other domains of client functioning, such as self-esteem (Lecomte et al. 1999). For example, a study led by British psychologist Philippa Garety found that, among persons presenting with a persistent form of schizophrenia that was resistant to medication, 50 percent showed a significant improvement in psychotic symptoms and a decrease in psychological distress (Garety, Fowler, and Kuipers 2000). And in a study of clients diagnosed with Bipolar I disorder, the investigators found that those in the cognitive-behavioural treatment group were 40 percent less likely to relapse (Lam et al. 2003).

One caveat concerns the comparability of studies, in that there has been an "apparent lack of uniformity regarding the therapies under the CBT appellation" (Lecomte and Lecomte 2002, 50). In other words, it is not always clear, at this point, what works with whom. However, since CBT approaches need to be tailored to the degree of disability and ability and "to the needs and circumstances of individual patients" (Norman and Townsend 1999, 246), it seems to be the case that a single, uniform approach is neither possible nor desirable.[5]

In considering the application of CBT with persons suffering from psychosis, the intractability of beliefs must be acknowledged; for some, unfortunately, neither medication nor cognitive techniques may be effective in shifting a fixed delusion. Another caution comes from evidence that clients need to have established some stability and supports in other areas of their life for CBT to be effective: a three-year study of clients in Pittsburgh who had received support and training in interpersonal skills and stress reduction found lower relapse rates and better social functioning among those in the treatment group, *except* for among the fifty-four individuals in the study who lived alone or with nonfamily members. The conclusion was that, for these persons, securing shelter, food, and clothing was so demanding that meeting other treatment requirements proved to be overwhelming (Hogarty et al. 1997).

Treatments for Children
Nonpharmacological treatments for children incorporate many of the same principles and techniques used in treating adults, with some adaptations (Bailey 2001). One adaptation concerns the method of communication: having children talk about upsetting experiences may be difficult, so approaches that permit them to draw, write, or use role play may be helpful. For example, a therapist may use cartoon figures and ask the child to fill in the thought bubbles above the figure. Playing along with children also affords the therapist an opportunity to establish rapport and to assess the child's functional abilities and ability to follow instructions.

For children with anxiety disorders, behavioural interventions (e.g., graduated exposure, relaxation responses, rewards) and cognitive techniques (e.g., thought-challenging) may be employed, with McClellan and Werry (2003, 1394) concluding that cognitive-behavioural therapies are in fact "the psychosocial treatments best supported by the literature, with effectiveness noted for a number of different illnesses and symptom states" (see also Manassis 2000). At the same time, these approaches can be stressful for the child, who may not understand the rationale behind the techniques, and for parents, who have to witness their child's distress. A document on the treatment of obsessive-compulsive disorder prepared by the Anxiety Disorders Association of British Columbia (n.d.) describes this dilemma:

[Children] often have trouble understanding why they need to cooperate with stopping the compulsive behavior. They become angry, upset and desperate and may even threaten to run away or hurt themselves or other people. Professionals trained in cognitive-behavioral approaches try to work with children to help them understand that the OCD is like a monster that is running their lives and they have to fight back. If we can help them to team up with their parents to fight the OCD, everybody feels successful and the OCD is brought under control. Sometimes the children need to be brought into the hospital to do this, because it is so hard for the parents to do at home.

The reference here to a "monster" is significant in that it highlights the importance of the use of *metaphor* in working with children. The monster metaphor is employed in a treatment model called Taming Worry Dragons, developed by two clinicians at the Mood and Anxiety Disorders Clinic of British Columbia's Children's Hospital. This model is described as follows:

> "Taming Worry Dragons" ... takes all the ideas of cognitive-behavioral treatments and adapts them with imaginative features that are appealing to children. Through some positive reframing, children learn that they have a "talent for creative worrying" and an "overactive alarm system" which work together to feed uncontrollable worries. When they worry, their body alarm goes off. This causes a racing heart, upset stomach and many other symptoms, which tell them that something terrible is going on. The creative imagination then conjures up bigger and more horrifying possibilities. The result is huge, scary, noisy and bossy "worry dragons" in their mind that then terrorize not only the child, but also the family. The challenge, therefore, is to tame these dragons by using a variety of tools.
>
> Children buy into this model which is consistent with their natural interest in fantasy and heroism. They are able to draw, describe, investigate and – eventually – tame their dragons. They use "trapping" tools of thought stopping (worry box, turning off the worry machine), compartmentalization with a schedule, and distraction tools such as exercise and activities. They then learn more sophisticated "taming" tools, including listening to and changing self-talk. Like all dragon-slayers they need to practice. They set a hierarchy of tasks for themselves in the training process, and determine how many units of "courage" would be needed to tackle each task. (Garland 2002, 29)

Changing Practices

There have been some promising developments in nonpharmacological treatments and supports for persons with serious, persistent mental disorders. At the same time, implementing these developing treatment modalities will be a challenge to public mental health programs in Canada, which have tended to rely on pharmacotherapy with physician-consultants and a limited form of case management by a primary worker who may have fifty to sixty individual clients in his or her caseload. It seems likely that training staff in newer treatment approaches and integrating these programs in the service delivery system will create tensions with respect to cost, efficiency, disciplinary boundaries, and individual worker interest.

Social Skills Training

Writing about social skills training programs, Liberman (1998, 6) notes: "Despite publishing books and treatment manuals and offering hundreds of workshops and apprenticeship opportunities for mental health professionals, we noted the limitations in the spread of this modality to the mainstream of services for the seriously mentally ill." In accounting for this state of affairs, the same author lists several "obstacles to dissemination" (5):

> (1) complexities in the treatment itself (in contrast to the ease of dissemination of new medications, which can be readily utilized by psychiatrists who are familiar with prescribing other medications) which often require special training programs; (2) conflicts between the innovative treatment and traditional, prevailing treatment philosophies in the host institution or agency; (3) lack of support and mandate from administrators and managers of treatment programs; (4) lack of "internal champions" (or local clinicians with formal or informal status and respect from colleagues) for the innovation; and (5) failure to convince clinicians that the innovation can be applied in ordinary practice settings.

In looking at ways to more effectively implement skills training programs, Wallace (1998, 17-18) suggests that "training curricula and methods should be refined, standardized and distributed in a format that allows them to be easily accessed and efficiently delivered" and that "clinicians may achieve better outcomes by focusing their efforts on delivering training rather than producing it" given that curriculum development is extremely time consuming.

A question remains, concerning the potentially wider implementation of skills training programs, as to who would provide the service delivery. Presently, this function is largely handled by rehabilitation specialists, either on mental health teams or at allied rehabilitation agencies. Nonrehab personnel may also run or assist in these programs, the result of personal interest rather than job requirement in most cases. Liberman (1998, 5), on the other hand, suggests that the ability to deliver social skills training should become one of the core, "generic" skills of any mental health clinician: "Clinicians must expand their repertoires, becoming expert teachers or trainers ... clinicians can overcome the learning disabilities of their patients so the latter can achieve their personal goals for higher levels of psychosocial functioning." There may be practical and political impediments to this vision, which also has ramifications for practitioners' undergraduate education across a number of disciplines. As well, it is unclear whether skills training would replace, or be added to, other core practitioner functions and, if the latter, how realistic this would be. As Wallace (1998, 18) concludes, "how best to accomplish these changes and then disseminate these techniques is yet to be determined."

Cognitive-Behavioural Therapy Ꞔkip

Similarly, the potentially more widespread implementation of cognitive-behavioural treatments by mental health teams raises a number of issues. As Norman and Townsend (1999, 251) note, one barrier will be cost effectiveness: "Cognitive-behavioral therapy is likely to prove significantly more labour intensive than many other approaches to treating psychosis. If the efficacy of CBT is further supported, it will be important to determine under what circumstances such approaches are cost effective, to identify the most important components of treatment packages, and to develop the most efficient methods of implementation."

One answer to this problem would be to carry out CBT with persons with psychosis in a group format, which is done with clients diagnosed with depression but which has not necessarily been the choice for CBT with persons suffering from schizophrenia (Lecomte and Lecomte 2002). Group treatments are presently more common in *inpatient* settings, which may have to do with the fact that there is a "captive audience" (Scheidlinger 1994). In addition to efficiency, groups offer the potential advantage of *normalization*: "In therapy, learning that one's problems are not unique is a powerful source of relief ... Cognitive-behavioral therapy, especially in a group format, validates the client's experience through the sharing of similar symptoms, distress and coping strategies" (Lecomte and Lecomte 2002, 54).

Persons with schizophrenia may express a dislike for groups and a preference for one-on-one sessions, although this preference is at least partly a result of service delivery traditions and the "institutionalization" of both the client and the practitioner. While the difficulty that some clients have with groups may be the result of negative symptoms, cognitive deficits, and a vulnerability to stress, which are disorder-related, it would be hoped that some of these difficulties could be overcome by skills taught in these groups. Acknowledging the difficulties in implementing group treatment modules, a "best practices" report nevertheless concludes that "group therapy needs to be 'sold' as effective and a fair way to make use of scarce resources" (British Columbia Ministry of Health 2002e, 33). Concerning the "selling" of groups, Lecomte and colleagues note that: "It is our experience that those who attend [groups] regularly have found a personal incentive which helps them overcome these difficulties; this is effective as long as the group addresses whatever their specific needs may be. It is therefore up to the mental health staff and group leader to insure that the group will be valuable to the client and, if so, work on convincing the client to attend at least one meeting before making a decision" (Lecomte, Leclerc, and Wykes 2001, iii).

On the matter of efficiency, a further question is whether group leaders would take over other medical and case management functions or whether the client would continue to get all services separately – undercutting cost effectiveness. A partial answer to this would be to offer CBT selectively – that is, to clients with medication-resistant, distressing symptoms – while having other clients continue to see case managers.

Another concern relating to the implementation of CBT in public mental health programs has to do with practitioner expertise. Traditionally, CBT has been taught and practised by clinical psychologists, although clinicians from other disciplines could get some exposure to these techniques in workshops or through postgraduate diploma programs. At the same time, psychologists may not be widely employed in many public mental health settings, finding work more in specialized clinics and private practice or, when part of a generic mental health team, performing assessments and psychological tests rather than doing ongoing clinical work. While one answer would be greater employment of PhD psychologists by mental health teams, the more likely scenario is training staff across disciplines in CBT, with ultimately a smaller number of staff being designated CBT specialists and mentors to the other staff.

Notes

1 This was not always the case in that some earlier evaluations of psychotherapy (most famously, a review by British psychologist Hans Eysenck in 1952) either showed outcomes no better than those achieved with placebo or, more often than not, were impossible to conduct because of difficulties in operationalizing the concepts under consideration.
2 For example, the Canadian Psychoanalytic Society (2001) notes that candidates for this treatment "may have already achieved important satisfactions – with friends, in marriage [and] in work," while the Gestalt Institute of Toronto (2004) observes that this approach has "been a means to achieve the personal growth of the *healthy individual*" (emphasis added).
3 Clients in some cases will receive medications with a *pro re nata* order: "take as needed."
4 The author is indebted to Pohsuan Zaide for assistance with the discussion in this section.
5 When selecting clients for CBT groups, factors such as age and functional ability are apparently more important considerations than diagnosis and symptom profile (Dr. Tania Lecomte, personal communication).

Other Resources

- The website of the Mental Health Evaluation and Community Consultation Unit at the University of British Columbia (http://www.mheccu.ubc.ca) has a number of downloadable documents, including the *Self-Care Depression Patient Guide*, which is a user-friendly introduction to cognitive approaches to depression.
- Self-help websites include http://www.mentalhealthrecovery.com (for people who experience "psychiatric symptoms"), http://www.power2u.org (website of the National Empowerment Centre), http://www.psychguides.com (a site with expert consensus guidelines on

psychiatric treatment written for clients and family members), and books about depression and mood disorders for nonspecialists that clients may find helpful include *The Feeling Good Handbook* by David Burns (1989), *Feeling Good: The New Mood Therapy* by the same author (1999), *The Depression Workbook* by Mary Copeland (1992), *On the Edge of Darkness* by Kathy Cronkite (1994), *Learned Optimism* by Martin Seligman (1991), *Your Depression Map* by Randy Paterson (2002), *Riding the Roller Coaster* by M. Bergen (1999), and *Darkness Visible* by William Styron (1990) (author of *Sophie's Choice*).

- The book *Getting to Sleep* by Ellen Catalano (1990) provides concrete suggestions for dealing with sleep difficulties.
- The website of the International Society for the Psychological Treatments of the Schizophrenias and Other Psychoses is at http://www.isps.org.

Rehabilitation and Recovery

While rehabilitation services have had a presence in mental health programs for some time, the pairing of rehabilitation with the *recovery* perspective is relatively new. Incorporating the concept of recovery – a vision of moving beyond symptom management to addressing broader existential concerns – has required a major shift in thinking, one with which some practitioners are still struggling. Although new in one sense, one can note several historical developments that laid the groundwork for this particular approach to mental health practice: (1) schools of psychotherapy emerging in the 1950s and 1960s that fell under the "humanist-existential" rubric, such as Rogerian or Client-Centred Therapy, which were noteworthy more for underlying values such as egalitarianism and self-determination than for specific techniques (Phares and Trull 1997); (2) grass-roots and self-help initiatives developed by clients themselves, who found community services to be either nonexistent or overly medically focused; (3) "labelling theory," a sociological perspective suggesting that the consequences of being diagnosed with a mental illness were more serious than the illness itself (see box next page).

Defining "rehabilitation" and "recovery" is not easy. Some authors emphasize a difference between the two, an example being Deegan (1988, 11), who suggests that "rehabilitation refers to the services and technologies that are made available to disabled persons so that they may learn to adapt to their world. Recovery refers to the lived or real life experience of persons as they accept and overcome the challenge of the disability." Another distinction is to see rehabilitation as a process and recovery as the *outcome* of this process (Jacobson and Curtis 2000). A further difference is a conception of rehabilitation as a practitioner-driven enterprise rather than as the client-driven, or collaborative, process that is intrinsic to (what is now called) the recovery model (Anthony 1993). While historically rehabilitation *has* been practitioner-driven, there has been growing dissatisfaction with this approach among clients; one writes that "it is important to understand that persons with a disability do not 'get rehabilitated' in the sense that cars get tuned up or televisions get repaired. They are not passive recipients of rehabilitation services. Rather, they experience themselves as recovering a new sense of self and of purpose within and beyond the limits of the disability" (Deegan 1988, 11).

Corrigan (2003, 346), on the other hand, suggests that "rehabilitation is *synonymous* with recovery: it means helping people get back to work and living on their own" (emphasis added). In trying to reconcile this with the preceding viewpoints, it might be said that to the extent that practitioners approach rehabilitation as a collaborative process and create the environments in which recovery can be fostered, the two concepts will converge. In fact, a Canadian report on "best practices" in psychosocial rehabilitation lists underlying principles that are very similar to those of the recovery model: client involvement, self-determination, personal choice, natural and peer supports, hope, and belonging (British Columbia Ministry of Health 2002f).

As noted, incorporating a recovery perspective into mental health practice has forced a reevaluation of practitioner attitudes. When first introduced into the mental health lexicon in the 1980s, the concept of recovery created some unease and confusion among clinicians for several interrelated reasons: (1) Many held a *symptom-based* definition of this concept, so the idea, for example, that persons with schizophrenia could be encouraged to work toward "recovery" when they continued to experience delusions and hallucinations seemed unrealistic and irresponsible. From the rehabilitation perspective, however, recovery is viewed much more broadly than in terms only of symptom management. (2) Based on the view that recovery, however defined, is not possible without initial medical stabilization, critics argue that resources will still need to be concentrated on the treatment – rather than the recovery – side of the ledger since many of those with psychotic illnesses lack insight – that is, do not believe there is anything wrong with them in the first place (Satel and Zdanowicz 2003).[1] (3) Historically, the socialization and experiences of mental health practitioners have tended to foster an attitude of *clinical pessimism;* after all, they are working with clients

In the Eye of the Beholder: Labelling Theory and Mental Disorder

A viewpoint in sociology that was popular in the 1960s, "labelling theory" (or societal reaction theory) shifted the focus away from individual psychology and genetic factors to *societal response* as a way of understanding how psychiatric disability is created. From labelling theory comes the concept of stigmatizing identities – such as "mental patient" or "criminal" – that form a *master status,* overriding all others in influencing how society responds to individuals. Another concept associated with the theory is *secondary deviance,* referring to entrenched behaviours and symptoms, which in this perspective are seen as resulting from institutional responses rather than from factors intrinsic to the individual.

Prominent adherents of labelling theory included Thomas Scheff, David Rosenhan, and Canadian sociologist Erving Goffman (who coined the term "total institution"). Goffman's field work at a psychiatric hospital in Washington, DC, formed the basis for his influential book *Asylums: Essays on the Social Situation of Mental Patients and Other Inmates* (1961), the thesis of which was that institutionalism stripped away individual dignity, fostered regressive behaviours and symptoms, and was the most important factor in creating the identity of a mental patient. A few years after this, David Rosenhan's provocative, often cited, and often criticized (e.g., see Spitzer 1975) study of "pseudo-patients," "On being sane in insane places" (1973), was published in the prestigious journal *Science.* This article reported on the situation of a number of "normal" persons who, after surreptitiously gaining admission to psychiatric hospitals, were never distinguished from the "real" patients by hospital staff, even though at no point after admission did they display any symptoms warranting psychiatric intervention. Rosenhan described the invisibility and "depersonalization" of institutionalized patients and concluded that "once a person is designated abnormal, all of his [*sic*] other behaviors and characteristics are colored by that label" (253).

Labelling theory has been criticized from a number of perspectives, with commentators questioning particularly the empirical support for this viewpoint (Davis 1987a; Gove 1970). While the "orthodox" version of the theory – with reference to "primary and secondary deviance" – has largely faded from view, it can be said that understanding some of the elements – the "stickiness" of psychiatric labels, the impact of stigma, and the negative consequences of our institutional arrangements – is as relevant now as ever. Indeed, it can be said that clients may become "institutionalized" even in the absence of large buildings by practice approaches that foster dependency and pessimism (Everett et al. 2003). Because of this, practitioners need to be cautious about hastily applying diagnostic categories and about retaining clients in care who could otherwise move on. Moreover, they need to be reflective about their role in expanding the scope and reach of psychiatry.

with "serious, persistent mental disorders." Because of this, there is a tendency to be very circumspect in discussions about prognosis and client self-determination (Bachrach 1996). Canadian author Arnold Kruger (2000), using the example of schizophrenia, reviews a number of factors that have contributed to this pessimism:

- Schizophrenia has been considered intractable *by definition:* from the outset it was conceptualized as a disorder with an inevitably downward or deteriorating course, initially by Emil Kraepelin (1856-1926) when it was known as *dementia praecox.* In their commentary, Harding, Zubin, and Strauss (1992, 27) note that, for Kraepelin, "prognosis confirmed diagnosis. If the person who had all the symptoms of dementia praecox improved, then Kraepelin routinely considered the patient to have been originally misdiagnosed – an interesting tautology." More recently, the *Clinical Manual of Supportive Psychotherapy* speaks of schizophrenia as "a *chronic illness* with a course of partial remissions and exacerbations" (Novalis, Rojcewicz, and Peele 1993, emphasis added). The current version of the American Psychiatric Association's (2000, 308-9) *Diagnostic and Statistical Manual (DSM)*, while acknowledging that the course of schizophrenia "may be variable," states that "complete remission is probably not common."
- Practitioners tend to see only the most disabled persons with this diagnosis, when, according to Harding and Zahniser (1994, 140), "such patients represent a small proportion of the actual possible spectrum." One estimate is that 17 percent of persons with schizophrenia and 40 percent of persons with psychosis go untreated (Ram et al. 1992), from which one may infer that a number of individuals are able to maintain themselves in the community "with minimal assistance" (Kruger 2000, 31).
- Follow-up studies of persons with schizophrenia have tended to be short-term. Longer-term studies have suggested that full or partial remission of symptoms may occur in later stages – that is, ten to twenty years after the onset of the disorder (see also Anthony, Rogers, and Farkas 2003).

To these factors one can also add the current paramountcy of the biological paradigm in psychiatry, wherein persons with schizophrenia are considered to be "hard-wired," so to speak. As well, it must be acknowledged that practitioner decision making, particularly with respect to client self-determination, will always be constrained by concerns about liability; a false positive – erring on the side of caution – is always preferable to a false negative from this perspective.

In reporting on the results of interviews conducted with thirty-two mental health clients, Killeen and O'Day (2004, 158-59) describe how low practitioner expectations – concerning returning to work in this case – are "imbedded in policies and programs":

> As we began to analyze the interviews ... we were struck by the degree to which their stories were saturated with negative messages and low expectations ... Some had been told by a doctor or a nurse in their initial hospitalization that they would never work again. Others, with college educations or solid work histories were placed by well-intentioned vocational rehabilitation counselors into unskilled low-wage positions and then encouraged to stay there ... rather than risk relapse by going after more challenging work. Often ignored was the possibility that the degree of stress created by a poverty-level lifestyle may be more destabilizing than the degree of stress engendered by challenging work ... Often an individual's talents, abilities and interests are simply forgotten or unwittingly relegated to the background by the concerned and well-intentioned individuals around them.

Recovery Principles: Theory and Practice

What exactly *do* we mean by recovery? A seminal article by William Anthony (1993) of Boston University's Center for Psychiatric Rehabilitation points out the multidimensional nature of this concept:

- Recovery can refer to recovery from the disorder itself – that is, remission of symptoms. *However*, in this conception recovery is possible even if some symptoms persist or return. Recovery, in other words, does not depend on the disorder being "cured."
- Recovery also refers to attempting to deal with and overcome the *stigma* associated with having a mental disorder, especially as it affects accessing education and employment. Practitioner attitudes can be instrumental in diminishing or contributing to this.
- Recovery also means dealing with diminished confidence and self-esteem resulting from lengthy periods of unemployment, and with feelings of loss that result from seeing ambitions for career, family, and companionship go unfulfilled.
- Recovery also refers to overcoming *iatrogenic* effects, such as medication side effects that result in movement disorders or impaired concentration, or practice approaches that have the effect of making the client overly dependent on health care providers. A Canadian Mental Health Association (CMHA) publication suggests that when clients are given no sense of personal responsibility by service providers, they reach a state of "learned helplessness and hopelessness," a state that practitioners contribute to by rewarding "easy to manage" clients – who do as they're told – and by

defining "insight" as the client's capacity to accept a bleak prognosis (Everett et al. 2003). These authors also note the negative effects of being labelled and processed: "Access to needed mental health resources comes only through 'certification of impairment and disability' ... a process that in effect *creates* the social category of psychiatric disability" (12, emphasis added).

In a more recent article Anthony (2003, 1) notes the importance, in the recovery vision, of the principle of "people first": "People with mental illnesses are people before they are cases, diagnoses or patients. They are not, as the mental health field has mistakenly emphasized, primarily defined and governed by their symptoms and their diagnoses. Rather, the principle of 'people first' assumes that people with severe mental illnesses primarily direct their own lives like their non-diagnosed brethren. That is, they are influenced by their own relationships with others, their own goals, their hopes, dreams and interests."

Anthony (1993, 18) gives a number of "basic assumptions of a recovery-focused mental health system." It is fair to say that several of these are contentious. The first assumption is that there are many pathways to recovery, meaning that recovery can occur without professional intervention; "professionals do not hold the key to recovery, consumers do" (18). Second, recovery is not a function of one's theory(s) about the causes of mental illness. That is, adopting a recovery vision does not commit a person to either side of the nature vs. nurture etiological debate. Third, it is acknowledged that recovering from the consequences of the disorder – stigma, iatrogenic effects, unemployment, poverty, discrimination, and social isolation – is often more difficult than recovering from the disorder itself. Fourth, recovery does not mean that the individual was not "really mentally ill" – that is, that their success was not a beacon of hope for others but rather an aberration or a fraud – an argument along the lines of the Kraepelinian tautology referred to earlier.[2] Finally, clients need to have someone present in their lives who believes in them: "People who are recovering talk about the people who believed in them when they did not even believe in themselves, who encouraged their recovery but did not force it, who tried to listen and understand when nothing seemed to be making sense. Recovery is a deeply human experience, facilitated by the deeply human responses of others. Recovery can be facilitated by any one person. Recovery can be everybody's business" (18). The importance of practitioners instilling hope is apparent from a number of client surveys and testimonials, as Bachrach (1996, 31) summarizes: "The patient authored literature reveals a number of relevant notions and ideas that are at best rarely given credence by professional program planners. Among these are the importance of hope to patients, their need for validation and encouragement, and their wish to be more fully involved in program planning efforts."

A brief comment should be made on what is arguably the most contentious assumption: that "recovery can occur without professional intervention." On this point, practitioners should try to be open-minded or at least pragmatic: "whatever works" is a maxim that more experienced clinicians often come to adopt. On the other hand, "professional" interventions should at least be considered before being ruled out. Given that psychotic disorders are potentially responsive to medication, it would be very tragic if clients, for whatever reason, were deterred by others from using this option. A better outcome would be to encourage persons to seek alternative approaches to healing – self-help, acupuncture, the creative arts – *alongside* professional treatment. It is possible that the alternative approaches chosen will conflict with "mainstream" programs, such as when clients pursue other, psychological therapies that conceptualize the mental health problem so differently as to create a "working at cross-purposes" situation. That being said, it is notable that a survey of 311 clients of professional programs, half of whom also used self-help services, found that the use of these services was associated with *greater* satisfaction with the professional mental health programs, leading the authors to conclude that "self-help and traditional mental health services can function complementarily, rather than in competition with one another" (Hodges et al. 2003, 1161).

Adopting a recovery perspective has a number of practice implications with respect to practitioner competencies as well as the design of mental health services. Concerning the individual practitioner, the ability to foster empowerment and recovery has now been identified as a core staff competency. A position paper on the topic details this expectation as follows (Coursey et al. 2000, 380-81): Staff should encourage independent thinking; support consumers' freedom to make mistakes; support choice and risk taking as leading to growth; avoid controlling behaviours; use a strength-based model; believe in the consumer's ability to recover; foster a sense of hope; shift from a stance of demoralizing pessimism to rational optimism; help foster the cycle of empowerment, hope, and independence; reframe relapses from "failure" to "opportunity to learn"; invite and foster the expression and enactment of individual goals and preferences; act in a way that fosters equalization and collaboration; use natural supports whenever possible; and accept legitimate feelings of sorrow, despair, anger, frustration, and excitement without pathologizing. There may be some question as to how, or whether, the attitudes and skills referred to here can be taught and evaluated and, if so, whether it should be the role of the human resources staff in mental health programs to train peer-support persons and/or practitioners "in the interpersonal skills necessary to facilitate this personal relationship" (Anthony 1993, 20).

Concerning the redesign of mental health services, Anthony (2000, 159) notes that this represents a radical paradigm shift, one where the accreditation standards used to evaluate health care organizations must be altered: "In the past, mental health systems were based on the belief that people with severe mental illness did not recover, and that the course of their illness was essentially a deteriorative course, or at best a maintenance course. As systems strive to create new initiatives consistent with this new vision of recovery, new system standards are needed." To this end, Jacobson and Curtis (2000, 335) suggest that incorporating a recovery perspective is potentially a difficult process in that, first, there is the danger of tokenism, where authorities may "simply rename their existing programs ... while the actual services offered remain the same," and, second, evaluating outcomes is problematic because "recovery" is an abstract concept not easily operationalized and measured.

An example of a practitioner dilemma, more prominent now in the era of recovery, concerns *goal setting*: program policies may require that goals be set in any involvement with a client and that, consistent with recovery principles, these goals be client-defined or driven; where the client declines to set goals, however, or where there is a disagreement between client and practitioner, there is still the danger that the goal set will not truly reflect the client's own interests.

Jacobson and Curtis (2000) go on to describe a number of strategies that may be used to implement recovery principles: (1) developing recovery vision statements; (2) developing recovery education for clients, family members, or practitioners, particularly the use of *cross-training*, where these different stakeholders join together as learners or educators; (3) employing consumers as board members, researchers, peer-support workers, and regular staff, recognizing the need for parallel organizational capacity building, which may include leadership training and workplace accommodations (see more on this below); (4) supporting client-run alternative programs, such as peer-support and self-help networks, drop-in centres, and wellness programs; (5) revising policies that may work against recovery – for example, practices that are insensitive to the experiences of trauma survivors and that may have the effect of retraumatizing these individuals (Harris and Fallot 2001).

With recovery as a philosophical underpinning, the discussion at this point moves to the goals, strategies, settings, and roles of psychosocial rehabilitation.

Psychosocial Rehabilitation: Goals, Strategies, Settings, and Roles

Corrigan (2003, 346) provides a framework for understanding the concept of psychiatric rehabilitation by referring to "four key structures": goals, strategies, settings, and roles.

Goals are the reasons why persons with psychiatric disabilities seek rehabilitation. These include: (1) *opportunity*, which is achieved by addressing prejudice, stigma, and discrimination through education and advocacy; (2) *inclusion*, which refers to experiences in housing, work, recreation, and social life, which are the same as among other members of the community, as opposed to separateness, manifested for example as "sheltered workshops" and psychiatric boarding homes; (3) *independence*, meaning the ability of clients to make decisions on their own; and (4) *quality of life*, which includes the satisfaction of basic needs and also refers to support networks, recreation, intellectual stimulation, and spiritual life.

Strategies are the tools that service providers use to help clients reach their goals. These include: (1) providing instrumental support, such as establishing linkages with community programs; (2) goal setting, so that the focus of rehabilitation is "driven by the consumer's perceptions of important needs" (Corrigan 2003, 350); (3) skills training; (4) transfer training, which refers to making skills learned more generalizable outside of the treatment setting – for example, by using homework exercises; and (5) family education and support.

Settings refers to the places where rehabilitation programs take place. One locale is the hospital, although given that in the post-deinstitutionalization era most hospitalizations are relatively brief, there may be some question as to how much rehabilitation programming can be provided in this setting. Nonetheless, brief hospital stays may still provide the opportunity for assessment of skills for independent living, some skills training (such as relapse prevention), and linkage with community programs. Community rehabilitation programs, which in the past tended to be physically separate and "sheltered," are increasingly provided *in situ*. An example of this is assertive community treatment (ACT), which in its earliest incarnation in the 1970s was referred to as "training in community living." While ACT is sometimes seen narrowly as a way of pulling hard-to-reach persons into treatment, it also has a teaching and skills training component that has the ultimate goal of greater client independence. Employment and education programs, discussed in more detail below, are also increasingly offered in competitive, integrated settings. Another example concerns the "day program," often operated as a hospital outpatient service, which provides structure, support, and skills training and in some cases takes over the clinical follow-up. (Hospital-based programs such as this may be on the decline, with commentators suggesting that services offered by day programs could be provided effectively in more normalized, integrated settings, such as supported employment programs [Drake et al. 1996]). Rehabilitation programs may also be of the self-help variety, the earliest post-deinstitutionalization example of this being the *clubhouse*, a setting where clients and service providers have equal status (ideally) and which offers social support and vocational rehabilitation: "Work provides the core healing process" (International Center for Clubhouse Development 2002, 1; see box).

Corrigan (2003, 354) suggests that "the various roles that describe providers of psychiatric rehabilitation are both multi-disciplinary and a-disciplinary" – that is, while practitioners may come from different professional backgrounds, they should "not permit the specialization of their discipline to suggest that some tasks are uniquely within their purview while the rest of the interventions are somebody else's work." While not all practitioners may be involved in rehabilitation in the sense of *services and technologies* – as per Deegan (1988), cited above – it is reasonable to suggest that they should appreciate the importance of the recovery perspective, referring to the *values and attitudes* that support rehabilitation.

The practice of psychosocial rehabilitation can be broken down into several "life-related domains" (British Columbia Ministry of Health 2002f, 3), which include personal life, work, and education. These domains are discussed separately below.

Personal Life

As was noted in the last chapter, mental disorders such as schizophrenia, because of the timing of their onset in the life cycle, the degree of impairment produced, and their duration, can result in life skill deficits. In some cases these skills are never learned; in some cases they are learned but fall into disuse, an outcome contributed to by any care providers who discourage independent thought and action.

The Clubhouse   SKiD

The genesis of the clubhouse model can be traced to the 1940s in New York, where a group of clients who had been patients at the same state hospital, and who had found little support in the outside world, formed a mutual-aid organization called WANA (We Are Not Alone). This eventually became Fountain House, whose mandate, described at its website (http://www.fountainhouse.org), is to provide programs "that facilitate recovery and rehabilitation." Fountain House has served as the model for a number of other organizations in the United States and Canada, which are usually run as non-profit societies. A clubhouse is defined as follows by the International Center for Clubhouse Development (ICCD) (2002, 1):

> A clubhouse is a place where people who have had mental illness come to rebuild their lives. The participants are called members, not patients, and the focus is on their strengths not their illness. Work in the clubhouse, whether it is clerical, data input, meal preparation or reaching out to their fellow members, provides the core healing process. Every opportunity provided is the result of the efforts of the members and small staff, who work side by side, in unique partnership. One of the most important steps members take toward greater independence is transitional employment, where they work in the community at real jobs. Members also receive help in securing housing, advancing their education, obtaining good psychiatric and medical care and maintaining government benefits. Membership is for life so members have all the time they need to secure their new life in the community.

The clubhouse is an example of a "separate" program, with respect both to physical space and mandate, catering just to mental health clients. This has its advantages in that the program may serve as respite or sanctuary for persons feeling overwhelmed as well as disadvantages in that a number of clients want normalized environments where they are not so clearly identified as "different" (Drake et al. 2003). It may be that the clubhouse fills a niche for those clients not ready for more competitive rehabilitation settings. On this point, a survey of Canadian clubhouses published by the Canadian Mental Health Association found that many clients valued the fact that the clubhouse was "a safe place for people with mental illness to come, have meals and get involved in social/recreational activities" (Hume 1997, 9). The survey found that while some clients were interested in skill development, others wanted "a place to go with no expectations" (9), raising the question of whether programs being run purely as drop-ins should use the clubhouse designation.

While the intention in the clubhouse model is that members and service providers will work side by side as equal partners, there is always the danger that organizations initially founded as self-help may be co-opted by professional or nonclient staff, leaving clients just token input into the decision-making process. To prevent this, the ICCD describes standards for clubhouse programs with respect to membership, relationships, house functions, and governance that may be used for accreditation purposes (see http://www.iccd.org).

Rehabilitation in the area of "personal life" refers to "services that help an individual gain or regain practical skills in the areas of personal care, home management, relationships and use of community resources" (British Columbia Ministry of Health 2002f, 3). "Personal life" may be partially captured by the concept/term "activities of daily living" (ADL). Components of personal life include the following:[3]

- *Personal care:* grooming and hygiene, physical health, relaxation, coping strategies and skills, fitness, nutrition, stress management, sleep, illness education (similar to relapse prevention), personal safety, drug and alcohol use, financial management, sexuality, smoking, and weight control.
- *Home management:* home safety, meal preparation, telephone skills, laundry, and household maintenance.
- *Relationships:* interpersonal skills, communication skills, self-advocacy, friendships, building social networks, assertiveness, anger management, sexuality (dating skills, healthy relationships), intimacy, and family relationships and support.
- *Community resources:* hearing about resources, transportation, local community resources – including health, social, and financial services – and accessibility issues.

Some problems with ADL may have more to do with resources than with personal failings. For example, a client's poor hygiene may be due to the fact that laundry facilities are inaccessible or unaffordable. This in turn speaks to the need to visit clients on their own "turf" in order to get an appreciation of the obstacles they face.

While practitioners will form general impressions of a client's skill deficits, there may be the need for a more systematic assessment – for example, when a hospital discharge is being planned. A number of life skill assessment instruments have been developed for this purpose – for the most part by and for occupational therapists (Asher 1996; Thomson 1992). The assessment method may involve a self-report, an interview, observation, a task, or a combination of these. For example, a "money management assessment," developed by the Occupational Therapy Department at Riverview Psychiatric Hospital in British Columbia, involves the following: (1) client self-report (clients are asked about how they manage their finances); (2) knowledge of currency (clients are asked to identify the name and worth of units of currency); (3) purchasing task, requiring calculation (staff persons give clients change from purchase, asking if amount given is correct); (4) knowledge of source of income (government pension, income assistance, inheritance, etc.); (5) description of assets and debts; (6) use of the banking system (name and location of bank, type of account, can client write a cheque, use a bank machine, etc.); (7) bill payment (can client identify what bill is for, amount, due date, and where payment is made); (8) budgeting (for essential and leisure items); (9) taxes (who prepares return, and where can you get assistance); and (10) comparison shopping (task involves comparing two items with different prices and sizes).

Practitioners need to be reflective and tactful when appraising the life skills of clients. The issues being addressed are very sensitive; none of us, after all, wants to appear incompetent. Further, clients should not be held to unreasonably high standards, standards that the average person does not always live up to. Practitioners have to balance, on the one hand, the need to encourage and model healthy behaviours with, on the other hand, the right of clients to be free from excessive interference and from the imposition of personal morality or excessive paternalism.

Skill deficits may be addressed in a number of settings, as noted earlier. Functional assessments may be performed by occupational therapists in hospitals or at community mental health clinics. Skills training may be offered by clinical and rehab staff at mental health clinics in either individual or group format. Skills training may also be offered through a number of community organizations, clubhouses, and self-help groups. The linchpin in all of this is the case manager, who, if not directly providing these services, should be alert to "personal life" problems, be aware of rehabilitation resources, and make linkages where appropriate.

Employment

The unemployment and underemployment rates for persons with a serious, persistent mental disorder have been estimated in North America to range from 70 to 90 percent (British Columbia Partners for Mental Health and Addictions Information 2003e; Eklund, Hansson, and Ahlqvist 2004; Killeen and O'Day 2004; McReynolds 2002; Rutman 1994). Since work is "central to self-identity, self-esteem and well-being" (Scheid and Anderson 1995, 164), unemployment may significantly impact the mental health of someone who is already struggling with the stigma associated with a psychiatric diagnosis. This struggle may be compounded by the attitudes of practitioners who, given the impairments associated with a disorder such as schizophrenia, may assume that high rates of unemployment are natural and inevitable. The counterargument is that people will tend to live up to expectations and that our expectations of clients have been consistently and unreasonably very low (Killeen and O'Day 2004; Kruger 2000). Cross-cultural studies that have found better outcomes in schizophrenia in the Third World[4] (as measured by periods of full remission) provide support for the view that employment and meaningful activity have therapeutic benefit and that, to this end, community expectations are crucial: "The structure of employment opportunities for people with psychiatric disabilities is very different in developing countries ... developing economies provide a naturally graduated ladder of work and recovery for people with psychiatric disabilities ... as much as people with disabilities are capable of doing ... their contribution is of use to the community and they are valued for it" (Kruger 2000, 34).

Clients themselves have for some time spoken about the importance of employment. A Canadian Mental Health Association report notes that "supports such as income, work and self-help, which are not usually provided by the mental health service system, are exactly the supports which consumers say are most important to them" (Trainor, Pomeroy, and Pape 1993, 12). One client writes as follows: "Told, upon the advent of my being diagnosed with bipolar affective disorder, that I may never work again, I rebelled. Whatever else I imagined myself to be before my diagnosis was contingent upon my ability to work and be a productive citizen. This fact was ingrained within the value system I inherited. It was part of myself that no doctor could diagnose away, or make disappear. This sense of who 'I' was in relation to myself and the world would prove stronger than any psychotropic drug I had ever ingested or any mental illness I supposedly had" (Molnar 2004, 7).

A review concludes that for mental health clients, "improvements in symptoms, lower hospitalization rates, greater social interaction, decreased anxiety, enhanced self-esteem and self-confidence and reduced stress are all potential benefits from engagement in a work setting" (British Columbia Ministry of Health 2002f, 17).

In addition to benefits to the clients themselves, employing persons with mental disorders can provide benefits to the organizations that employ them, particularly when these are mental health programs. As reviewed by Bainbridge (1998, 23), these include the dispelling of negative myths about clients, the fact that "acknowledgement of the value of consumer roles in service provision makes explicit statements about the overall worth of consumers," and the positive influence that clients can have on service philosophy and practice. On this last point, the present author found that mentoring a client peer-support worker led to more careful reflection about the ethical and clinical foundations of mental health practice, and that the mentor learned and grew at least as much from the experience as the client did.

The remainder of this section reviews types of employment potentially supported by mental health programs, barriers to the successful employment of clients, and accommodations that can be made to support client involvement in the workplace.

Types of Employment

In considering employment services potentially offered through, or supported by, mental health programs, two broad categories can be identified: preemployment and employment (British Columbia Ministry of Health 2002f). As noted above, earlier approaches to vocational rehabilitation in mental health followed set steps, with the individual typically starting in a sheltered workshop, where the work involved "light industrial tasks done in a workshop setting for token wages" (Trainor and Tremblay 1992, 65). Critics of this approach argue that clients "become stalled in some of the intermediate steps that are presumed to facilitate their progress toward regular community activities and do not get to the desired endpoint" (Drake et al. 2003, 436). While "sheltered" models still exist, there is increasingly a consensus that vocational programs should be based on a competitive, rather than sheltered, model of work.

Preemployment services include the following:

- *Vocational assessment and career counselling.* Here the target group is persons who are defining or redefining vocational goals.
- *Preemployment and work readiness training.* In this area clients are given skills training, work experience, and job search services; goals are to increase confidence and "work tolerance" and to help individuals "grow into" a job (British Columbia Ministry of Health 2002f, 22-23).
- *Volunteer work.* Compensations here are not financial (apart from honoraria) but rather may be in the form of verbal and written recognition or enhancement of an individual's sense of purpose and self-esteem. Volunteer work may be an end in itself or an opportunity to develop skills and gain work experience in a safer environment. Mental health programs may partner with existing volunteer services or develop their own service.
- *Transitional employment.* This is defined as a "time-limited series of placements in community jobs for the purpose of gaining work experience and building self-confidence" (British Columbia Ministry of Health 2002f, 26). Placements usually involve on-the-job training, and participants are paid at the going rate. This has traditionally involved a partnership between a mental health clubhouse program and an employer, with positions being held for mental health clients who, if unable to work for a period, would be replaced by another client from the clubhouse (thus alleviating the problem of staff turnover for the employer) (Johnson 1997).

Under the heading "employment" are the following models:

Supported employment, which involves individuals working "for pay, minimum wage or better, as regular employees in integrated competitive settings," with "ongoing, long-term, adequate support" being offered (British Columbia Ministry of Health 2002f, 29). Support would include ongoing assessment and skill development, as needed. Evaluations of supported employment programs have found long-term benefits in terms of job tenure, job competitiveness, and self-esteem (Salyers et al. 2004).

■ *Peer support*, which may involve peer mentoring, advocacy and education, and running peer-support groups.[5] Increasingly, peer support is being recognized as a valuable service largely because of the experience that the client service provider brings to his or her role in working with other clients: "Consumers have an in-depth knowledge of the system and can share insights with non-consumer providers and clients from the position of having been there. The consumer provider's credibility is magnified in the eyes of clients when they can relate a specific issue to their own personal experience. Also high on the list of benefits is the role modeling for clients of success, recovery and healing" (Bainbridge 1998, iii).

■ *Client-run businesses and services*, described in one article as "collective efforts to create work which is meaningful by virtue of the individual's stake in the enterprise" (Trainor and Tremblay 1992, 65). In an article detailing the genesis of A-Way Express Couriers, a nonprofit client-run courier service in Toronto, the authors recall how the founding members "wanted an empowering workplace in which the employees could be supported in becoming more independent" and "felt very strongly that they no longer wanted make-work projects or handouts" (Shragge et al. 1999, 46). It is noted that whether these operations are totally consumer-driven or supported by mental health staff, "it is vitally important to have strong support from stakeholders with business experience in areas such as the preparation of business plans, finding funding, marketing and other sound business fundamentals" (British Columbia Ministry of Health 2002f, 32). Since the advent of client-run businesses in the 1970s, local initiatives in Ontario have been supported by the Ontario Council of Alternative Businesses, established in 1994, which provides development assistance, education, and training (Shragge et al. 1999). Concerning the mental health benefits of employment, a survey of the staff at five Ontario client-run businesses found that tenure with these companies was associated with a reduction in hospital admissions, inpatient days, and contacts with crisis services (Trainor and Tremblay 1992).

Barriers

As noted, practitioner expectations, or lack of same, may present a barrier to supporting employment for mental health clients, which has been the impetus in some cases for clients to go outside the system in order to set up their own projects and businesses. Concerning positions that are created for clients within the mental health system, there is the potential for resentment among nonclient staff who may fear affirmative action hiring policies that would result in job displacement (Mowbray et al. 1996). There is the further danger of nonclient staff viewing client appointments as tokenism and minimizing or trivializing client roles and responsibilities (Fox and Hilton 1994). Nonclient staff may question the skills and "professionalism" of client coworkers, such as the ability to maintain confidentiality (Mowbray et al. 1996). In this author's own experience, great trepidation was initially expressed by agency personnel at the thought of client employees overhearing discussions in the staff room or having access to client files.[6] With respect to making inroads when nonclient staff are nervous about change, one author suggests: (1) that staff should be allowed to express their fears and concerns; (2) that management needs to be clear about what is expected; (3) that management may initially need to work with the most motivated staff; (4) that new people should be hired who already have the attitudes and skills to foster client involvement; and (5) that change be brought about gradually (Reidy 1992).

There may also be tensions for peer-support workers with respect to their relationships with other clients (Mowbray et al. 1996). These can include the prejudice, among client service recipients, that only a "qualified" professional can assist them or the view that client service providers are no longer true "peers" once they become employees. There may also be mistrust stemming from a perception that the peer-support worker has in some sense "sold out" to the authorities. In the worst-case scenario, the client employee becomes marginalized from both reference groups – professionals and peers.

Other potential barriers concern inflexible employment and income assistance policies. For example, if 100 percent of additional earnings are clawed back by the government from clients on income assistance, this may act as a disincentive for those who work part time or who are seeking a graduated return to employment. Clients will be deterred from vocational rehabilitation if they believe that this will mean a loss of disability benefits. The cost of transportation alone can become prohibitive if remuneration is inadequate. Employee contracts may also need to take account of the fact that relapses (perhaps involving hospitalization) are "episodic and unpredictable in nature" (Rutman 1994, 18).

Finally, the individual client employee may face a number of challenges having to do with the impact and consequences of having a mental disorder. As one author summarizes, "persons with psychiatric disability often exhibit cognitive, perceptual, affective and interpersonal deficits intrinsic to or resulting from the mental illness" (Rutman 1994, 17). Impairment may be caused by the disorder itself or by side effects of the medications used to treat the disorder. Because their lives and careers have been interrupted by a psychiatric disorder, clients in many instances "lack [the] normal life experiences and roles that are the foundation of one's vocational identity" and may be (as one author puts it) "vocationally immature" (17). Job applicants face the problem of gaps in their resumes and of not having references, in addition to the decision about whether to disclose their identities as mental health clients. Clients may, not unrealistically, have a host of worries and doubts about employment, such as fears about their work performance, fear of failure, fear of the unknown, a feeling that they cannot contribute anything of value, role strain, and even a fear of success in some cases (Mowbray et al. 1996; Valentine and Capponi 1989; Wilson 1996).

Accommodations

The intent of accommodations is to provide a more supportive workplace for persons with disabilities.[7] As reviewed by Bainbridge (1998, 31)," accommodations" for client employees include flexible scheduling, which can refer to allowing more time for orientation and for the completion of specific tasks and to allowing time off to accommodate medical and counselling appointments – "difficult to arrange, but often the most successful accommodation" (see also Secker et al. 2003). The employer may also need to consider providing coverage for absences due to hospitalization, a feature of the transitional employment model (see above). Other considerations include the provision of an advocate for advice and support, a job coach, or an employee willing to act as a mentor. Concerning organizational culture, acceptance and inclusion need to be the guiding philosophies of practice for programs to be considered inclusive (Bainbridge 1998). To help achieve these ends, Curtis and Smith (1996) suggest that there be: (1) clarity and consistency in ethical and practice standards, which are communicated clearly and often through words and action; (2) an acceptance of ambiguity; (3) open discussions about boundaries and ethical issues in safe forums; and (4) opportunities for collegial support.

In assessing the effect of accommodations, Fabian and colleagues (1993) reviewed job retention among thirty adults with serious mental disorders in a supported employment program in Maryland. Accommodations included modifying job tasks, work schedules, work procedures, and performance expectations, and providing orientation and training to supervisors and coworkers. The authors found a direct correlation between the number of accommodations and job tenure – that is, during the study period participants with five or more accommodations (five being the mean for the study) had a median retention period twice as long as that for those with fewer accommodations (twenty-four compared to twelve months). It was found that the two most important factors were *employer education* and the presence of *on-site job coaches,* who were able to negotiate on behalf of the employee.

Supported Education

Supported education "involves the integration of people with severe mental health disabilities into post-secondary education, and the provision of the supports that these individuals require in order to be successful in an education environment" (Neuman 2003, 6). Supported education is "relatively new to the field of psychosocial rehabilitation" (British Columbia Ministry of Health 2002f, 5) and grew out of the field of special education where students with "special needs" were first identified (Weiner 2003).

Three models for supported education have been identified: *self-contained, on-site,* and *mobile support.* "Self-contained" classrooms are ones where all the students have psychiatric disabilities, and the curriculum is specifically designed for the benefit of this population. Courses in this model are often noncredit, with the emphasis being placed on "personal development, vocational planning and academic upgrading" (Weiner 2003, 4). Some programs offer certificate training leading to competitive employment, such as tourism and office assistant work (British Columbia Ministry of Health 2002f). In general, self-contained programs are seen as something to build from "to help [students] achieve access to higher education in a manner in which [they] can experience success" (Weiner 2003, 4).

"On-site" refers to students with psychiatric disabilities attending regular university classes with additional support provided. A variation of this model is "mobile support," which involves support being provided to the student by external mental health practitioners, in addition to or instead of accommodations being provided by the educational institution. One government report concludes that "supported education services are to a large extent dependent on partnerships" between mental health services and educational institutions, that "development of these partnerships is critical and ... relies on excellent communication," and that "a shift in attitude [may be] required among educational and mental health staff to further develop this key service" (British Columbia Ministry of Health 2002f, 16). For their part, mental health practitioners may perform a valuable role in educating administrative and instructional staff at postsecondary institutions.

For persons with diminished confidence and self-esteem, which is often the case when struggling with a mental disorder, the prospect of returning to school can be daunting. Potential barriers also include the attitudes of mental health practitioners, teachers, and administrators as well as how education programs are structured and delivered. Barriers may also have to do with the effects of the disorder itself:

> People with psychiatric disabilities often exhibit cognitive, perceptual, affective and interpersonal deficits intrinsic to or resulting from the mental illness. In addition, there can be feelings of anxiety, hopelessness and guilt combined with perceptual problems, difficulty in processing and/or retaining information, effects of learning disabilities and limited attention span. Individuals with serious mental illnesses cannot predict when they might become ill or how long they might be away from a classroom setting because of relapse. When medications are prescribed, it frequently takes time to determine the dosage that is most effective at allowing full participation in an educational setting. (British Columbia Ministry of Health 2002f, 14)

For all these reasons, consideration of accommodations for students with mental disorders is important. Accommodations are usually arranged through a campus disability office and involve the student meeting with a counsellor and providing documentation from a physician (in most cases). Professors do not need to know the diagnosis but rather are informed about functional limitations. Accommodations can take various forms (Vagnerova 2003b; Weiner 2003) and include:

- Preparation courses and orientation sessions for persons with disabilities.
- Classroom accommodations, such as preferential seating (e.g. away from other students for an agoraphobia sufferer), permitting beverages (to help with medication side effects such as sedation and dry mouth), and assistance with note taking (such as having another student or a friend take notes, or allowing use of a tape recorder).
- Studying accommodations, such as texts on tape, tutoring, mentoring, and the creation of peer-support groups.
- Assignment accommodations, such as delays granted due to hospitalization (or other mental health concerns) and assistance in completing assignments during hospitalization.
- Examination accommodations, such as altering the format, allowing the use of a computer if handwriting is made difficult because of side effects, allowing more time to write the exam, allocation of a separate room, and giving a (different) take home exam.

- Administrative accommodations, such as flexibility in determining full-time status for the purposes of financial aid and health insurance as well as offering an incomplete grade, rather than a failure, if the student suffers a relapse.

One of the most significant potential barriers is the cost of education, with tuition fees rising significantly in Canada in recent years ("Fees limit access," 2003; McKee 2003). While this applies to any student, it is especially a concern for mental health clients, who typically have more limited financial resources. As reviewed by McCormick and Martel (2003) funding options include bursaries made available for persons with psychiatric disabilities by individuals, mental health agencies, and provincial governments and also include the Canada Student Loan Program, the Canada Study Grant for Students with Permanent Disabilities, the Canada Millennium Scholarship Foundation, a fund for vocational rehabilitation for persons receiving Canada Pension Plan Disability Benefits, and the Federal Permanent Disability Benefits Program.

Notes

1 In this article, published by the conservative American online journal *National Review*, the authors conclude that: "The problem with the recovery vision is that it is a dangerously partial vision. It sets up unrealistic expectations for those who will never fully 'recover,' no matter how hard they try, because their illness is so severe" (Satel and Zdanowicz 2003).

2 By way of example, American psychiatrist Daniel Fisher, who went on to complete an MD and PhD after being diagnosed with schizophrenia, notes that the typical response to his own recovery is for people to assume that he must have been misdiagnosed or, if "truly" schizophrenic, be incompetent to perform his professional duties (Fisher 1999).

3 This section is adapted from a document produced by the Personal Life Committee, a group of occupational therapists employed by the Vancouver Coastal Health Authority.

4 See Leff et al. (1992); Thara (2004); and Chapter 9 in Whitaker (2002).

5 At the time of writing, sixty-five clients were employed part time as peer-support workers at the author's agency, Vancouver Community Mental Health Services.

6 By policy, clients could not be hired as workers by the same team or unit where they themselves were clients.

7 Mental health clients have some qualified protections under law in the area of employment. Under Canadian federal and provincial human rights legislation, as well as Section 15 of the *Charter of Rights*, employers may not discriminate against employees or potential employees on the basis of mental disability, although these provisions do not apply to "bona fide occupational qualifications." In other words, refusing to hire someone who cannot perform the duties of a job because of mental disability would not infringe human rights legislation (Robertson 1994). Human rights legislation also imposes a duty to provide workplace accommodations for persons who are otherwise qualified, although this duty is "not limitless ... [and] must be balanced against the right of an employer to conduct its business in a safe, economic and efficient manner" (the "undue hardship" standard) (D'Andrea 2003, s.4, p.69).

Other Resources

- A publication by the British Columbia division of the Canadian Mental Health Association (CMHA), *Visions,* issue number 17 on supported education, is available at http://www.cmha-bc.org./content/resources/visions/issues/17.pdf
- The Psychiatric Dis/Abilities Program at Toronto's York University has its website at http://www.yorku.ca/cdc/pdp/index.htm.
- The recovery website for Hamilton County, Ohio (http://www.mhrecovery.com), has articles, links, and best practices guidelines related to recovery from mental illness.
- The federal government operates a website with information on disability-related programs and services in Canada (see http://www.pwd-online.ca).
- The website of the International Center for Clubhouse Development (http://www.iccd.org) has a directory of programs in different countries, information on accreditation, and links to library resources.
- The website of the British Columbia division of the CMHA (http://www.cmha-bc.org/inventory) provides an employment services database "that is oriented toward the unique needs of people with mental health issues."

The Legal and Ethical Context of Mental Health Practice

As we have seen, mental health practitioners in the course of their work may interfere with the liberty of individuals, such as when they arrange for the involuntary detention and treatment of someone in a hospital psychiatric ward or when they are supervising a community treatment order. At this point we turn to the legal and philosophical basis for curtailing freedom, asking "how is it justified?"

Some would argue that it is rarely if ever justified. This extreme version of civil libertarianism – epitomized by the writings of American author Thomas Szasz (see box on next page) – relies on the premise that persons exhibiting apparently disordered thinking are in reality competent agents exercising free will, notwithstanding the fact that some observers may find the behaviour to be upsetting. A less extreme viewpoint is that, while we may at times have to interfere with the liberty of individuals, "interference always stands in need of justification" and that "the onus of justification always lies on those who want to interfere" (Browne et al. 2002, 285). This view is associated with English philosopher John Stuart Mill, who in his famous essay *On Liberty*, published in 1859, argued that state intervention, no matter how well intentioned, leads inevitably to the *infantilization* of the subjected person. Mill recognized that the state had a right to intervene – referred to as the government's **police powers** – in order to prevent harm from coming to *others*. Further, Mill saw that not all adult citizens could be held to the same standard of responsibility, that some were "encumbered" due to lack of information, duress, or particular emotional states (Browne et al. 2002).

If one assumes, then, that a mental disorder constitutes a form of encumbrance that may compromise a person's ability to care for him or herself, there is still the question "at what point do we intervene?" A problem with focusing on the *prevention* of harm is that it necessitates the prediction of future behaviour, an exercise fraught with difficulty. Indeed, some – often family members – complain that this requirement may mean waiting until it is "too late" (Hardin 1993; Hall 2000). For these reasons, an alternative position is that mental health practitioners have an obligation to look after individuals who, simply put, are unable to look after themselves, even if there is no imminent risk of harm to the individual or to others. This is referred to as the *parens patriae* (government as parent) powers of the state.

Debates about when to intervene have proven contentious for family members, clients' rights advocates, practitioners, and legislators – who must craft the criteria to be included in mental health statutes. Intervention decisions can be seen as falling somewhere in a continuum from a *narrow* standard for intervention (e.g., imminent physical danger to self or others) to a *broad* standard for intervention, which may refer to the "welfare" of the individual, need for treatment, "best interests," or the potential for future deterioration (see box on next page). The standard that any jurisdiction adopts must be viewed in historical, social, and political context. A number of North American jurisdictions that in the 1970s adopted legislation reflecting an emphasis on civil rights have in more recent years seen the pendulum swing back to *broadening* the standard for intervention (Gray, Shone, and Liddle

Thomas Szasz and the Myth of Mental Illness

In considering psychiatry and civil rights, it is impossible not to refer to the views of American author Thomas Szasz, who, although himself a psychiatrist, has been a steadfast critic of psychiatric practices. In a number of publications (e.g., *The Myth of Mental Illness* [1974]; *Schizophrenia: The Sacred Symbol of Psychiatry* [1976]; *Psychiatric Slavery* [1977]) and on his website (http://www.szasz.com), he has argued that "mental illness" has no basis in physical reality and that labelling individuals "schizophrenic" is simply a means by which society controls persons exhibiting undesirable behaviour. This position appears to fly in the face of increasing evidence that disorders such as schizophrenia do have a biological basis (see Chapter 2) and has also been criticized as a heartless stance in that the logical outcome is the abandonment of individuals who cannot look after themselves (Gray, Shone, and Liddle 2000). In Szasz's writings there is an emphasis on personal accountability and a dismissal of the idea of mental illness as an excuse for unacceptable behaviour. Notably, his website is called the "Cybercenter for Liberty and *Responsibility*" (emphasis added). Szasz is still cited as an authority by critics of psychiatry and some psychiatric consumers (e.g., Shimrat 1997), although an opponent suggests that his theories finally "have been relegated to the shelf of quirks of medical history" (Torrey 1988, 165).

2000). Critics suggest that these more recent legislative developments, which include community treatment orders (see below), are the product of an increased preoccupation with "protection of the public" and that media accounts of violent behaviour by psychiatric patients have swayed popular and political opinion (Davis 2002). Notwithstanding legal parameters, it must be emphasized that there will also be variance at the level of *individual practitioners* as to their own "risk tolerance," where they sit on the intervention continuum, and consequently how legislative standards will be interpreted.

The *Charter of Rights*

Before looking at Canadian mental health statutes, it is necessary to consider the impact of the *Charter of Rights and Freedoms*. Enacted in 1982, this is Canada's supreme law, one that, with some exceptions,[1] takes precedence over other existing federal and provincial statutes, including mental health laws. Several sections of the *Charter* may have application in considering the reasonableness of laws that permit the involuntary detention and treatment of mentally disordered persons. These include:

- s. 7: Right to life, liberty, and security of the person.
- s. 9: Right not to be arbitrarily detained.
- s. 12: Right not to be subjected to any cruel and unusual punishment.
- s. 15: Right to equal protection of the law without discrimination, including discrimination based on mental disability.

If a law appears to infringe one or more of the *Charter* rights and a challenge is made, the government must be able to show that any infringement was in accordance with the principles of fundamental justice, procedural fairness, and a balancing of the interests of the individual and society or that the law can be "saved" by Section 1 of the *Charter*, which states that the rights therein are "subject only to such reasonable limits prescribed by law as can be demonstrably justified in a free and democratic society." In practice, Section 1 refers to a legal test developed in a court case called *Oakes*,[2]

Decisions about intervention: A continuum

<--->

Imminent physical danger	"Welfare" of client
(narrow standard,	(broad standard, preemptive
intervention as last resort)	intervention)

which requires the following: the infringing law must pursue an objective that is "pressing and substantial"; there must be a rational connection between how the law works and its objective; the law must infringe upon *Charter* rights as little as is reasonably possible; and there must be proportionality between the effects of an infringing law and the objective of the law.

In anticipation of the potential impact of the *Charter*, in 1987 an interprovincial committee drafted a *Uniform Mental Health Act* to comply with *Charter* guarantees, with the hope that this would lead to greater standardization of the various provincial and territorial mental health acts (Davis 1995b).[3] Notwithstanding this measure, the different acts still vary somewhat with respect to substantive and procedural aspects.

Provincial Mental Health Acts and Involuntary Hospitalization

With health care a provincial jurisdiction in Canada, each province and territory has an act that governs the involuntary detention ("committal" or "certification") and treatment of persons presumed to have a mental disorder. This section reviews (1) the criteria for involuntary admission, (2) the procedures used in committals, (3) the issue of treatment refusal, (4) community treatment orders, and (5) legal protections for the patient. The reader is cautioned that the laws referred to here were current as this book went to press but that the relevant statutes would need to be accessed concurrently regarding possible revisions.

Criteria for Involuntary Admission

Canadian mental health acts make reference to "safety," "protection," or "harm" (to self or others) as the basis for intervening with mentally disordered persons, although court decisions to clarify the interpretation of these terms have sometimes been required.

As noted above, in the 1970s, with increasing recognition of the civil rights of psychiatric patients, detention criteria were narrowed in some jurisdictions so that *dangerousness* became the key consideration. It was felt, by some, that certifying patients for their own "welfare" when their behaviour was no immediate threat to anyone reflected an overly broad and paternalistic standard. Thus in 1979 Ontario adopted the physical dangerousness standard in its *Mental Health Act*, the first province to do so (Gray, Shone, and Liddle 2000). British Columbia dropped the "welfare test" (although not until 1987), leaving only the "protection" standard. The standard in the Yukon and the Northwest Territories currently is "serious bodily harm."

Gray, Shone, and Liddle (2000) offer a number of critiques of physical dangerousness as the sole basis for involuntary hospitalization. They point out that this may mean ignoring the needs of an individual who is deteriorating physically and mentally but more gradually. There is also evidence from a number of (mainly American) studies that clinicians end up "bending the rules" in any case by continuing to commit to hospital persons who (apparently) would benefit from treatment but who may not meet the dangerousness criterion; this is based on the finding that in jurisdictions that narrowed committal standards, patients continued to be sent to hospital at the same rate as they had been prior to the change in the law (Appelbaum 1994). This sort of decision making may be supported by judicial opinion; Gray, Shone, and Liddle (2000, 118) report that "Ontario courts have interpreted serious bodily harm/imminent and serious physical impairment relatively broadly."

By contrast, several Canadian jurisdictions – Manitoba, Saskatchewan, and British Columbia – include prevention of mental or physical deterioration as a basis for involuntary hospitalization in their mental health statutes. Interestingly, Ontario, first to enact the physical dangerousness standard, subsequently broadened the committal standard in its *Mental Health Act* (in 2000) to include "deterioration" but added the qualification that this criterion could be used only when there was an established history of successful psychiatric treatment.

While in some provinces the committal criterion is further defined or qualified (the Ontario *Mental Health Act* refers to *"serious bodily harm"*), in others the criterion is left unqualified. In Prince Edward Island the standard is "safety" of self or others, which one legal analyst argues can, and has, been interpreted more broadly to include nonphysical harms (Robertson 1994). In Alberta the standard is "danger" to self or others. Concerning the possible ambiguity of this term, an Alberta government task force concluded that it would be best not to qualify the meaning of "dangerousness"; rather, there should be "latitude for the exercise of professional discretion and clinical acumen" (Government of Alberta 1983, 56). In British Columbia the standard of "protection" was challenged in the 1993 BC Supreme Court case *McCorkell v. Director of Riverview Hospital Review Panel*,[4] where the plaintiff argued that the standard was "vague and overbroad" and that, consequently, committed persons were being denied their liberty and subjected to arbitrary detention, contrary to *Charter of Rights* guarantees. In dismissing this action, Justice Donald wrote that "given the purpose of the *Act* – the treatment of the mentally disordered who need protection and care – the language must permit the exercise of some discretion." He further stated that "protection" could refer to "social, family, vocational or financial harm" (beyond simply physical danger), thereby giving a very broad interpretation of the committal standard. The BC *Mental Health Act* was undergoing a process of revision at the time, and this court decision was seen as a victory for those concerned about restricting access to treatment for the mentally ill (Davis 1995b).

In looking at certification standards, some comment must be made on how decision making is affected by resource availability. As noted earlier, in many larger urban centres in Canada, there is great pressure on psychiatric beds in general hospitals. Consequently, it has become more difficult to get patients admitted, and hospital staff feel more of an onus to move patients out as new cases arrive at the front door. Doctors in the community are of course aware of this and know that even though a particular patient might be certifiable by the letter of the law, he or she may not be detained or may be discharged quickly if there are others arriving at the hospital who are apparently more in need. In other words, while a particular certification standard – such as that adopted by British Columbia following the *McCorkell* decision – may appear broad in theory, a narrower standard will be applied in practice if hospital beds are in short supply.

Procedures Used in Committals

There are three mechanisms by which a person can be hospitalized involuntarily in Canada. The first and most frequent method is a certificate signed by a physician (not necessarily a psychiatrist). In all jurisdictions, except Nova Scotia, only one certificate is required.[5] Exceptions have been made in the Yukon and the Northwest Territories, presumably because of limited access to physicians, where in the former a nurse and in the latter a psychologist can arrange a certification if no other alternatives are available. The single certificate authorizes detention of the person for twenty-four to seventy-two hours, depending on the jurisdiction. Beyond this time, a second certificate must be signed at hospital for the person to be detained longer. Statutory or common law provide for involuntary treatment of the patient during this initial period if the circumstances can be considered an emergency (Gray, Shone, and Liddle 2000).

The second method of involuntary hospitalization is apprehension by a police officer. This typically occurs in evenings or on weekends when medical offices may be closed. There is a presumption that accessing a physician in these cases is impossible or impractical. A somewhat narrower statutory standard for police apprehensions is applied in some jurisdictions; for example, there is reference to "danger" in the case of British Columbia, Alberta, and Nova Scotia.

The third method, available in all Canadian jurisdictions, is a judge's warrant. This method, used presumably because no other mechanisms are available, involves a citizen approaching (depending on the jurisdiction) a judge, magistrate, or justice of the peace and making a statement that a person is apparently mentally ill and apparently meets the certification criteria. A warrant may then be issued to the police.

The Issue of Treatment Refusal

Canadian provinces handle the question of involuntary treatment differently. In some provinces the committal process allows the attending physician to go ahead and treat the patient (typically with medication) with or without consent; this is the case in British Columbia, Saskatchewan, Newfoundland, and Prince Edward Island. "Requiring/needing treatment" is, in fact, a criterion for committal in the BC and Saskatchewan statutes.

In other provinces treatment is considered a separate issue, and involuntary treatment decisions are handled by a tribunal or court, in the case of Quebec and New Brunswick, or by a substitute decision maker, in the case of Ontario, Alberta, Manitoba, the Yukon, and the Northwest Territories. In this latter group a hierarchy of potential decision makers is approached in turn, ending with the public trustee if no other qualified person can be found.

How did these different approaches come about? Historically, the right to refuse treatment was not addressed in mental health statutes; rather, the discretion to impose treatment involuntarily was granted as part of the authority to commit persons to hospital. Following the 1960s, however, more legal protections were built into mental health acts, a reflection of greater societal recognition of patients' rights. It was noted that psychiatric treatments could have deleterious effects – electroconvulsive therapy (ECT), in particular, received a lot of bad publicity – and, further, that *non*psychiatric patients had the right to refuse medical treatments and procedures, notwithstanding their potential benefits and necessity. It was also argued that the question of competency in one area of decision making should not automatically extend to another – that is, that despite being committed to a psychiatric facility, a patient could still make reasonable decisions about his or her treatment, particularly in the case of previously expressed wishes. Legal analysts have suggested that statutes, such as British Columbia's *Mental Health Act*, that do not provide a mechanism for considering the competency of patients concerning their treatment wishes, are likely in violation of *Charter* guarantees, such as the rights to life, liberty, and security (s. 7) and to freedom from discrimination on the basis of mental disability (s. 15) (O'Neill 1990; Verdun-Jones 1988).

In provinces that use substitute decision makers, three distinct standards can be identified (Gray, Shone, and Liddle 2000). The first, used in Alberta, is "best interests," where the substitute makes treatment decisions based on what he or she believes are the best interests of the patient without necessarily any consideration of the patient's previously expressed wishes. The second standard, used in Manitoba, has been called "modified best interests." In this case the substitute is to take into account the patient's previously expressed wishes, made when competent, but can resort to the "best interests" standard if the substitute believes that the patient's wishes "would endanger the physical or mental health or safety of the patient or another person" (Manitoba *Mental Health Act*, s. 28.4). The third standard, used in Ontario, the Yukon, and the Northwest Territories, is "capable wishes." Here the patient's previously expressed wishes not to be treated, made when competent, must be adhered to. There are also review processes, such as Ontario's, where the substitute or the psychiatric practitioner may approach a board of review for permission to override the patient's previously expressed wishes.

The question of involuntary treatment and substitute decision making was considered in the 1991 Ontario Court of Appeal case *Fleming v. Reid*.[6] Under the *Mental Health Act* at that time, a review board would receive the expressed wishes of the patient, made when apparently competent, but was not obliged to follow the wishes (in the case of treatment refusal) and instead could apply a "best interests" standard. The court ruled in this case that the relevant provisions in the *Act* were in violation of the *Charter* and thus invalid. The judgment read: "Although the right to be free from non-consensual psychiatric treatment is not an absolute one, the state has not demonstrated any compelling reason for entirely eliminating this right, without any hearing or review."

The idea that patients committed to a psychiatric facility should have a (qualified) right to refuse treatment has been criticized, predominantly by clinicians (O'Reilly 1998). Several points have been raised. One is that, since the days of *One Flew Over the Cuckoo's Nest*, conditions in hospitals have improved, as have treatments, the latter with respect to both efficacy and side effects. A second argument is that the comparison with treatment refusal by *non*psychiatric patients is spurious since in the case of psychiatric patients the organ that is used to make decisions – the brain – is the very one impaired by illness. Another critic points to "the danger of advance directives being applied in a circumstance that a person could not foresee" (Hoffman 1997, 84). Finally, perhaps the most compelling argument is that not offering treatment to a hospitalized patient may mean that the individual will have to be detained longer than would otherwise be the case and that further mental and physical deterioration, and greater risk to staff and other patients, will be the result (Kelly et al. 2002; O'Reilly 1998). One group of Ontario authors refers to this practice as the "right to remain psychotic" (McCaldon, Conacher, and Clark 1991).

A more recent case concerning the right to refuse treatment was the Supreme Court of Canada's decision in *Starson v. Swayze* (2003). The respondent in this case, Scott Starson, had appealed an Ontario review board's decision to permit his involuntary treatment during a hospitalization that had resulted from his being found "not criminally responsible" for uttering death threats (see section on "mental disorder and the *Criminal Code*" on p. 284). Diagnosed with bipolar disorder, Starson was a gifted amateur physicist who claimed that medications impaired his ability to write scientific papers. The statute in question, the Ontario *Health Care Consent Act*, permitted involuntary treatment on the grounds of *incapacity*, with **capacity** being defined as (1) the ability to understand information relevant to making a treatment decision and (2) the ability to appreciate the "reasonably foreseeable consequences" of the decision or lack of one. The Consent and Capacity Board's finding of incapacity was overturned by the provincial Superior Court, a decision upheld by the Court of Appeal. This was appealed further to the Supreme Court of Canada, which in a 6-3 decision determined that Starson was by law capable of making decisions about his psychiatric treatment, finding that the statutory test for incapacity had been misapplied by the Consent and Capacity Board. The court also concluded that the onus should be on the doctors to prove why medication is needed rather than on the patient to make a case against it. The Supreme Court's ruling was criticized by family support groups and by the respondent's own mother, who in a newspaper interview stated that "without his medication   he will be institutionalized for the rest of his life" (Tibbetts 2003, A3).

Conditional Leave and Community Treatment Orders

Historically, "certification" has referred to *inpatient* status. However, in recent years, there has been greater utilization of – and debate about – statutes that provide for *outpatient* certification. Provisions of this sort have been implemented in a number of British Commonwealth countries, including Canada, as well as in the United States (Davis 2002; Swartz and Monahan 2001; Torrey and Kaplan 1995). While they go by different names, the main distinction is between **conditional (extended) leaves**, whereby involuntary patient status, commenced during hospitalization, is continued after hospital discharge, and community treatment orders, which authorize the initiation of involuntary status in the community.

Regarding conditional leaves, New Brunswick and Saskatchewan have provisions for time-limited leaves, with the intention that the patient return to hospital afterward. British Columbia, Alberta, Manitoba, Prince Edward Island, and the Yukon provide for indefinite leaves, where the patient may be returned to hospital if the leave conditions are "breached," but otherwise remains on leave or is discharged absolutely while in the community. In 2000 Ontario enacted a conditional leave provision with a three-month maximum duration. The conditions in this type of order typically require that the patient attend appointments at the treatment setting and take psychotropic medication as prescribed. Procedurally, extended leave involves a transfer of care from the hospital to the community, with the attending community physician then renewing the involuntary status – or not – on a schedule similar to that followed in the hospital.

The use of extended leave is usually justified as a way of preventing the "revolving door syndrome." The following quotation is taken from the *Guide to the Mental Health Act* (British Columbia Ministry of Health 1999, 42-43): "Reasons for using extended leave can include assisting patients who, despite sensitive care, are unable to maintain themselves on medication; placing a person in the community on a trial basis; or providing long-term support or assistance in managing everyday activities. Since stopping medication can result in relapse, such patients may end up in the 'revolving door' of involuntary hospitalization – becoming recommitted and discharged when the medication takes effect. As repeated episodes of acute psychiatric illness can harm a patient's recovery, extended leave can offer the patient a better prognosis."

Two provinces, Saskatchewan (in 1993) and Ontario (in 2000), have introduced provisions whereby a treatment order can be initiated in the community. Some evidence of treatment "failure" is required before such an order can be started: two hospital admissions or more than thirty days in hospital during the preceding three years in the case of Ontario, and three admissions or more than sixty inpatient days during the preceding two years in the case of Saskatchewan. At the time of writing, the province of Alberta was also considering legislating community treatment orders.

The use of outpatient certification remains an issue that has produced strong divisions of opinion. Supporters argue, as noted above, that community treatment orders are effective in reducing rates of rehospitalization, a claim that seems to have some empirical support (Fernandez and Nygard 1990), and that they are, by definition, less restrictive than hospitalization since the person remains in the community. Indeed, several provinces make explicit reference to the "less restrictive" status of outpatient certification in the language of the legislation (Gray, Shone, and Liddle 2000).

On the other hand, critics have raised a number of concerns (Allen and Smith 2001; Everett 2001). One has to do with the implication, and stereotype, that the mentally ill are so dangerous that they need tight controls. It is noteworthy, for instance, that the Ontario community treatment legislation was called "Brian's Law," after the name of a sportscaster who was killed by an apparently mentally ill assailant. (Similar pieces of legislation in New

York and California were referred to, respectively, as "Kendra's Law" and "Laura's Law.") Another criticism concerns resource availability, with some suggesting that the move to community treatment orders is a cynical way of trying to deal with the fact that there are insufficient treatment and rehabilitation services in place (Stainsby 2000); as one analyst puts it, "coercion will not lead to more effective treatment if the treatment system itself is inadequate" (Diamond 1996, 60). Others have challenged the claim that outpatient certification is in fact "less restrictive," pointing to the indefinite length of the orders. There have also been concerns among mental health practitioners about the extra pressure on hospital beds if patients are "recalled," and about how community orders change the therapeutic relationship when the policing function of the worker's role necessarily becomes emphasized (Davis 2002).

Despite these concerns, there is evidence of increasing utilization of community treatment orders in Canadian jurisdictions. In Vancouver, British Columbia, for example, the number of cases of persons required to report to a mental health team as a condition of extended leave more than doubled in a three-year period to at least 254 as of January 2005.[7]

Legal Protections
Provincial and territorial mental health acts provide some safeguards and protections whereby involuntary treatment or detention is reviewed and may be challenged. As noted above, some jurisdictions provide for a qualified right to refuse treatment, while others authorize treating personnel to unilaterally override treatment refusal (in the case of British Columbia, such treatment decisions are "deemed to have been given with the consent of the patient"). The patient may request a second medical opinion in Manitoba, British Columbia, and the Northwest Territories, although implementation of these opinions relies on the discretion of the treating facility.

The most common method by which a patient may challenge certification is by an application to a review board or panel, which is available in all Canadian jurisdictions (except the Northwest Territories, where a court performs this function). The review board is supposed to function as an independent tribunal, which does not cost the patient anything and which is normally less formal than a court hearing. The composition of, and procedures used by, these boards vary somewhat from jurisdiction to jurisdiction (Gray, Shone, and Liddle 2000). In some provinces periodic reviews of detention are mandatory.

A number of empirical studies of the review board process have been conducted in Canada. One survey of Ontario hospitals, for example, found that while only 9 percent of review board applications resulted in the certificate being rescinded, in 25 percent of cases the treating physician changed the patient status to voluntary after an application was made, suggesting – perhaps – an aversion to dealing with the "red tape" of tribunal proceedings (Komer et al. 1999). Data from British Columbia show that in 2004 patients successfully appealed their detention in 23 percent of cases when the appeal was heard; however, two-thirds of review applications never got to that stage, being suspended, rejected, or cancelled instead (British Columbia Ministry of Health Services 2005).

A second, less common method of challenging certification is through the courts. Patients may be deterred from this approach because of the time and potential cost involved, although some advocacy organizations may take on cases without charge. Most jurisdictions considering these appeals may examine both the facts of the case and points of law. Another method involving the courts is to challenge the certification by way of habeas corpus, which may make use of a procedural violation, such as the certificate's having been filled out incorrectly or having expired (Savage and McKague 1987).

One final point concerns how patients are informed of their rights in the first place. Critics have complained that, notwithstanding statutory provisions, treating personnel may be less than enthusiastic in carrying out this task and that comprehension on the part of the patient may be limited by various factors, such as mental disorder, sedation, literacy, and ethnicity.[8] In recent years patients' rights organizations have taken a more proactive stance on this issue – for example, going on-site at psychiatric facilities to educate patients about legal protections.

Competency and Adult Guardianship

Apart from mental disorder (putting aside for the moment the problem of adequately defining this term), an individual's decision-making abilities may be compromised by other conditions. For instance, an elderly person may become increasingly unable to manage his or her affairs because of progressive dementia. Another example would be the plight of a young man with a serious head injury who is consequently unable to make decisions about his treatment, rehabilitation, and residential placement. Or one could cite the situation facing an individual and her family where she had suffered a stroke and could not make financial decisions. These examples refer to the question of **competency**, which Silberfeld and Fish (1994) define as having sufficient ability to perform a specific task, as opposed to actions that are beyond an individual's control. Examples of decisions that are affected by competency include choosing a residence, making a will, financial planning, end-of-life care and health care in general, and instructing a lawyer. With competency referring to a *series* of abilities, it can be seen that some individuals could be competent in one area, such as financial planning, but not in another, such as the safe operation of a motor vehicle.

Mental health practitioners may be called in to assess competency in situations like those described above. When this arises, Silberfeld and Fish (1994) suggest that an informal assessment be done first partly because the consequences are less onerous; a formal assessment may necessitate restrictions of that individual's liberty, restrictions that can be wide-ranging. Being *wrongly* found incompetent can cause considerable psychological and practical harms for the individual so assessed.

A more formal assessment involves a consideration of risk (discussed in more detail later in this chapter) and typically has both (1) a medical-psychiatric component, involving a mental status exam and other structured instruments (see Chapter 10), and (2) a functional component, involving task-specific tests, preferably done in vivo at the person's residence (see Chapter 12). In the case of assessing financial competence, criteria used may include (1) ability to communicate, (2) sufficient knowledge of assets and expenses, (3) ability to handle day-to-day transactions, (4) directive ability (identifying appropriate individuals who could assist with financial decisions), (5) consistent expression of preferences, (6) ability to understand and weigh options, and (7) ability to rationalize choices (Silberfeld et al. 1993). Depending on the gravity and complexity of the decisions, competency assessments may be multidisciplinary conferences that include an ethicist. Should a person be found incompetent, someone else, either an individual or a public agency, can be appointed as a **guardian** by a judge to make decisions on behalf of that person, with the individual or agency then being under a legal duty to safeguard the interests and wellbeing of the incompetent person.

In recent years a number of provinces have reformed adult guardianship, consent to treatment, and adult protection laws, "formaliz[ing] the common practice of relatives, or someone appointed by a person when capable, making health decisions if the person becomes incapable" (Gray, Shone, and Liddle 2002, 8). A number of developments have provided the impetus for these legal reforms (Gordon and Verdun-Jones 1992): (1) that the population in Canada is aging, making the care needs of the elderly more prominent and pressing; (2) deinstitutionalization, with more of the elderly disabled now being cared for in community settings; (3) a greater awareness of the issues of abuse and neglect of the elderly; (4) the advent of the *Charter of Rights* and the need for laws to conform with these guarantees; and (5) criticisms of the existing laws. Analysts note that earlier guardianship laws, for instance, had more to do with protection of estates than persons, that they provided no guidelines to practitioners by which competency could be assessed, and that competency was defined in an "all or nothing" fashion rather than in a manner reflecting the current vision of guardianship as limited in scope and tailored to the individual case (Gordon and Verdun-Jones 1992).

Concerning the particular provisions of guardianship legislation, readers may refer to more specialized texts, such as Gordon and Verdun-Jones (1992), bearing in mind that the law is often in a state of flux. Using British Columbia as a brief example, one can note that the relevant provisions are contained in a number of different statutes:

- *Adult Guardianship Act:* provides (in part) designated agencies with the mandate to look into reports of abuse or neglect.
- *Representation Agreement Act:* provides for adults who want to appoint someone to manage their financial affairs and to make personal care and health care decisions if they become incapable of doing so themselves. Representation agreements, also known as *advanced planning* or **"Ulysses"** agreements, provide guidelines to a support team, which may include practitioners and family members, and take on particular importance in cases where the client is a parent and child care decisions need to be made in the event of the parent becoming unwell.
- *Power of Attorney Act*: provides for the appointment of someone to manage an individual's financial affairs (only).
- *Health Care (Consent) and Care Facilities (Admission) Act*: codifies the common law and customary practices with respect to consent and substitute consent to health care for those who don't have representation agreements. Establishing informed consent requires a test of the client's **capacity** – that is, the ability to understand the nature of a health care intervention, risks, benefits, and alternatives.
- *Public Guardian and Trustee Act*: provides for a substitute decision maker of last resort and for a system to monitor the activities of those who are making decisions for others.
- *Patients Property Act*: provides for the public guardian and trustee to act as a surrogate financial manager for incapable adults who are patients of a psychiatric facility.

While guardianship laws give mental health practitioners the authority to, for example, remove an individual from a residence and place him or her elsewhere when there is evidence of abuse or neglect, there is recognition, reflected in the law, that this type of action should be carried out only as a last resort – that is, after other, less intrusive supports have been considered (Gordon and Verdun-Jones 1992). Increasingly, protocols developed by community mental health programs are specifying that, before any action is taken, there should be a presumption of competency and that self-determination and minimal intrusiveness should be the guiding principles.

One can see that there are definite similarities between the powers given under adult guardianship laws and those given under mental health acts as they relate to the assessment, hospitalization, and treatment of persons apparently incapable of making decisions for themselves. In fact, some have suggested that with developments in adult guardianship in Canada, it is no longer necessary to have separate mental health legislation (Gordon 1993; Szmuckler and Holloway 1998). Gray, Shone, and Liddle (2000) suggest some reasons why use of guardianship laws would be preferable to reliance on a mental health act: (1) the person most involved and concerned with the client is making decisions rather than a paid practitioner who may not know the client well; (2) guardianship laws have more broad powers (e.g., authority in the area of finances), making assistance more comprehensive; (3) inpatient admission can be obtained for people who do not meet the involuntary admission criteria of mental health acts. These authors also point out potential barriers: (1) guardianship means arranging lawyers, assessors, and court time, which may be costly, time-consuming, and unappealing to practitioners and others; (2) guardianship may cause more tension and strife among family members if the order is contested; (3) guardianship requires the presence of a competent, concerned decision maker. If guardianship is not widely used at present in Canada, it may be because of unfamiliarity with new legislation and because certification under a mental health act is a quicker, more expedient option for practitioners, albeit one that offers mainly short-term benefits.

Mental Disorder and the *Criminal Code*

The *Criminal Code*, a federal statute, contains a number of provisions concerning persons before the criminal courts who are apparently suffering from a mental disorder. The need for such provisions becomes more apparent when one considers the evidence that substantial numbers of the seriously mentally ill in Canada are, unfortunately, being caught up in the criminal justice process, as was discussed in Chapter 9.

To begin with, the *Criminal Code* gives a judge the authority to order a psychiatric assessment of an accused person, which is intended to address that person's **fitness to stand trial** and/or whether they may be not criminally responsible by reason of mental disorder (NCRMD).[9] This assessment may be done in custody, usually at a psychiatric facility. The *Code* stipulates that in-custody fitness assessments should not be more than five days' duration, although there are provisions for extending this period.

"Fitness to stand trial" refers to the accused person's mental state while at court and whether he or she can competently participate in an adversarial criminal proceeding. The test, according to the *Criminal Code*, is whether the accused can understand the nature or object of the proceedings, understand the possible consequences of the proceedings, or communicate with defence counsel. Canadian courts may try to avoid applying too high a standard of fitness in such cases because of the delays and possible deprivations of liberty that may ensue given that a finding of unfitness may result in the accused being held in custody until fitness is restored (Tollefson and Starkman 1993). Of particular concern are those individuals suffering from apparently intractable conditions such as fetal alcohol syndrome, since there is the prospect that once declared unfit they will never be found competent to stand trial (Department of Justice Canada 2003). The *Criminal Code* also authorizes, following a finding of unfitness, involuntary psychiatric treatment of the accused to restore fitness, an unusual exception to the rule that psychiatric treatment is to be governed by provincial or territorial statutes.

Historically, the pretrial psychiatric assessment, while ostensibly addressing fitness, has been used in Canada as a mechanism whereby mentally ill persons charged with less serious offences have been "diverted" – that is, transferred to psychiatric facilities with charges being dropped. This is a practice that has had both its proponents and its critics and one that may be on the decline partly because of the downsizing of psychiatric hospitals and partly because of changes to the *Criminal Code* in 1992 that restrict the duration and scope of pretrial assessments (Davis 1994b, 1994c).

The court (or the accused) may also request an assessment of criminal responsibility. The test here is that the accused, at the time of the act or omission, must have been suffering from a mental disorder "which made him or her incapable of appreciating the nature and quality of the act or omission, or of knowing that it was wrong" (*Criminal Code*, s. 16.1). For judicial interpretations of this test, the reader is referred to more specialized texts (e.g., Verdun-Jones 2002). Historically, defence lawyers in Canada have been reluctant to use (what was then called) the "insanity defence," particularly for lesser offences, because it could result in a lengthy detention in a psychiatric hospital, a longer period in many cases than typical jail sentences for similar offences (Davis 1994a). The *Criminal Code* at that time mandated the *automatic* and *indeterminate* detention of an insanity acquittee and did not provide specific criteria by which the person's status, including consideration of discharge, would be reviewed. These provisions were found to be in violation of the *Charter of Rights* and were ruled invalid in the landmark 1991 Supreme Court of Canada decision in *Regina v. Swain*.[10] This decision necessitated the passage of new legislation in 1992. Now, for people found

NCRMD, the *Criminal Code* specifies that a review board must make a disposition that is the "least onerous and least restrictive to the accused" and that if the accused is not deemed to be a "significant threat" (*Criminal Code*, s. 672.54) to the safety of the public, he or she is to be given an absolute discharge. Persons not given an absolute discharge may be detained in hospital or may be granted a conditional discharge where they report periodically to an outpatient clinic. With the consequences of being found NCRMD now less onerous, analysts have suggested that the mental disorder defence has become a "more attractive option" in Canada (Verdun-Jones 2000), and in fact there is evidence that the use of this defence has increased since 1992 (Grant 1997; Livingston et al. 2003).

Apart from the questions of fitness and criminal responsibility, an individual's mental state may be an issue at the point of sentencing. In particular, there may be a requirement, as a condition of probation, that the person attend for psychiatric treatment. In some instances this order has been written as a requirement to "take medication"; however, this practice – enforcing medication compliance through a probation order – was found in a 1990 British Columbia Court of Appeal decision[11] to be "an unreasonable restraint upon the liberty and security of the accused person" (s. 7 of the *Charter*) and thus unlawful. In this ruling the judge stated that accused persons would still be responsible for maintaining their mental health and that a refusal to take medication could result in an order to report more frequently to a probation officer for monitoring (Davis 1995b).

In looking at barriers to treatment, it can be said that mental health practitioners are often very reluctant to deal with persons under a court order unless they are mandated to do so (i.e., work at a specialized forensic unit). Indeed, clients with histories that combine "madness" and "badness" are often doubly stigmatized, both by the public and sometimes by treating professionals.

Ethical Decision Making

The Current Environment
The decision making of mental health practitioners is circumscribed, as we have seen, by laws such as the *Charter of Rights and Freedoms* and other federal, provincial, and territorial statutes, although this statement is qualified by the observation that professionals can in some cases "work around" the law (Davis 1994b) and by the finding that *extra*legal factors – such as resource availability – are commonly crucial to understanding intervention decisions. However, the statutes and case law referred to here can provide only rough guidelines for clinical practice and will necessarily be a patchwork. Most clinical decisions are not underpinned by clear legal mandates

but represent the exercise of practitioner discretion. Further, the key decision of certification – sending someone involuntarily to hospital – which may provide temporary comfort to the practitioner or family member, is a "last resort" type of action that may not always be applicable and that may provide only a short-term "solution." For all these reasons, it is necessary for practitioners to apply an ethical framework in the appraisal of decisions concerning clients with complex needs.

Arguably, the ethical decisions facing mental health practitioners, particularly the tension between client autonomy and practitioner paternalism, are more challenging at present than they have ever been. As was discussed earlier in this book, mental health services have been increasingly influenced by the consumer empowerment movement and the recovery paradigm, which emphasize consumer-driven initiatives while offering a critique of practices that reinforce professional authority and hierarchy (Anthony 1993; Curtis and Hodge 1995; Davis 2002). For example, an article on practitioner competencies in the *Psychiatric Rehabilitation Journal* lists the following as desired attitudes or approaches with respect to fostering client empowerment: encouraging independent thinking, supporting consumers' freedom to make their own mistakes, supporting choices and risk taking as leading to growth, and avoiding controlling practitioner behaviours (Coursey et al. 2000).

At the same time, practitioners must contend with initiatives that are not easily reconciled with a consumer empowerment movement – that is, program and policy developments that appear to signal a move to *greater* practitioner paternalism. These developments include a broadening of committal criteria in some jurisdictions, a greater reliance on community treatment orders, a greater reliance on "aggressive" methods of intervention such as assertive case management (Dennis and Monahan 1996), and a move to accommodate stakeholders such as family support groups who may advocate for greater access to treatment and more coercive practices. In a report by the mental health advocate for the Province of British Columbia, the potential conflict between the agenda of family advocates and an empowerment perspective is highlighted: "Self-advocates, peer advocates and formal advocates for people with mental illness did not always have the same perspective as family advocates ... The central and most controversial point was the role of coercion in the treatment system. Relatives of ill people, typically with schizophrenia, tended to see their family member as having little insight into his or her illness and requiring compulsory treatment. Consumer advocates, on the other hand ... saw coercion as a strategy that reduces self-esteem and dignity and ultimately drives people out of the treatment system" (Hall 2000, 20).

In another area of practice, the increasing use of assertive community treatment (ACT) programs presents ethical challenges to the practitioner. As we
have seen, ACT programs are used in many North American centres to supplement traditional, office-based services (see Chapter 7). ACT programs target
"harder to reach" clients, are outreach based, involve more frequent and
prolonged client contact, deal with the "nitty-gritty" activities of daily living, and emphasize pragmatism – "whatever works" (Davis 2002). While
there is evidence that these programs have been effective in preventing rehospitalization, critics have argued that the approach used is overly controlling and paternalistic and "flies in the face of the progress which has been
achieved [concerning empowerment] in recent years" (Spindel and Nugent
1999, 2). One analyst notes that when first conceived in the 1970s "consumer empowerment was not a serious consideration [with ACT programs]"
since ACT "was designed to 'do' for the client what the client could not do
for himself or herself" and that while times have changed, "a clear articula-
tion of the underlying ethical principles of these 'new teams' [still] does not
yet exist" (Diamond 1996, 53).

In confronting these and other challenges, a systematic application of ethical principles and guidelines is necessary. In particular, it can be argued that
greater attention needs to be paid to the development of guidelines specific
to more coercive forms of practice, such as community treatment orders and
ACT programs (Davis 2002; Everett 2001). Apart from guidelines, a *process*
also needs to exist so that discussions of applied ethics can take place – that
is, an organizational structure and culture that encourage open group discussion and feedback regarding complex and difficult treatment scenarios.
Curtis and Hodge (1995, 54-55) note that "managers have a responsibility
to help line staff make thoughtful decisions, and to develop an environment where staff can safely and comfortably raise such questions [about
ethical decisions] ... In some organizations, it is difficult for many staff to raise
questions about ethics or relationship boundaries, or even to admit they
have concerns, since doing so may imply a failing in judgment."

Applying Ethical Principles
The helping professions, such as medicine, nursing, psychology, social work,
and occupational therapy, provide members with codes of ethics, from which
certain core principles can be identified.

The first of these is *autonomy*, which refers to self-determination and re-
specting people's preferences. Another core principle is *nonmaleficence*, or
"do no harm." The flip side of this is iatrogenesis, where a "helper" inadvert-
ently creates or worsens a problem, such as when surgery is done poorly or
when it may not have been necessary in the first place. In mental health,

there are a number of ways that a treatment approach may be harmful, despite the best intentions of the practitioner. For instance, the psychotropic medications given may produce such severe side effects that the client is deterred from using them. It may also be the case that a particular style of interaction, such as being very confrontational, will retraumatize persons who have suffered childhood abuse (Harris and Fallot 2001). Another area of concern may be that assertive community treatment programs that do a lot *for* the client – in terms of activities of daily living – may actually make the client more, rather than less, dependent. As one ethicist puts it, "if adults are prevented from making their own decisions, they revert to being children" (Browne et al. 2002).[12] The corollary of nonmaleficence is *beneficence*, "do good." More accurately, this principle refers to the prevention, avoidance, or removal of harms and, using the example of severe medication side effects, may involve the consideration of the "minimum therapeutic dose" or the application of a cost-benefit analysis.

The next principle is *justice*, which refers to fairness and nondiscriminatory practices (i.e., treating like cases alike). Another way of looking at this is to ask whether we hold clients to a different standard than other people. For example, someone may recommend that an individual continue to have outreach workers visit him or her because the person keeps a messy place or perhaps because he or she has a poor diet, mainly ordering in pizzas. But should messiness alone warrant the intrusion of an outreach worker when nonclients are permitted to be messy? It may also be the case that we hold older persons to a higher standard, particularly concerning risky behaviour. For example, should your elderly grandfather be restrained from going hang-gliding, something he has always longed to do? The answer would depend on a number of factors, but the key question is whether the individual's age *alone* should be the reason for the restraint. In considering the justice principle, the practitioner should ask *whose* standards, or values, are being upheld.

Another core principle is *veracity*, "tell the truth." Practitioners may sometimes withhold or distort information because they feel that the client may not be able to handle it or, in fact, because of their *own* comfort levels (Kirk and Kutchins 1992). Consent of the client may not truly be informed consent. This author has experienced situations when doctors have been uncomfortable in sharing a diagnosis of schizophrenia with a client; this stems from weighing the stigma of the label (and more generally from the limitations of diagnosing – see Chapter 3) against the client's right to know what is being written in his or her file. This tradition, of the practitioner as aloof authority figure, has been challenged with the move to models of practice that involve the client as collaborator. Related to veracity is the principle of *fidelity*, "keep your promises." For example, clients may need to hold the hope that at some point they will be tapered off the medications that they are now being prescribed or that they will have their community treatment orders rescinded, and practitioners will agree to these expectations without any real intention of fulfilling them. Practitioners should keep their promises or at least not promise what they cannot deliver.

Finally, there are the twin principles of *utility* and *futility*. Simply put, should practitioners persist with an intervention, and the harms that may incidentally arise from it, when there is no evidence of effectiveness?

These principles may, in some cases, provide a course of action for the practitioner. Often, however, more information is needed. In the case of the hang-gliding grandfather, for example, one might ask how physically frail this individual is or whether there is any cognitive impairment. In approaching this task, a decision-making framework articulated by Browne and colleagues (2002) will be used.

To begin with, when considering an intervention that an individual might not agree with – such as preventing the grandfather from hang-gliding – there must be some question of *risk*. Without any apparent risk, it is exceedingly difficult to justify any interference. Risk can be seen as a function of both the degree of harm that may result and the probability that it will happen. For example, concerns about an elderly relative falling in her apartment may be related to the frequency with which this occurs, but even when the event is infrequent, concern may be raised if the individual has osteoporosis and is likely to sustain a serious injury. Risk is seen as applying to *specific* situations – for example, risk of starting a fire, risk of being evicted, or risk of malnutrition. In assessing risk, Silberfeld and Fish (1994) suggest that care providers consider several factors, such as: Is the risk new or old? Are there concrete instances of harm? Is the risk imminent or remote? Can the assessment be considered "objective?" Is the risk *chosen* or accidental? And is the risk to self or others? Regarding this last point, as was noted at the beginning of this chapter, a different standard is applied if the risk is to someone else; conversely, if the risk is to self and the decision maker is competent, interference is not justified. Concerning risk to others, Browne and colleagues (2002) note that, for example, "worry to relatives" is insufficient to support an intervention unless it can be argued that the individual's actions are not voluntary due to some form of impairment and, similarly, that an unhealthy lifestyle in and of itself cannot be the basis for interference because of the justice principle.

Assuming that the existence of risk has been established, the practitioner needs to consider whether the client's actions are voluntary or whether there is "encumbrance." Encumbrance can refer to the acute phase of a mental illness or to incompetence due to dementia, intoxication, duress (coercion or manipulation by a third party), or inaccurate or incomplete information. If an individual is unencumbered and apparently acting against his or her "best interests," practitioners may try to explain and argue for a change in behaviour – what ethicists refer to as "soft" paternalism – but, in this framework, should stop short of pressuring and physical coercion – "hard" paternalism (Brown et al. 2002).

Narrative Example: David

David is a forty-year-old man diagnosed with schizophrenia. He has been followed by a mental health team for some years and is on antipsychotic medication, usually in the form of an injection. He does not strenuously resist taking this medication but doesn't necessarily agree with the need to take it, nor with his diagnosis. He appears to suffer from thought-blocking and auditory hallucinations, which are sometimes present even when he is on medication. At times he appears "spaced out" and at other times can be seen laughing to himself. These symptoms are not sufficient for him to be certified for hospitalization in the opinion of the psychiatrist on the mental health team.

David lives in a skid-row area where there is a lot of illicit drug activity. He uses a lot of street drugs himself, mostly crack cocaine, and appears to have no motivation to change. Attempts to get him into detox or drug treatment programs have mostly been unsuccessful. He has been neglecting his personal hygiene and nutrition and has lost some weight. This is likely due to the effects of the cocaine and to the fact that any financial resources he has go toward purchasing drugs. When his mother buys him new clothes, he can be seen a short time later attempting to sell these on the street.

His mother is very worried about David. She would like him to be certified under the *Mental Health Act* "for his own protection," particularly given his neglect of self-care and what she sees as his risk of disease transmission (e.g., HIV if he is using drugs with others and sharing their equipment). His psychiatrist will not certify him, stating that he is not acutely psychotic and that his cocaine use is the result of his being a drug addict, not the schizophrenia. The mother disagrees, arguing that schizophrenia makes people more vulnerable to drug addiction and that her son is not capable of making decisions for himself. She is very angry with the mental health team for, as she puts it, not doing their job of looking after her son and has complained about this to a family support group. The mother and a representative of the support group want to meet with you, the case manager, to talk about this.

Finally, when considering intervening with someone who is encumbered, the practitioner should try to ensure that the intervention will be effective (utility), that the benefits will outweigh the costs (beneficence), that any interference is the mildest possible (nonmaleficence), and that any interference be nondiscriminatory (justice). Implementing these principles when working with older adults will mean trying to maximize the independence of the person in question and to avoid, if possible, placing the individual in a facility and thus having that person lose his or her residence. In practice this involves building in supports such as respite care, homemaking, "meals on wheels," physical accommodations, and alert signalling devices, and may also mean putting in place power of attorney or trustee arrangements to protect the individual's assets and make sure that bills are paid. As well, practitioners will often get involved with informal support networks, including neighbours, friends, and family. In working with *younger* adults the same principles apply, although options may be more limited because the situation will often be one where the client has a psychotic illness but is refusing treatment. In these cases decision making typically boils down to a question of whether the practitioners involved feel the client is certifiable or not – whether the risk is intolerable with respect to both legal parameters and personal comfort levels – bearing in mind that involuntary hospitalization may damage the client-worker relationship and that it is not a long-term solution. Risk will sometimes be exacerbated by drug abuse, with the client being in a "pre-contemplative" state, thus unlikely to agree to placement in a detox or addiction treatment program. Short of certification, practitioners may attempt persuasion, and may also consider more coercive approaches such as assertive outreach or outpatient committal. While it may seem crass to talk about "carrots and sticks," experience shows that workers will often achieve some headway, or credibility, if they can be seen to be acquiring some tangible benefit for the client. In these difficult situations worker perseverance, a nonjudgmental attitude, and an emphasis on maintaining the relationship are all important factors. It must be borne in mind that persons working in community mental health settings will always be dealing with some degree of risk, and that the appropriate goal is risk reduction, not elimination.

To conclude this chapter, the reader is given a narrative involving a client, David (see box on previous page). After reading this passage, consider the following questions: What are your initial feelings and reactions to this situation? What assumptions or biases may be in operation on your part? What ethical principles may apply? What is the nature and degree of risk, if any, in this scenario? If you were the worker involved, what would your course of action be?

Notes

1 For instance, the "notwithstanding clause," although rarely used, permits the federal or provincial governments to declare that a law shall remain in force despite the *Charter*.
2 *R. v. Oakes*, [1986] 1 S.C.R. 103.
3 The new Canadian territory of Nunavut (created in 1999) has imported its *Mental Health Act* from the Northwest Territories.
4 *McCorkell v. Riverview Hospital Review Panel*, [1993] 8 W.W.R. 169, 81 BCL.R. (2d) 273 (S.C.).
5 In the last revision of the British Columbia *Mental Health Act* (1999), the number of physicians required to certify was changed from two (unaffiliated) to one, which was interpreted as a progressive move by some and as a retrograde move by patients' rights advocates.
6 82 DLR (4th) 298 (Ont CA).
7 These figures were kept by an individual team director, rather than more systematically (as with an online information system), and may be an underestimate.
8 A survey of previously hospitalized clients in New Brunswick found that one in eight did not know whether they had been admitted involuntarily (Miedema 1994).
9 Previously referred to as "not guilty by reason of insanity."
10 (1991), 63 C.C.C. (3d) 481 (C.C.C.).
11 *R. v. Rogers* (1990), 61 C.C.C. (3d) 481 (BCC.A.).
12 In the same vein, Canadian psychologist Tana Dineen (2000, 159) suggests that the "psychology industry" promotes "encouraged dependency" and "externalized responsibility."

Other Resources

▪ The Representation Agreement Resource Centre, a Canadian website, provides information and publications on various aspects of representation agreements (see http://www.rarc.ca).

Diversity and
Cultural Competence

14

Canada has seen a number of demographic shifts in relatively recent times and is increasingly a land of cultural and ethnic diversity. Data from Statistics Canada show how immigration patterns have changed:[1] among immigrants surveyed in 1996, the vast majority of recent arrivals were from Africa, Asia, the Middle East, Latin America, and the Caribbean (over 800,000 arrivals between 1991 and 1996, compared to about 52,000 arrivals prior to 1961). Conversely, the number of immigrants from "traditional" source countries in the United Kingdom and continental Europe declined over this same period: of those surveyed in 1996, 942,000 had arrived prior to 1961, compared to 197,000 between 1991 and 1996. Data from the 2001 Canada Census reveal the following:

- 5.4 million persons were immigrants, about 18 percent of the total population. Of this number, one-third (1.8 million) had been in the country fewer than ten years. Percentages were much higher in the larger urban centres: in Metropolitan Toronto 43.5 percent of residents (about 2 million persons) had been born in other countries, with about 40 percent of this number having arrived in the previous ten years. In Metropolitan Vancouver 37.5 percent of residents were immigrants, with 43 percent of this number having arriving within ten years of the survey.
- In Metropolitan Toronto 39 percent of residents – nearly two in five – did not have English or French as a mother tongue; in Metropolitan Vancouver the equivalent figure was 37 percent (rising to 50 percent in the City of Vancouver "proper").
- 13.4 percent of the national population was defined as "visible minority." Again, this figure was much higher in the larger urban centres – that is, 36.8 percent in Metropolitan Toronto and 36.9 percent in Metropolitan Vancouver. A subsequent report from Statistics Canada (2005) predicts that the visible minority figure will grow to between 19 and 23

percent nationwide by 2017 and to about 50 percent in Toronto and Vancouver.

The changing face of Canada has not necessarily been reflected in how mental health services are organized and delivered. In particular, it can be argued that our diagnostic systems and treatment modalities show an ethnocentric bias and that in many cases we either do not understand alternative conceptualizations of mental disorder or clumsily apply ethnic stereotypes that do not account for the diversity *within* cultural groupings. Further, there is the problem of language barriers and the fact that translation services are not always available. This resulting "lack of fit" may result in minority clients not accessing, or disproportionately dropping out of, mental health treatment (Deiser 2002; McCabe and Priebe 2004; LaRoche 2002). For example, in 1998 it was found that members of Vancouver's large Chinese community were utilizing services of community mental health teams at only 62 percent of the rate expected based on their representation in the population (Greater Vancouver Mental Health Service Intercultural Committee 1999).

This chapter reviews the particular mental health concerns of immigrants, First Nations persons, and persons of other sexual orientations; existing barriers to service provision and help-seeking; and practice developments and philosophies that have arisen in an effort to make services more effective and accessible.

The Mental Health of Minorities[2]

Immigrants and Refugees

As noted, Canada's urban population includes a large number of recent immigrants, most of whom will speak English or French as a second language. Trying to get a sense of the nature and prevalence of mental health problems among this group is complicated by the limitations of the available data (Hyman 2001); on this point, one group of authors suggests that there has been "frequent unjustified exclusion" of minority groups from clinical and epidemiological studies (Flores et al. 2002, 82). Any assessment of needs is also confounded by differences in help-seeking behaviour. For some immigrant groups, the stigma of mental disorder is particularly acute because of the sense of shame or failure that it may bring to the family; consequently, families may be more likely to keep their unwell relative at home and to seek help only as a last resort. Reluctance to seek help may also be influenced by the perception that service providers will not be sensitive to their particular cultural needs and traditions. Estimating the prevalence of mental disorder is also complicated by the misinterpretation of symptoms: it has been noted that for some immigrants, based on experiences in their country of origin, maintaining a certain level of suspiciousness is normal and adaptive, whereas this may be interpreted as paranoia by practitioners in the new country (Ganesan 2000; see also Whaley 1998 concerning the African American experience).

The mental health needs of immigrant groups may vary in relation to the length of time that they have been in the new country. It has been hypothesized that immigration is a process characterized by initial feelings of joy and relief, followed by a period where there are regrets, feelings of loss, and adjustment difficulties, and ultimately ending with a stage where there is some reconciliation (Pedersen 1995). In this conception the risk for developing mental disorders increases following an "incubation" period that may last one to two years (Beiser and Hyman 1997), a prediction that was borne out in a study of psychiatric disorders among Iranian immigrants to Canada (Bagheri 1992).

There is evidence that refugee groups in Canada suffer from higher rates of psychological problems resulting from past trauma and adjustment to the new community. A study of adolescents from refugee families in Montreal found that rates of depression and anxiety were one and a half to two times higher in the refugee group than in the general public due to refugee camp experiences and family separation (Tousignant 1997). A study of children of Southeast Asian immigrants in Vancouver found, compared to other youth in the area, higher rates of depression, which interviews showed to be associated with communication problems at school, intergenerational conflicts at home, ambivalence about ethnic identity, and perceived discrimination (Hyman, Beiser, and Vu 2000). Practitioners need to be alert to the possibility of post-traumatic stress disorder (PTSD) among refugees escaping war-torn countries; for example, the prevalence of PTSD has been reported to be as high as 90 percent among groups such as Cambodians fleeing the Pol Pot regime (Kinzie et al. 1990).

In Canada a task force was established in 1986 to look at mental health issues affecting immigrants. In its published report, the task force concluded that it was not immigration per se but the contingencies *surrounding* immigration that affected mental health status:

> Pre-migration stresses such as catastrophic experiences, refugee camp internment, together with post-migration stresses such as poverty, unemployment and separation from family (frequent components of the refugee and resettlement process) jeopardize mental health. Personal resources such as fluency in the host country language, ethnic pride and positive attitudes toward acculturation, together with social resources, such as family and

ethnic community support and a positive reception by the host country, not only exert a beneficial effect on mental health, but may buffer the impact of stressful experience. Socio-demographic characteristics such as age, gender, education and ethnicity affect the chances of being exposed to stressful situations, as well as the availability of personal and social resources. (Hyman 2001, 42)

Concerning socio-demographic variables, it is suggested that adolescents and the elderly may be more vulnerable groups, along with persons who have experienced a greater initial drop in economic status (Ganesan 2000). Concerning economic status, a survey of first-generation immigrants in British Columbia found about half of recent immigrants (residents for fewer than five years) and one-quarter of all immigrants to be living below the poverty line, compared to 11 percent of nonimmigrant families (Greater Vancouver Mental Health Service Intercultural Committee 1999). This study concluded that "immigrant and refugee families have to wait a long time before their financial situation is similar to that of Canadian-born families" (4).

The First Nations
According to the 2001 Canada Census, there were just under one million First Nations persons in Canada, referring to North American Indians,[3] Inuit, and Metis. There is considerable diversity within this population: the First Nations in Canada represent "11 major language groups, more than 58 dialects and some 596 bands residing on 2284 reserves, cities and rural communities" (Kirmayer, Brass, and Tait 2000, 6).

In Canada persons of First Nations ancestry suffer from a range of health problems at higher rates than the rest of the population (Health Canada 2004b). Life expectancy is substantially shorter among the First Nations due to higher infant mortality, accidents, and suicides (Kirmayer, Brass, and Tait 2000). A 2004 report produced by the Canadian Population Health Initiative determined that in addition to higher suicide rates and shorter life expectancy (by five to ten years), Aboriginal peoples in Canada had three times the rate of diabetes and sixteen times the rate of tuberculosis compared to the general public (Branswell 2004). A random survey of Inuit residents of an Arctic community found current rates of depression and alcohol abuse to be 26.5 percent and 30.6 percent, respectively, numbers that the authors found "troubling" in that they are among the highest reported in North America and also because solutions appear to be elusive (Haggarty et al. 2000, 361). Substantially higher rates of fetal alcohol syndrome are reported among Aboriginal Canadians compared to other groups (Shah 2004). Even among other disadvantaged groups, First Nations persons fare more poorly on a number of health indicators: for instance, a study of injection drug users on Vancouver's skid row found Aboriginal persons becoming HIV positive at twice the rate of non-Aboriginal persons (Craib et al. 2003).

Suicide rates among young First Nations persons in northern, more remote communities are among the highest in the world and have created something of an international scandal for Canada (Elliott 2000; Kirmayer, Boothroyd, and Hodgins 1998; McAndrew 1999; Mittelstaedt and Haggart 1999). According to Health Canada (2004b) First Nations suicide rates are two to five times that of the general public, with the highest rate occurring among the Inuit – 70 per 100,000. In reviewing the historical accounts, one author concludes that the higher suicide rates seen in First Nations communities is a consequence of colonialism: "The general consensus is that self-inflicted events among Aboriginal people were, at the time of European contact, extremely limited" (Leenaars 2000, 58).

In examining the high rates of suicide seen in Native communities, investigators have looked at associated factors at both the individual and social/structural level. One study involving the Inuit in northern Quebec found that risk factors for suicide included male gender, personal or parental history of substance abuse (particularly solvents), a history of physical abuse, and feelings of alienation from the community. That males in the study were more likely to both attempt and complete suicide – a different pattern than that seen among non-Natives – led the authors to conclude that "there has been greater disruption of traditional roles for males resulting in profound problems of identity and self-esteem" (Kirmayer, Brass, and Tait 2000, 11). A study of First Nations persons in British Columbia concluded that there was a link between lower suicide rates and "local control" – that is, community control of police, fire, education, health, existence of local facilities for cultural activities, self-government, and involvement in land claims (Chandler and Lalonde 1998). The authors found that the absence of these variables was associated with a higher rate of suicide in communities without local control. A study conducted in Nunavut (Harckham 2003, 74) involving interviews with Inuit residents of the community of Arviat found a number expressing the belief that "an individual cannot be mentally healthy without taking responsibility for their actions," leading the author to speculate that, over time, "colonialism [had] eroded a belief in self-sufficiency and encouraged a sense of dependency." Subjects in this study also suggested that to have a healthier community, there should be more role models to look up to, which would represent proof of the "community's ability to foster and support healthy lifestyles and choices" (78).

Concerning approaches to healing, one observer points out that in North America colonization has had the effect of eliminating traditional practices that "offered Native peoples a complex and effective system of healing ... based on a holistic approach which attempted to balance the physical, mental, emotional and spiritual aspects of people" (Leenaars 2000, 59). There are clear indications here of the need to restore Native healing practices, which is occurring in a number of settings in Canada.

Montreal psychiatrist Laurence Kirmayer and colleagues suggest that, regarding the needs of the First Nations, "mental health services and promotion must be directed at both individual and community levels" (Kirmayer, Brass, and Tait 2000, 16). Concerning community-level interventions, a provincial government report concludes that "'ecological' approaches (i.e., intervening with families, schools, local governments, systems, and communities) hold greater promise than individual, clinic-based interventions," implying that practitioners will require "a new and different set of skills" in the areas of community development and public education (Mussell, Cardiff, and White 2004, 32).

Barriers to Service Provision

In considering the mental health needs of Canada's culturally diverse population, one can identify a number of potential barriers to establishing and maintaining a constructive relationship between service providers and minority clients. These barriers include language, different worldviews as to what constitutes mental disorder and mental health, stigma, mistrust, and how services are designed and allocated.

Language

Language differences potentially represent a fundamental barrier to accessing and effectively utilizing mental health services, a barrier that may be underestimated by practitioners. In an article on the role of professional interpreters in mental health, a McGill University researcher notes that "language is central to a person's cultural identity and is the most basic means through which people encode and express their emotions and their most complex thoughts, beliefs and values. Although it seems obvious that, in any clinical encounter, the ability to communicate effectively is essential, the underutilization of interpreters by health professionals working with clients from ethnocultural communities with language barriers remains surprisingly common. Of concern is that most studies of immigrants in Canada find that one, if not the greatest, barrier to access to care is the lack of interpreters or of bilingual service providers" (Blake 2003, 21). This author observes that reluctance to use interpreters can come from the perception that the process will be too costly in terms of time and effort; it is also noted that there may be a misunderstanding of the role of the interpreter.

The temptation to use untrained interpreters can lead to other difficulties with respect to accuracy and objectivity. Blake (2003, 22) suggests that "the use of informal interpreters represents a lack of recognition of the skills required to act as a competent interpreter. Mechanical word-for-word translation is often insufficient to convey meaning. Often, words cannot be literally translated from one language to another, owing to a lack of clear correspondence between the words of the two languages. Cultural 'idioms of distress' and the context or meaning of a symptom can be lost in attempts at literal translation."

Culture-Specific Syndromes
The criticism has been made that the American Psychiatric Association's *Diagnostic and Statistical Manual (DSM)* is an ethnocentric document, similar to other artifacts that reflect the particular cultures that produce them. Some categories given in the *DSM* are not well known in other parts of the world (an example being anorexia nervosa), while at the same time there are syndromes or states of mind not historically included in Western classification systems that carry a particular metaphorical power for people in other, non-Western societies. In more recent editions of the *DSM*, some concessions have been made, including an outline for "cultural [diagnostic] formulation" and a "glossary of culture-bound syndromes," albeit as appendices. Examples from the latest revision of the *DSM* (American Psychiatric Association 2000) include *amok*, originally identified in Malaysia, which is characterized by a period of brooding followed by aggressive outbursts, and *pibloktoq*, seen among the Inuit, described as an abrupt dissociative episode, which may be followed by seizures and coma.

The existence of culture-specific syndromes poses something of a challenge to Western psychiatry since the credibility of the biological paradigm rests to some extent on the idea of the *universality* of mental disorders. One author notes that from this perspective there may be an assumption "that cultural differences are a superficial 'mask' – a layer that must be peeled away to reveal the real, biological 'fact' underlying the disorder" (Hamid 2000a, 5; see also Kleinman and Cohen 1997). An example of this comes from an article on practitioner competencies where it is noted that clinicians should be able to "*separate* cultural aspects from the person's psychopathology" (Coursey et al. 2000, 388, emphasis added). In short, there may be a tendency to assume that culture-specific syndromes are simply *DSM* categories under a different name or to dismiss them altogether. The danger in doing this, however, is that symptoms may be misinterpreted and treatment approaches misapplied. Hamid (2000a, 8) gives the example of *taijin kyofusho*, seen among Japanese people, which is a state of "intense fear that one's body, body parts or bodily functions are displeasing, embarrassing or offensive." At first glance, this appears to be a description of social phobia, as per the *DSM*; however, in Japan, where there is a greater emphasis on *group* obligations, the focus is on the potential embarrassment that may be caused for *others* rather than for the individual in question. Hamid (2000a, 6) concludes, "Even if there are *some* universal mental disorders, that doesn't mean that there are *only* universal mental disorders with variations only in name. When dealing with human culture, it is much more complex than that. Biology and environment are too intertwined. A failure to understand this complexity can lead to misdiagnosis and inaccurate research" (emphasis in original). Concerning differing conceptions of mental disorder, the authors of a British study – wherein it was found that white subjects, compared to second-generation, nonwhite subjects, were more likely to support biological explanations of mental disorder – note that "dissonance between patients' and professionals' explanatory models may affect help-seeking behaviour, treatment compliance, satisfaction and culturally sensitive clinical practice" (McCabe and Priebe 2004, 25).

Treatment Approaches

Sometimes the practitioner's beliefs about treatment goals and procedures may not coincide with those of persons from another culture. One example is the idea that personal growth is contingent upon individuation and independence from the family of origin and that "enmeshment" is an "expression of family dysfunction" (Goldenberg and Goldenberg 1980, 48). This North American perspective may clash with the views of immigrants and First Nations persons who value the interconnectedness of families. A practitioner working with the Hispanic community notes that parents contacted by the mental health system fear "that they themselves or their child-rearing practices will be blamed for the child's problem" and that "their parental authority could be undermined by a professional who does not understand the family cultural background" (Sanchez 2000, 10). In a different area, beliefs about the body may conflict with treatment procedures. For example, some Chinese persons may be worried about how medications may affect the body's homeostasis or be reluctant to have blood tests because one's vitality may be diminished when this "vital" agent is removed (Woo 2000).

Stigma

While being involved with the mental health system is stigmatizing for anyone, it may be particularly so for some immigrant and minority groups. Family shame and the concept of karma – how deeds performed in a past life affect the current life – may be relevant to understanding attitudes toward mental disorder in Asian communities and have been identified as primary barriers to accessing mental health services (Li and Browne 2000). A Vietnamese practitioner notes that "the notion of mental illness is quite dreadful to the Vietnamese people, who believe that there is a very remote chance of recovery. Along the way the person also brings shame and disgrace to the family due to, as culturally believed, possible bad deeds in a past life – even though nothing was done wrong in the present" (Van Le 2000, 9). Similarly, in Chinese communities the attitude may be that "family troubles stay in the house" (Li and Browne 2000, 150) since removing a mentally ill person from his or her family is often perceived as a failure or loss of control by the other members. In addition, there may be concern about how an acknowledged mental illness will affect the marriage prospects of siblings (Macnaughton 2000; Woo 2000; see also Pyke et al. 2001 regarding the Afro-Canadian experience). On this point, the author of a longitudinal survey of persons diagnosed with schizophrenia in India found that "in almost all cases, the fact that the bride suffered from mental illness was not disclosed to the groom or his family" (Thara 2004).

Accessing outside services may also be discouraged when group cohesion is paramount, such as in orthodox religious communities. A study of the prevalence of depression among an Amish community found relatively high levels of this disorder but concomitantly high levels of reluctance to seek treatment from mental health providers; the author concluded that "boundary maintenance was achieved through two social control mechanisms: religious-based stigmatization of depression, and the construction of mental health providers as illegitimate help agents" (Reiling 2002, 428).

Service Allocation

It is acknowledged that in Canada there is a lack of mental health services in northern and more remote areas, which disproportionately affects First Nations communities (Hall 2001; Harckham 2003). Where services are provided, the mandates of these programs may not reflect the needs of minority groups. For example, a number of refugees and First Nations persons may be experiencing the psychological effects of trauma, yet mental health units may not see this as a "serious, persistent mental illness" or may not have staff trained in the assessment and treatment of this type of problem.

Mistrust

Practitioners need to be sensitive to the fact that many immigrants and First Nations persons have had less than positive experiences with "the authorities" and may therefore have some apprehensiveness and ambivalence about the role of mental health service providers. Immigrants may also fear, not unrealistically, that their immigration status will be adversely affected by a mental health designation.

Changing Practices

Practitioner Competencies

Increasingly, **cultural competence** is being recognized as a core skill for mental health practitioners in agency mission statements (Pyke et al. 2001), in professional and academic publications (Coursey et al. 2000; Lo and Fung 2003; Sue, Arredondo, and McDavis 1992; Thakur 2003), and in the codes of ethics and practice guidelines of professional associations (American Psychological Association 1990; Canadian Counselling Association 1999). The following discussion draws from these sources.

One area of competence refers to attitudes and beliefs as well as the ability of the practitioner to be reflective, self-aware, and open-minded. Sue, Arredondo, and McDavis (1992) suggest that culturally skilled counsellors are aware of how their own cultural background, experiences, and values influence psychological processes; are aware of their own communication style and of any stereotypes and negative emotional reactions held toward other ethnic groups; and are able to respect other, different belief systems and helping practices.

A second area of competence refers to knowledge: "The knowledge we use to inform our efforts should not be limited to the western biomedical model, but should include experiential knowledge gained from the person with the illness ... and also should include concepts of mental health or illness that come from different cultural traditions" (Macnaughton 2000, 14). To this end, practitioners need to actively seek out education and training experiences to enhance their understanding of the minority experience and worldview, which may in part be achieved by forging links with organizations representing these other communities. Practitioners also need to recognize the limits of their own expertise and seek consultation and/or make referrals as necessary. Knowledge may also refer to awareness of the limitations or bias of assessment and treatment procedures, especially those that have been "standardized": "Counsellors [should] proceed with caution when judging and interpreting the performance of minority group members and any other persons not represented in the group on which the evaluation and assessment instruments and procedures were standardized. They [should] recognize and take into account the potential effects of age, ethnicity, disability, culture, gender, religion, sexual orientation and socio-economic status on both the administration of, and the interpretation of data from, such instruments and procedures" (Canadian Counselling Association 1999, 12).

As well, practitioners need to have knowledge of the socio-political context of minority clients, how discrimination may affect the manifestation of psychological disorders and help-seeking behaviour (perhaps within the practitioner's own agency), and how a "problem" personalized by the client may in fact stem from racism or bias.

A third area of competence refers to practice skills. This could include awareness of the different meanings of nonverbal communications such as gestures, silence, and eye contact, awareness of the limitations of a particular helping style, and an ability or willingness to engage in other "verbal/non-verbal helping responses" (Sue, Arredondo, and McDavis 1992, 48). The practitioner also needs to be careful about using psychological jargon and to be sure that the client understands the meanings of terms. Using the language requested by the client is desirable: there is evidence that bilingual counsellors are better able to retain clients in treatment and obviate the use of crisis response teams (Ziguras et al. 2003), an assertion supported by a survey of seniors from the Chinese and Tamil communities in Toronto, which found that having an "ethnospecific," fully bilingual mental health service provider was clearly preferred by the subjects interviewed (Sadavoy, Meier, and Ong 2004). The practitioner who is unilingual should consider referral to or consultation with a translator or bilingual associate (see more on this point below) and should also be open to consulting with traditional healers – such as those from the First Nations, who are establishing alternative treatment and healing programs in a number of mental health and institutional settings in Canada. Practitioners may also need to possess or develop advocacy skills for systems-level interventions when there is evidence that the client's "individual" concerns are a result of institutional barriers, biases, and gate-keeping arrangements.

In attempting to come up with a more systematic approach to culturally informed practice, psychiatrists affiliated with the University of Toronto (Lo and Fung 2003, 166) have suggested a *cultural analysis* framework as a "hypothesis-generating strategy" for the practitioner. Within this framework there are three broad domains: (1) "self," which refers to "cultural influences on psychological aspects of the self" (166), such as the manifestation of somatic rather than psychological symptoms seen among some groups; (2) "relations," which refers to cultural influences on client perceptions of relationships with family, the community, and nature, such as the view that wellness is a state of being in harmony with, as opposed to in control of, one's environment; and (3) "treatment," referring to elements of therapy that may be especially influenced by culture, such as the use of alternative treatments (e.g., herbs and acupuncture) and the role of the healer as authoritative versus collaborative.

Structural Arrangements

In addition to consideration of practitioner competencies, mental health service providers need to look at how their programs are structured and delivered with respect to potential clients from minority groups. This usually requires a conscious decision on the part of officials to make diversity and service equity "key issues for the agency to address" (Pyke et al. 2001, 182). Multicultural organizational change may be achieved through a number of approaches, including (1) recruitment and promotion of staff from diverse ethnic groups, (2) community outreach, (3) cultural events, (4) sensitivity training, and (5) developing partnerships that will facilitate improved attitudes between mainstream and other ethnic groups (Williams 2001).

In moving to the level of service delivery, Kirmayer and colleagues (2003, 146) note that three main models have been developed to better meet the needs of minority clients: (1) the training of clinicians in generic approaches to cultural competency, (2) "ethnospecific" mental health services or clinics, and (3) the use of specially trained mental health translators and "culture brokers." Given fiscal restraints and the great diversity seen in Canadian urban centres, the development of ethnospecific clinics may be precluded, which "suggest[s] the potential value of a consultation-liaison model as a mechanism to address the impact of cultural diversity on mental health problems" (151). These cultural consultations may take three forms: (1) direct contact with the client by the consultant, usually with the referring person present; (2) a discussion with only the referring clinician, covering recommendations about treatment options and resources; and (3) education sessions or conferences with a number of representatives of the referring organization, who may present recurring problems, questions, and concerns.

Kirmayer and colleagues (2003) describe a cultural consultation service (CCS) established in Montreal in 1999 at a general hospital. Personnel included two part-time psychiatrists as well as psychologists, social workers, psychiatric nurses, and medical anthropologists. Referring sources most frequently made requests for help in clarifying diagnosis or the meaning of specific symptoms (58%), for assistance in treatment planning (45%), and for information or a link to resources related to a specific cultural group (25%). Issues raised in the consultations were most commonly as follows:

- variations in family systems, roles, and value systems (e.g., patriarchal families)
- identity issues related to age and gender roles (e.g., the importance of marriage and child-bearing)
- the impact of exposure to torture and war
- the stressful impact of the refugee claimant process

- the impact of immigration on intergenerational tensions
- the effects of covert racism or biases in service provision
- the prevalence of dissociative and somatoform symptoms that were initially misdiagnosed
- previous experiences with healers in the country of origin
- the importance of religious practices for coping and social support.

A preliminary evaluation of the program revealed positive outcomes as well as ongoing challenges. It was found that cultural consultation "often facilitated the therapeutic alliance between the referring person and the patient ... [particularly when] the consulting clinician was present during the clinical interview carried out by the culture broker" (Kirmayer et al. 2003, 150). On the other hand, it was found that, while having a culture broker from a similar background to the client could be positive, in some cases clients expressed concerns that being seen by someone from their own community compromised their privacy, a realistic concern for clients "from small cultural communities with high degrees of stigmatization of mental health problems" (150).

A somewhat different, more limited version of a consultation-liaison program has existed in Vancouver since 1992. In this program there are five culture brokers, referred to as multicultural mental health liaison workers, representing the Chinese, Indo-Canadian, Southeast Asian, Latin American, and First Nations communities, dispersed among the eight city mental health teams. The program focuses on "indirect or facilitative services such as education, consultation and training, service brokerage and service coordination" (Peters 2000, 19). While there is some direct clinical service, this is usually in the form of cotherapy with the referring clinician. The mandate of these workers is to "act mainly as systems change agents – the goal is to increase the capability of all staff within the mental health system to work effectively with the full range of people in the community they are mandated to treat" (19).

With all of these programs the goal should be a two-way flow of information between practitioner and client rather than the establishment of a process for "converting" the client's worldview to one consistent with the medical model (see Turbett 2000).

Sexual Orientation

Including sexual orientation in a chapter that deals with ethnic diversity may at first glance seem to be an awkward fit; however, it can be argued that many of the same issues and concepts that apply to working with people from diverse ethnic backgrounds – stereotyping, prejudice, ethnocentrism, minority status, mistrust – can also be applied to work that is undertaken with persons of varied sexual orientations. This section briefly reviews some of the mental health needs specific to these persons and some of the barriers to care.

One preliminary caution concerns terminology: one cannot assume that there is a consensus as to the definition or usage of words such as "homosexual," "gay," or "transgendered." For example, a number of people are uncomfortable with the term "homosexual" because it may appear too clinical or because it connotes a narrow focus on sexuality. In the case of "transgendered," some use the term to refer to persons contemplating or who have undergone a sex-change operation, while others, such as an association of international educators, define it more broadly as an "identity of gender that is at variance with society's assigned gender roles" (Spellman 2000). Some professional publications have adopted the acronym GLBT (gay/lesbian/bisexual/transgendered) when referring, more globally, to non-heterosexual orientations, and this term will be used here (Paterson and Bishop 2000).[4] In any case, practitioners must be very sensitive about the language that they use, consider letting the client drive the discussion in this area, and, if and where terms must be used, have clients self-define their orientation. Other misunderstandings may arise over the tendency to view sexual orientation as a dichotomy (gay vs. straight), when the best evidence indicates that it is better understood as a *continuum*, ranging from exclusively same-sex-oriented to exclusively opposite-sex-oriented (Haslam 1997). In another conceptualization, three overlapping dimensions of sexual orientation have been identified. These are same-gender (1) sexual behaviour, (2) desire, and (3) identity (Laumann et al. 1994). Thus, concerning point (1), some individuals will engage in sexual behaviour with members of the same gender but may continue to publicly and privately identify themselves as heterosexual.

Mental Health Needs

While a number of the mental health needs of GLBT persons will be similar to those seen among other groups, there are some particular challenges faced by this community. Intolerance and homophobia still exist in our society, as illustrated by a 2003 *New York Times*-CBS poll of American residents, which found that 49 percent answered "no" to the question "do you think homosexual relations should be legal?" (O'Neill 2003). Canadians may not be any more enlightened, as evidenced by a large-scale 2005 telephone survey wherein 49 percent of respondents stated that homosexuality is an "abnormal" condition (Sutherland, 2005). The issue of same-sex marriage in particular has caused bitter divisions of opinion and some acrimonious public debate in Canada. Concerns about intolerance mean that "coming out," for young persons in particular, can thus be a difficult decision and one that is further complicated by familial and cultural factors. Thoughts of suicide and self-harm may result from the internal conflict over orientation and disclosure and because of interpersonal conflicts, including personal attacks within the family and at school (Remafedi 1994). Studies conducted in the United States have found the lifetime prevalence of suicide attempts in gay and bisexual adolescents to be about 30 percent (Herrell et al. 1999). While some of these studies have been criticized for having nonrepresentative samples and confounding variables (such as substance misuse), subsequent investigations using population-based samples and multivariate models have concluded that "same-gender sexual orientation is significantly associated with suicidality" (Herrell et al. 1999, 867).

Similar results were found in a survey of GLBT teenagers in urban settings in British Columbia (McCreary Centre Society 1999),[5] which noted that, because of their "different" status, respondents in many instances experienced rejection, isolation, self-doubt, and low self-esteem. Seventeen percent of respondents had been assaulted at school, 9 percent assaulted outside school, 34 percent threatened with violence at school, and 80 percent subjected to homophobic remarks at school. None of the youth in the survey gave high ratings to the quality of their family relationships. The study also found that GLBT youth were more likely to engage in substance misuse than were non-GLBT youth.

Among older GLBT individuals there are other challenges. For example, there is the question of parenting and how society regards nonheterosexual persons as parents. Loss and bereavement are prominent issues: GLBT persons may have to deal with the loss of their own status and standing in some cases, estrangement from family members, and the loss of friends and loved ones because of the HIV epidemic. For persons who are HIV positive, the physical and psychological toll of dealing with complex and changing medication regimens and their side effects is a significant issue.

For practitioners, a significant concern is the less obvious forms of systemic discrimination that GLBT individuals experience in the social service, health care, and mental health systems, which can have the net effect of causing the person to withdraw rather than seek help.

Barriers to Care and Practice Implications
In considering the mistrust that GLBT individuals may feel with respect to the mental health establishment, one should recall that in earlier versions of the *DSM*, homosexuality was classified as a "sexual deviation." This was dropped in the 1970s, although the diagnosis "ego-dystonic homosexual-

ity" was retained until the 1980s (Shorter 1997). The idea that sexual orientation is ego-dystonic – referring to a state of dissatisfaction or an incompatibility with one's self-concept – has been used as justification for "conversion therapies" (which are still attempted today).[6] Concerning young persons, prior to the 1990s children could be certified for admittance to a psychiatric facility for "gender normalization." This unfortunate legacy has necessitated the creation of professional practice guidelines to reaffirm the non-pathological status of sexual orientation (Paterson and Bishop 2000).[7]

Other barriers to effective therapeutic engagement include practitioner beliefs that every psychological problem must be linked to sexual orientation, or assumptions about homogeneity within the GLBT community, both of which remind us of the need to avoid stereotyping and to look past the "designation" of the client with whom we are working. Sexual orientation, after all, is only one attribute of an individual (and may be a separate issue from gender identity and gender expression). Practitioners may be uncomfortable with references to sexuality and avoid these areas of discomfort; inevitably, this discomfort will be perceived by the client, which will affect any therapeutic alliance. Alternately, some practitioners may believe that the GLBT client should be seen "somewhere else," and if deflection from mainstream mental health services is happening, this means that mental health issues having nothing to do with sexual orientation are being missed. Practitioners need to be very reflective and honest with themselves about unexamined feelings regarding GLBT clients. As one clinician notes, "Any gay person approaching any health care setting comes with a sense of self that may be built on a bedrock of shame. Health care professionals have the power to increase or decrease that shame" (Halstead 1998, 5).

In determining whether a practice environment is welcoming to GLBT clients, the procedures and documents used need to be considered. For example, do forms refer to marital status or other exclusionary categories? Are same-sex partners recognized, or, as has been reported in some hospital settings, are they denied access to their partners because they aren't "family?"

To forge stronger links with the GLBT community, Paterson and Bishop (2000) suggest that practitioners consider doing outreach with GLBT groups, that program posters be placed in GLBT venues, that programs have GLBT role models and representatives on committees, and that naive practitioners become knowledgeable about the resources available in this community.

Guidelines have been developed to assist mental health practitioners working with GLBT clients, guidelines that address the importance of attitudes, skill sets, and knowledge base – for example, an understanding of the distinctions and intersections within the realms of sex, gender, and sexual orientation – issues not always covered in practitioner training or curricula. On this matter, interested readers are directed to guidelines developed by the American Psychological Association (2005) and by Paterson and Bishop (2000).

Notes

1 The data referred to here are from the 1996 and 2001 Censuses, available at http://www.statcan.ca. "Metropolitan" refers to "census metropolitan area," which is the city proper plus surrounding municipalities.
2 "Minority" here refers to persons of other than European descent.
3 "North American Indian" is the term used by Statistics Canada.
4 An alternate acronym, used particularly with young persons, is GLBN (gay/lesbian/bisexual/not sure) (Garofalo et al. 1999).
5 Website: http://www.mcs.bc.ca.
6 For example, the website of the National Association for Research and Therapy of Homosexuality (http://www.narth.com) talks about making "effective psychological therapy available to all homosexual men and women who seek change" and classifies as "myths" the beliefs that "homosexuality is normal" and that "homosexuals cannot change." On the issue of changing sexual orientation, a *New York Times*-CBS poll (referred to earlier) found that 44 percent of all respondents, and over three-quarters of conservative Christians, believed homosexuality to be a "choice" or a "lifestyle decision" (O'Neill 2003, A5).
7 Currently the *DSM* includes "gender identity disorder" and "transvestic fetishism" as mental disorders.

Other Resources

- The website of McGill University's Division of Social and Transcultural Psychiatry in Montreal (http://www.mcgill.ca/tcpsych/) has a number of downloadable reports.
- The website of the Centre of Excellence for Research on Immigration and Settlement (CERIS) (http://ceris.metropolis.net) has a number of downloadable reports and links to other sites and resources on immigration topics. CERIS is a partnership program that includes Toronto area universities and social service agencies.
- The Statistics Canada website (http://www.statcan.ca) has census data and reports on immigration patterns and the ethnocultural makeup of Canada.
- The University of California, San Francisco, has a webpage entitled "Primary Care Clinical Practice Guidelines Cross Cultural Resources," which includes a number of useful links and publications on cross-cultural medicine (see http://medicine.ucsf.edu/resources/guidelines/culture.html).
- The website of Multicultural Mental Health Australia (http://www.mmha.org.au) has a number of resources, links, and documents pertaining to cultural competence in mental health practice.
- The Stanford Geriatric Education Center has a number of online modules designed to assist practitioners in providing culturally sensitive care to ethnic elders (see http://sgec.stanford.edu/training).
- Transcend, a Canadian website, offers support, education, and resource information for transgendered persons and interested others (see http://www.transgender.org/transcend). This website also gives more detailed information on "trans" language and terminology.

Afterword: Future Challenges

At this point a brief overview is given of some of the more important challenges still facing mental health practitioners. In "taking stock" of where we are in community mental health in Canada, there is reason for optimism and cause for concern. More stakeholders have been given a voice, although some would argue that theirs is but a token input. There is greater recognition of consumer choice, but in many cases the actual availability of these choices is limited. After a period of almost exclusive reliance on pharmacotherapy, there is increasing evidence that nonpharmacological approaches to treatment – cognitive-behavioural therapies, self-management, peer support – are also effective, although barriers to their implementation exist. The recovery model has made inroads, even though not all practitioners have accepted it. To reiterate a comment from the introduction, these are interesting times for mental health practitioners and, potentially, a time of opportunity.

Best Practices: Rhetoric and Reality
There is by now a large "best practices" literature, putting aside debates about the quality of the evidence supporting it. What is less clear, however, is the extent to which mental health systems in Canada are meeting these standards.

One problem, as this is being written, is that there appears to be a shortage of evaluation research to answer this question. Drawing from the American experience, research conducted in the late 1990s found that the mental health systems investigated were meeting best-practice standards in only a minority of cases: a study of programs for persons with schizophrenia in two states found that clients "were highly unlikely to receive effective services" such as psychoeducation and supported employment (Torrey et al. 2001, 46), with another, population-based survey concluding that only 25 percent of service users were receiving treatment consistent with evidence-based guidelines

(Wang, Berglund, and Kessler 2000). In Canada, a 2004 study of early psychosis services at provincial inpatient and community programs, sponsored by the BC Schizophrenia Society (2004), found that "public education was found to be occurring in fewer areas than would be anticipated" (16), and that "half of respondents reported a lack of training for ER staff in early psychosis and limited improvement in handling these cases in recent years" (27). Despite these observations, and the fact that the response rate to the survey was only 48 percent, the author concluded that overall the province rated a "C+." To some extent program quality is addressed through periodic accreditation reviews, with accrediting bodies now recognizing to a greater extent, for example, the need for consumer involvement and choice in the treatment process. It is also possible that the impetus to improve practice may ultimately come from fear of liability, with governments in Canada now recognizing that failure to meet standards may leave them more vulnerable to litigation (Kines 2004). In any case, barriers to program evaluation – whether these are bureaucratic, fiscal, or political – need to be addressed.

A second, even more fundamental problem concerns the question: why, at the clinical end, is there so little "uptake" of evidence being produced at the research end? In an article titled "So much research evidence, so little dissemination," Canadian psychiatrist Charlotte Waddell (2001) considers this conundrum and notes that even "packaging" findings in clinical practice guidelines and systematic reviews has had only a moderate impact on actual practice, and that more "active dissemination approaches are needed" (p. 3). Observing that currently "it is nobody's job to disseminate research evidence" (Waddell, 2001, p. 5), this author suggests, among other strategies, the employment of "knowledge brokers," persons who are both research literate and savvy about the needs of practitioners and administrators, as a way to bridge these different solitudes.

Cost Containment

An overriding concern for stakeholders is the issue of cost containment in the public health care sector (e.g., Lee 2004). While this is a concern for all providers and recipients of health care services, it is a particular worry for those in the mental health system. Now situated in regional health authorities, mental health programs – the "orphan child" of Medicare in the words of the Romanow Report – are especially vulnerable to these cost pressures, with the ever-present fear, based on previous experience, that dollars allocated to mental health will be channelled elsewhere, such as to acute care (Goering, Wasylenki, and Durbin 2000).

A reduction in the availability of hospital psychiatric beds – supported by the best-practices principle of "decreas[ing] use of more ... costly services" (British Columbia Ministry of Health 2002e, 10) – has not in most cases been compensated for by a necessary increase in community services, particularly adequately staffed clinics, supported housing, outreach, and peer support. While we have seen the development and partial implementation of newer programs such as shared care, assertive outreach, acute home treatment, and early psychosis intervention, these initiatives cannot compensate if core services are insufficient (Davis 1996). All this speaks to the need for advocacy not just by support organizations such as the Canadian Mental Health Association (CMHA) and the Schizophrenia Society of Canada (SSC) but by practitioners themselves in concert with other stakeholders. Practitioners often have the skills to advocate at a microlevel – that is, to acquire resources for individual clients – and should consider developing these skills and applying them to systemic concerns.

Defining the Priority Population

Notwithstanding the advent of designations such as "serious and persistent," clinical and administrative staff at mental health programs continue to struggle with the eligibility criteria for their services, a tension that may be heightened by the lobbying activities of groups representing persons, such as those with anxiety disorders and trauma-related conditions, who believe that they have been historically underserved. How should we respond to individuals whose problems apparently do not reach the "serious" threshold? Any idea of expanding mandates must confront the reality of limited resources: hospital outpatient programs, which have treated persons with "less serious"/nonpsychotic disorders, are also under budgetary pressures, and other potential avenues such as psychological counselling are generally not funded by provincial Medicare programs. Psychiatrists in private practice typically see persons with less serious conditions; however, these practitioners are in relatively short supply and often have lengthy waiting lists. There are also attitudinal barriers concerning the provision of services to other diagnostic groups: for many practitioners, the apparently willful behaviour of persons diagnosed with substance misuse and personality disorders is evidence of a "less-deserving" status.

Redefining the target population has implications for practitioner training, as a Canadian psychiatrist notes: "Our claim for expertise based on adequate training has always been uneven between diagnoses. Other medical colleagues and allied mental health professionals are now scrutinizing this training and challenging our claim. The training received during residency in the management of affective [mood] disorders or schizophrenia stands in sharp contrast in quantity and quality to the limited training received in the management of substance abuse ... personality disorders, or eating disorders" (el-Guebaly 1997, 3-4).

The question remains as to whether it is realistic to talk about having "generalist" practitioners and case managers or whether other approaches – such as better general screening and subsequent assignment to on- or off-site specialists – are more feasible.

Treatment Approaches: Business as Usual?
Treatment by public mental health teams has historically involved a triad: the client, a physician-consultant who is in charge of medical management, and a case manager who provides supportive counselling and linkage with other resources. The utility and sustainability of this arrangement has been called into question in recent times by increasingly large caseloads and by the development of other treatment models, notably cognitive-behavioural therapies (CBT), which are accumulating a large evidence base supporting their efficacy. Outside of psychology most practitioners have had only limited exposure to CBT until recently, which obviously raises a training issue. On the question of practitioner training, the usual practice of a workshop with no follow-up is clearly inadequate; Latimer (2005, S49) suggests that this "spray and pray" method should be bolstered by periodic meetings with a skilled consultant over a period of years.

Since CBT is delivered in a group format, it is potentially a more efficient form of service delivery. However, group formats are not a panacea, and there will always be the necessity of one-on-one work to deal with the needs of individual clients. At the same time, the difficulty in implementing group treatments speaks to the significance of service traditions as well as practitioner and client mindsets as barriers to change. Practitioners and managers must take a serious look at the service delivery method and whether it should be "business as usual."

Accommodating Stakeholders
Increasingly, other stakeholders, such as clients, family members, and the organizations representing them, have been able to voice their concerns about mental health policies and systems of service delivery in Canada. To what extent these stakeholders are actually being accommodated, however, is another matter. That there is now "an increasingly explicit commitment to consumer empowerment and participation in the mental health field" (Dickinson 2002, 381) is not easily reconciled with new, coercive methods of service delivery involving community treatment orders and assertive out-

reach, demands from family advocates for easier access to treatment, and a reliance on pharmacological treatments that are administered by an expert/ authority within a medical model. Practitioner decision making is further constrained, in many cases, by management that, at the end of the day, is more concerned about liability should something go wrong, notwithstanding the lip service paid to "client empowerment." The challenge of accommodating stakeholders is also complicated by the reality that there is no clear consensus of interests within stakeholder groups, let alone between them; as Dickinson (2002, 384) notes, "the various stakeholders ... don't necessarily agree on the nature of the problem ... nor ... on the best solution to it."

While there is no easy answer to this conundrum, two observations will be made here. First, the stereotype of psychiatric reductionism is, unfortunately, true in many instances. In their focus on symptom management, practitioners have been guilty of not *really* listening to what their clients are saying about recovering from a mental disorder, of not trying to understand their needs, hopes, and fears. Even if we ultimately must "agree to disagree" with our clients, we must hear them out and consider seriously their larger existential concerns. Second, practitioners must realize that while we can be part of the solution, we can also be part of the problem. A proportion of the disability and dependency that goes along with having a mental disorder is created by how the system responds to this situation, by how we process, categorize, and indoctrinate the client population. Thus, while not diminishing the importance of accessible, comprehensive mental health treatment services, practitioners need to be reflective about the effects of clinical pessimism, of keeping clients in a dependent position, and of not allowing people to take chances.

Glossary

Acute home treatment. Acute care provided in the home for a limited period to treat acute psychiatric symptoms that would otherwise require inpatient admission.

Assertive community treatment (ACT). A type of service delivery that attempts to combine psychiatric treatment, case management, and rehabilitation through frequent outreach by a multidisciplinary team. The target group is clients who have a high degree of functional impairment and/or are "intensive users of the system of care" (British Columbia Ministry of Health, 2002a, 6.)

Atypical antipsychotics. Newer-generation drugs that have a better side-effect profile with respect to "extrapyramidal symptoms" (see below) than older-generation products.

Best practices. Exemplary mental health services. While not easily defined, the term refers to practices that are evidence-based and that produce outcomes superior to those of other interventions. Indicators of better outcomes are usually quantitative, with hospitalization frequency (lower) and duration (shorter) being two common examples.

Capacity. A concept that is similar to "competency" (see below). "Capacity" has been used in Canadian law to refer to the ability to make decisions about one's own psychiatric treatment, particularly to understand information presented and to appreciate the consequences of decisions or nondecisions.

Case management. A term that refers to a role – rather than to a particular professional background or discipline – where the focus is on *linkage* with resources and *coordination of care*, not necessarily on direct provision of services. Effectiveness in case management is related to knowledge of resources, perseverance, advocacy, and accountability.

Certification. Involuntary hospitalization, a procedure authorized in most cases by a physician. Also known as "committal."

Client. In this book, the term used for a person who uses mental health services.

Cognitive-behavioural therapy (CBT). A very broad range of psychological techniques, some more "behavioural" (e.g., systematic desensitization) and some more "cognitive" (e.g., recognizing, challenging, and replacing distorted patterns of thinking). While originally used for persons with mood disorders, CBT has become increasingly influential and has been used with children as well as adapted and applied in cases of adults with personality and psychotic disorders.

Committal. See certification.

Community treatment order (CTO). (Also known as outpatient commitment.) A legal provision whereby a mental health client can be treated involuntarily while in the community (as opposed to involuntary *inpatient* status). These orders usually have conditions requiring the person to seek psychiatric care and to take medication. Unlike "conditional/extended leaves" (see below), the initiation of a CTO does not require that the person be in hospital.

Competency. Having sufficient ability to perform a specific task, as opposed to actions that are beyond an individual's control. A person making financial and health care decisions while suffering from dementia would be an example of a situation where a competency assessment might be required.

Conditional/extended leaves. Similar to community treatment orders, conditional/extended leave is a legal provision whereby a mental health client can be treated involuntarily while in the community. These special leaves are initiated when the person is still in hospital.

Criminalization. Based on the observation that mentally disordered persons are overrepresented in correctional settings, this refers to the hypothesis that troublesome behaviour that would have presumably been dealt with previously by the mental health system – usually by hospital detention – is now being dealt with by the criminal justice system in the post-deinstitutionalization era.

Cultural competence. "A specific set of values, attitudes, knowledge and skills that sensitize and improve sharing of information and assistance between people of different cultural orientations" (Mussell, Cardiff, and White 2004, 7).

Deinstitutionalization. Defined by Bachrach (1994, 24) as "the replacement of long-stay psychiatric hospitals with smaller, less isolated community-based service alternatives for the care of individuals with schizophrenia and other major mental illnesses."

Delusion. An apparently false belief, held despite evidence to the contrary.

Differential diagnosis. A reference to other psychiatric conditions that need to be ruled in or out before a more specific diagnosis can be made in a particular case.

Diversion. The suspension of criminal charges on the understanding that the accused person will instead receive prompt treatment within the mental health system.

DSM. The *Diagnostic and Statistical Manual* of the American Psychiatric Association. This system of classifying mental disorders is used in most community mental health settings in Canada.

Duty to warn. A legal/ethical duty, not well defined for practical purposes, under which a practitioner may breach client confidentiality if there is specific information concerning the potential for serious physical harm to a third party as a consequence of the client's actions.

Early psychosis intervention (EPI). Stage-sensitive programs specific to the treatment and rehabilitation of persons experiencing a "first break."

Electroconvulsive therapy (ECT). Widely used in earlier times, ECT is now used mainly as a treatment for depression when other methods have failed. The procedure involves inducing a minor brain seizure by the application of a brief electric current to sites on the scalp. How the therapeutic effect is achieved is still not fully understood.

Etiology. A medical term referring to the presumed cause of an illness or disorder.

Evidence-based. Practices or interventions that have received systematic evaluation demonstrating their superiority to other interventions or to no intervention (placebo). The "gold standard" in evaluation is the "experimental design" (see below), which involves random assignment of subjects to treatment and control groups.

Experimental design. A data source underpinning evidence-based practice that is considered the "gold standard" in medicine, if not all of mental health, but a standard that is difficult to achieve. The logic is that by ensuring intergroup equivalency (through randomization) and by isolating the independent variable (the presumed cause) in research designs, one can best rule out confounding factors and make causal inferences.

Expressed emotion. A concept used in the study of schizophrenia. In this hypothesis, relapse – a breakthrough of symptoms – is more likely when there is emotional overinvolvement or excessive critical comments in the individual's immediate social environment.

Extrapyramidal symptoms (EPS). Movement disorders that are the side effects of medication, particularly older antipsychotic drugs.

Fitness to stand trial. A legal term referring to an accused person's mental state at the time of trial (not at the time of the offence; see "not criminally responsible" below). Accused persons may be found "unfit" to participate in this adversarial process if, as the result of a mental disorder, they are unable to understand the nature or object of the proceedings, to understand the possible consequences of the proceedings, or to communicate with defence counsel. The trial is delayed until the accused is found fit, unless the accused is diverted from the criminal justice process.

Forensic psychiatry. A branch of the mental health system that provides assessment and/or treatment as mandated by the courts.

Guardian. In mental health this term refers to an individual or public agency appointed (usually by court order) to make decisions on behalf of a person found to be in some respect incompetent. The guardian has a legal and ethical duty to safeguard the interests and wellbeing of the incompetent person.

Hallucination. A false perception, such as auditory hallucinations (which are a common symptom of schizophrenia).

Harm reduction. According to the Centre for Addiction and Mental Health in Toronto (2002a, 2), harm reduction is "any program or policy designed to reduce drug-related harm without requiring the cessation of drug use." Examples of this are needle exchange programs, intended to reduce the transmission of diseases such as HIV among injection drug users, and treatment programs that do not require abstinence since the alternative might be the client's leaving the program. By contrast, criminalized drug use is seen as having created *greater* harm by marginalizing drug users, enlarging black markets and organized crime, and corrupting law enforcement officials.

Iatrogenic. A term that refers to treatments, attitudes, and traditions in mental health that cause harm or create greater disability among clients.

Index of suspicion. In assessing drug abuse without direct evidence or reliable self-reports, practitioners may apply a checklist of behavioural indicators that presumably reflect problems with substance use, such as housing instability, difficulty budgeting, prostitution, sudden unexplained mood shifts, employment problems, suicidal behaviour, hygiene problems, weight loss, and legal difficulties.

Labelling theory. A viewpoint in sociology, popular in the 1960s, that emphasized the role societal and institutional responses play in creating psychiatric disability, shifting the focus away from individual psychology and biological factors.

Mental status examination (MSE). An assessment conducted by a trained clinician that involves considering the client's appearance, behaviour, thought form, thought content, mood, and orientation.

Mobile crisis team. A seven-day-a-week service with some after-hours capacity that provides brief crisis intervention through telephone contact or home visits.

Motivational interviewing. A counselling approach that starts from an assumption of ambivalence and takes into account a client's degree of willingness to change. The helper tries to develop discrepancy in the client's position without being confrontational. Originally used in the field of addictions.

Neurotransmitters. Chemicals that transmit nerve impulses across the synapse (gap) between nerve cells by attaching to receptor sites (receiving cells) on the neighbouring cell. The activity of neurotransmitters is altered by psychotropic medications.

Not criminally responsible by reason of mental disorder (NCRMD). A special verdict in criminal trials based on the test that the accused, at the time of the act or omission, was suffering from a mental disorder "which made him or her incapable of appreciating the nature and quality of the act or omission, or of knowing that it was wrong" (*Criminal Code*, s. 16.1). Persons found NCRMD are usually initially detained in a secure hospital or given a conditional discharge, both of which require them to report to a review board.

Not in my back yard (NIMBY). Refers to hostile public attitudes with respect to (in this case) persons with mental health problems, particularly the desire not to have these individuals residing in the same neighbourhood.

Parens patriae. "Government as parent." This term refers to the right of the state to intervene in the case of individuals who are unable to look after themselves, even if they present no immediate threat to their own safety or to that of others. As applied to mental health legislation, *parens patriae* powers constitute a broad basis for intervention (see also "police powers" below).

Patent protection. Legislation that limits the production of cheaper, generic medication by rival drug companies.

Police powers. The right of the state to intervene in order to prevent harm from coming to others. As applied to mental health legislation, "police powers" constitute a *narrow* basis for intervention (see also *"parens patriae"* above).

Primary care. The first and most frequent point of contact with the health care system, which for many persons will be their family physician. While primary mental health care may be provided through community mental health clinics or private psychiatrists, the available evidence indicates that this service is more often than not provided in Canada by general practitioners.

Primary diagnosis. Defined alternately as (1) the condition that is the main focus of attention or treatment, (2) the condition that causes the greatest disability, or (3) the condition that precipitated admission to a psychiatric facility. Use of this term/concept has been problematic in the case of persons with co-occurring psychiatric and addictive disorders, with Minkoff (2001b) arguing that in this case both conditions should be considered "primary."

Prodrome. A term that refers to (1) the signs and symptoms seen in younger persons before the initial manifestation of a mental disorder (especially psychotic disorders) and (2) the signs and symptoms seen prior to a relapse (Ehmann, Hanson, and Friedlander 2004). The initial prodrome is usually diagnosed retrospectively. Attempts to identify the onset of a psychotic disorder at this early stage are complicated by the fact that symptoms are often nonspecific.

Psychodynamism. A group of theories and therapeutic techniques that have in common the following tenets: (1) early childhood experiences, particularly the relationship with one's family of origin, are crucial to understanding the development of personality and mental health problems; (2) early, unresolved conflicts may be *repressed* into the *unconscious* and may manifest themselves later – in a different form – as symptoms of a mental disorder (e.g., a phobia); (3) unconscious conflicts are accessed and ultimately resolved by psychotherapy, the "talking cure."

Psychosis. A mental condition indicative of a clear break with reality, characterized by the presence of delusions (false beliefs) and/or hallucinations (false perceptions).

Psychotropic. The name for the medications used in psychiatry, which include antipsychotics, antidepressants, mood stabilizers, anti-anxiety agents, stimulants, and antiparkinsonian agents.

Recovery. As used in recent years in the field of psychiatric rehabilitation, this term refers to a model of service delivery that (1) looks beyond symptom management to the client's broader existential concerns; (2) recognizes that recovering from the consequences of the disorder, such as stigma, is often more difficult than recovering from the disorder itself; (3) recognizes that there are many pathways to recovery; and (4) emphasizes the recovery process as one that should be collaborative or client-driven rather than practitioner-driven. The recovery concept emphasizes the importance of conveying hope to clients, of restoring self-esteem, and of attaining meaningful roles in society.

Refractory. As per *Webster's Dictionary*, "resisting ordinary methods of treatment." In psychiatry this term is most commonly used to denote persons whose symptoms do not respond to medication.

Relapse prevention. A strategy that involves a client's recognition of the "early warning signs" of a particular disorder, the avoidance of high-risk situations that may exacerbate the disorder, and putting into action early intervention strategies that may head off potential problems.

Secondary care. Services provided in a general hospital psychiatric unit.

Self-management. A term and set of concepts borrowed in part from the "chronic disease model" that has been applied to the treatment of persons suffering, for example, from asthma, diabetes, or arthritis. Self-management refers to the provision of education and skills training to persons with mental disorders, and emphasizes that clients must have a central and active role in determining their own care.

Serious, persistent mental disorder. While it is generally acknowledged that persons with serious mental disorders should be the priority group in public community mental health programs, defining the term "serious" (or "severe") has been difficult. Most definitions refer to (1) diagnosis, with schizophrenia and bipolar disorder always being included, (2) a substantial degree of functional impairment, and (3) persistence of symptoms.

Shared care. Collaborative activities between family physicians and psychiatric services designed to improve mental health care for clients.

Skills training. Techniques, either cognitive or behavioural, that assist an individual in coping with or managing the effects of a mental disorder. "Effects" refer both to particular symptoms and to social situations that may be made difficult or more stressful because of deficits created by the disorder or because of responses by others to the disorder.

Stakeholder. A term that refers to individuals or groups who would expect to be consulted, or to have some say, in policy development.

Stress-vulnerability. A theoretical model acknowledging that the expression of a mental disorder is a function of both vulnerability (e.g., genetic factors) and stress (e.g., a relationship breakdown).

Symptom substitution. From psychoanalytic theory, the hypothesis that treating symptoms without tracing them back to their psychic origin is ineffective and leads to their appearance in another form.

Tardive dyskinesia. An irreversible movement disorder – often manifested in the facial muscles, such as the lips and tongue – associated with long-term use of older antipsychotic drugs.

Telepsychiatry. The use of electronic communication and information technologies to provide or support clinical mental health care at a distance (American Psychiatric Association 1998), particularly video conferencing.

Tertiary care. This term refers to (1) inpatient programs that accept admissions only from other hospitals, (2) long-stay inpatient programs, or (3) most commonly, specialized inpatient programs for persons whose needs are more complex.

Tolerance. An aspect of drug dependency referring to the need to keep increasing the dose in order to achieve the same effect.

Transinstitutionalization. The process of shifting the care and containment of individuals with mental disorders from one institution to another – for example, from the psychiatric hospital system to the criminal justice system.

"Ulysses" agreements. A type of representation or advanced planning agreement that gives guidelines to a client's support team in areas such as finances, child care, and health care should the client become unwell due to a mental disorder. Ulysses was a legendary king of ancient Ithaca who, fearing the bewitching effect of the "sirens," bade his shipmates to ignore his pleas while under their influence.

References

Abidi, S., and S. Bhaskara. 2003. "From chlorpromazine to clozapine: Antipsychotic adverse effects and the clinician's dilemma." *Canadian Journal of Psychiatry* 44: 749-55.

Abramson, M. 1972. "The criminalization of mentally disordered behavior: Possible side effects of a new mental health law." *Hospital and Community Psychiatry* 23: 101-5.

Acorn, S. 1993. "Mental and physical health of homeless persons who use emergency shelters in Vancouver." *Hospital and Community Psychiatry* 44: 854-57.

Adler, R. 2003. "New dynamic imaging techniques provide a deeper look at Alzheimer's and schizophrenia." *The Boston Globe,* 6 May, B11.

Alberta Mental Health Board. N.d. Provincial Forensic Psychiatry Program. http://www.amhb.ab.ca/programs/calgary_target.html.

Allen, M., and V. Smith. 2001. "Opening Pandora's Box: The practical and legal dangers of involuntary outpatient commitment." *Psychiatric Services* 52: 342-46.

Allen, T. 2000. *Someone to Talk To: Care and Control of the Homeless.* Halifax: Fernwood.

Ambrosia, E., et al. 1992. "The street health report: A study of the health status and barriers to health care of homeless women and men in the City of Toronto." Unpublished manuscript.

Amenson, C., and R. Liberman. 2001. "Dissemination of educational classes for families of adults with schizophrenia." *Psychiatric Services* 52: 589-92.

American Association for the Advancement of Science. 2003. "Cognitive therapy for schizophrenia: Hope for those whom drugs haven't helped." http://www.eurekalert.org/pub_releases/2003-02/aaft-ctf020503.php.

American Psychiatric Association. 1998. APA resource document on telepsychiatry via video conferencing. http://www.psych.org/psych_pract/tp_paper.cfm#def.

–. 2000. *Diagnostic and Statistical Manual (DSM).* 4th ed., with text revision. Washington, DC: American Psychiatric Association.

–. 2003. "Practice guidelines for the assessment and treatment of patients with suicidal behaviors." Arlington, Virginia: American Psychiatric Association.

American Psychological Association. 1990. "APA guidelines for providers of psychological services to ethnic, linguistic, and culturally diverse populations." http://www.apa.org/pi/guide.html.

–. 2005. "Guidelines for psychotherapy with lesbian, gay, and bisexual clients." http://www.apa.org/pi/lgbc/guidelines.html.

Andrews, G., et al., eds. 2000. *Management of Mental Disorders.* Canadian edition. Vancouver: Mental Health Evaluation and Community Consultation Unit, University of British Columbia.

Angell, M. 2004. "The truth about the drug companies." http://www.nybooks.com/articles/17244?email.

Angermeyer, M., M. Beck, and H. Matschinger. 2003. "Determinants of the public's prefer-ence for social distance from people with schizophrenia." *Canadian Journal of Psychiatry* 48: 663-68.

Angst, J. 1999. "Major depression in 1998: Are we providing optimal therapy?" *Journal of Clinical Psychiatry* 60, supplement 6: 5-9.

Anthony, W. 1993. "Recovering from mental illness: The guiding vision of the mental health service system in the 1990s." *Psychosocial Rehabilitation Journal* 16, 4: 11-21.

–. 2000. "A recovery-oriented service system: Setting some system level standards." *Psychiatric Rehabilitation Journal* 24: 159-68.

–. 2003. "Expanding the evidence base in an era of recovery." *Psychiatric Rehabilitation Journal* 26: 1-2.

–, E. Rogers, and M. Farkas. 2003. "Research on evidence-based practices: Future directions in an era of recovery." *Community Mental Health Journal* 39: 101-14.

Antony, M., and R. Swinson. 1996. "Anxiety disorders and their treatment: A critical review of the evidence-based literature." Ottawa: Health Canada.

Anxiety Disorders Association of British Columbia. N.d. "Obsessive-compulsive disorder: Causes, complications and cures." http://www.anxietybc.com.

Appelbaum, P. 1994. *Almost a Revolution.* New York: Oxford University Press.

Appignanesi, R. 1979. *Freud for Beginners.* New York: Pantheon Books.

Arboleda-Florez, J. 1998. "Mental illness and violence: An epidemiological appraisal of the evidence." *Canadian Journal of Psychiatry* 43: 989-96.

–. 2003. "Considerations on the stigma of mental illness." *Canadian Journal of Psychiatry* 48: 645-50.

Arkar, H., and D. Eker. 1992. "Influence of having a hospitalized mentally ill member in the family on attitudes toward mental patients in Turkey." *Social Psychiatry and Psychiatric Epidemiology* 27: 151-55.

Asher, A. 1996. *Occupational Therapy Assessment Tools: An Annotated Index.* 2nd ed. Bethesda, MD: American Occupational Therapy Association.

Associated Press. 2005. "Tsunami too much for some survivors; psychiatrists worry more will suffer." http://healthandfitness.simpatico.msn.ca/Bell.Sympatico.CMS/Print.aspx?type=feed.

Aubrey, T., and J. Myner. 1996. "Community integration and quality of life: A comparison of persons with psychiatric disabilities in housing programs and community residents who are neighbors." *Canadian Journal of Community Mental Health* 15: 5-19.

Bachrach, L. 1994. "Deinstitutionalization: What Does It Really Mean?" In *Schizophrenia: Exploring the Spectrum of Psychosis,* ed. R. Ancill, S. Holliday, and J. Higenbottam, 21-34. Chichester, UK: John Wiley and Sons.

–. 1996. "What Do Patients Say about Program Planning? Perspectives from the Patient-Authored Literature." In *Schizophrenia: Breaking Down the Barriers,* ed. S. Holliday, R. Ancill, and G. MacEwan, 17-37. New York: John Wiley and Sons.

Bagheri, A. 1992. "Psychiatric problems among Iranian immigrants in Canada." *Canadian Journal of Psychiatry* 37: 7-11.

Bailey, K. 2004. "Should nurses prescribe?" *Journal of Psychosocial Nursing* 42: 14-19.

Bailey, V. 2001. "Cognitive-behavioural therapies for children and adolescents." *Advances in Psychiatric Treatment* 7: 224-32.

Bainbridge, L. 1998. *Consumer Involvement in the Workplace: A Literature Review.* Report prepared for the Greater Vancouver Mental Health Services Society.

Ballou, M., and L. Brown, eds. 2002. *Rethinking Mental Health and Disorder: Feminist Perspectives.* London, UK: Guilford.

Barak, G., and R. Bohm. 1989. "The crimes of the homeless or the crime of homelessness? On the dialectics of criminalization, decriminalization and victimization." *Contemporary Crises* 13: 2-14.

Barer, M. 2004. "Should Canada permit direct-to-consumer advertising of prescription pharmaceuticals?" *Healthcare Quarterly* 7: 24.

Barkhimer, R. 2003. "Breaking the silence of stigma." *Schizophrenia Digest* (Spring): 22-28.

Barlow, D., and M. Hersen. 1984. *Single Case Experimental Designs: Strategies for Studying Behavior Change.* 2nd ed. New York: Pergamon.

Barry, K., et al. 2003. "Effect of strengths model vs. assertive community treatment model on participant outcomes and utilization: Two year follow-up." *Psychiatric Rehabilitation Journal* 26: 268-77.

Bassett, A., D. Addington, P.E. Cook, R. Dickson, J.O. Goldberg, W. Honer, L. Kopala, and A. Malla. 1998. "Canadian clinical practice guidelines for the treatment of schizophrenia." *Canadian Journal of Psychiatry* 43, supplement 2: 25-40.

Beck, A., et al. 1979. *Cognitive Therapy of Depression.* New York: Guilford.

Beck, C., et al. 1999. "Psychostimulant prescriptions higher than expected: A self-report survey." *Canadian Journal of Psychiatry* 44: 680-84.

Beierle, A. 1996. "High anxiety." http://www.emory.edu/EMORY_MAGAZINE/winter96/virtreality.html.

Beiser, M., and I. Hyman. 1997. "Southeast Asian Refugees in Canada." In *Ethnicity, Immigration, and Psychopathology,* ed. I. Al-Issa and M. Tousignant, 35-56. New York: Plenum.

Bekelman, J., Y. Li, and C. Gross. 2003. "Scope and impact of financial conflicts of interest in biomedical research." *Journal of the American Medical Association* 289: 454-65.

Bell, C., ed. 2000. "Psychiatric aspects of violence: Issues in prevention and treatment." *New Directions for Mental Health Services* 86 (Summer).

Ben Noun, L. 1996. "Characteristics of patients refusing professional psychiatric treatment in a primary care clinic." *Israel Journal of Psychiatry* 33: 167-74.

Bentley, K., and J. Walsh. 2001. *The Social Worker and Psychotropic Medication.* Belmont: Brooks/Cole.

Bergen, M. 1999. *Riding the Roller Coaster.* Kelowna, BC: Northstone Pub.

Best, J. 2001. *Damned Lies and Statistics: Untangling Numbers from the Media, Politicians, and Activists.* Berkeley, CA: University of California Press.

Bhullar, J. 2000. "Consumer-run housing options." *Visions: BC's Mental Health Journal* 10: 16-17.

Bilsker, D. 2003. "Self-management in the mental health field." *Visions: BC's Mental Health Journal* 18: 4-5.

Birchwood, M., P. Todd, and C. Jackson. 1998. "Early intervention in psychosis: The critical period hypothesis." *British Journal of Psychiatry* 172, supplement 33: 53-59.

–, and K. Brunet. 2004. "Delay in secondary mental health services constitutes a major component of DUP in the UK" Paper presented at the 4th International Conference on Early Psychosis, Vancouver, BC, 29 September.

Bisetty, K. 2004. "One-third of police killings are 'suicide by cop': Study." *Vancouver Sun,* 4 October, A1-A2.

Blackwell, T. 2005. "US official: Canadian pot no soft drug." *Vancouver Sun,* 11 March, A1-A2.

Blake, C. 2003. "Ethical considerations in working with culturally diverse populations: The essential role of professional interpreters." *Canadian Psychiatric Association Bulletin* 35: 21-23.

Bland, R. 1997. "Epidemiology of affective disorders: A review." *Canadian Journal of Psychiatry* 42: 367-77.

–. 1998. "Psychiatry and the burden of mental illness." *Canadian Journal of Psychiatry* 43: 801-10.

–. 1999. "Editorial: Precursors to schizophrenia." *Canadian Journal of Psychiatry* 44: 335-49.

Blin, O. 1999. "A comparative review of new antispychotics." *Canadian Journal of Psychiatry* 44: 235-44.

Bogart, T., and P. Solomon. 1999. "Procedures to share treatment information among mental health providers, consumers and families." *Psychiatric Services* 50: 1321-25.

Bonner-Jackson, A., et al. 2005. "The influence of encoding strategy on episodic memory and cortical activity in schizophrenia." *Biological Psychiatry* 58: 47-55.

Borum, R. 1996. "Improving the clinical practice of violence risk assessment." *American Psychologist* 51: 945-56.

Bose, R. 1997. "Psychiatry and the popular conception of possession among the Bangladeshis in London." *International Journal of Social Psychiatry* 43: 1-15.

Bourgeois, M., et al. 2004. "Awareness of disorder and suicide risk in the treatment of schizophrenia: Results of the international suicide prevention trial." *American Journal of Psychiatry* 161: 1494-96.

Bowman, M. 1999. "Individual differences in posttraumatic distress: Problems with the DSM-IV model." *Canadian Journal of Psychiatry* 44: 21-33.

Boydell, K., and B. Everett. 1992. "What makes a house a home? An evaluation of a supported housing project for individuals with long-term psychiatric background." *Canadian Journal of Community Mental Health* 10: 109-23.

–, B. Gladstone, and E. Crawford. 2002. "The knowledge resource base: Beginning the dialogue." *Canadian Journal of Community Mental Health* 21: 19-33.

Bradley, G. 1991. "Intensive case management and the multi-problem client: An evaluation of the inter-ministerial project." Master's thesis, School of Social Work, University of British Columbia.

Brand, J. 1968. "The United States: A Historical Perspective." In *Community Mental Health: An International Perspective*, ed. R. Williams and L. Ozarin, 18-43. San Francisco: Jossey-Bass.

Branham, D. 2003. "Drugs for kids need scrutiny." *Vancouver Sun*, 12 December, B2-B3.

–. 2004. "6200 BC children on unapproved medication." *Vancouver Sun*, 4 February, A1.

Branswell, H. 2004. "First Nations, Inuit peoples still have significantly shorter life expectancy." http://mediresource.sympatico.ca/channel_health_news_detail.asp?channel_id=11&menu_item_id=4&news_id=3461.

Breggin, P. 1991. *Toxic Psychiatry*. New York: St. Martin's Press.

Briere, J. 2002. "Treating Adult Survivors of Severe Childhood Abuse and Neglect: Further Developments of an Integrative Model." In *The APSAC Handbook on Child Maltreatment*, ed. J. Myers et al., 175-202. 2nd ed. Newbury Park, CA: Sage.

Briggs, K., T. Choptiany, and R. Steinberg. 1997. "Treating teens: Evaluation of a newly developed adolescent day hospital." *Canadian Psychiatric Association Bulletin* 29: 79-81.

British Columbia Ministry of Health. 1999. *Guide to the Mental Health Act*. Victoria: BC Ministry of Health.

–. 2002a. *Best Practices: Assertive Community Treatment*. Victoria: BC Ministry of Health.

–. 2002b. *Best Practices: Consumer Involvement and Initiatives*. Victoria: BC Ministry of Health.

–. 2002c. *Best Practices: Family Involvement and Support*. Victoria: BC Ministry of Health.

–. 2002d. *Best Practices: Housing*. Victoria: BC Ministry of Health.

–. 2002e. *Best Practices: Inpatient/Outpatient Services*. Victoria: BC Ministry of Health.

–. 2002f. *Best Practices: Psychosocial Rehabilitation and Recovery*. Victoria: BC Ministry of Health.

British Columbia Ministry of Health Services. 2003a. *Historical Perspective: Mental Health Resource Utilization in British Columbia (1997/98 to 1999/00) prior to Health Authority Restructuring in 2001*. Victoria: BC Ministry of Health Services.

–. 2003b. *Historical Perspective: Mental Health Service System in British Columbia (1997/98 to 1999/00) prior to Health Authority Restructuring in 2001*. Victoria: BC Ministry of Health Services.

–. 2005. *Mental Health Act Review Panel's Statistical Report: 2004*. Victoria: BC Ministry of Health Services.

British Columbia Partners for Mental Health and Addictions Information. 2003a. "Concurrent disorders: Addictions and mental disorders." http://www.cmha-bc.org/content/resources/primer/32-stigma.pdf.

–. 2003b. "Housing for people with mental disorders and addictions." http://www.cmha-bc.org/content/resources/primer/35-housing.pdf.

–. 2003c. "Mental disorders toolkit: Information and resources for effective self-management of mental disorders." http://www.heretohelp.bc.ca/publications/toolkits/mdtoolkit.pdf.

–. 2003d. "Stigma and discrimination around mental disorders and addiction." http://www.cmha-bc.org/content/resources/primer/32-stigma.pdf.

–. 2003e. "Unemployment and mental health and addictions." http://www.cmha-bc.org/content/resources/primer/32-stigma.pdf.

British Columbia Reproductive Care Program, Reproductive Best Practices Working Group. 2003. *Best Practice Guidelines Relating to Reproductive Mental Health.* Vancouver: BC Reproductive Care Program.

British Columbia Schizophrenia Society. 2000. "Questions to ask the psychiatrist." http://www.bcss.org/support/psychiatrist.html.

–. 2004. "A quiet revolution: Early psychosis services in BC, a survey of hospital and community resources." Richmond: BC Schizophrenia Society.

Brook, P. 2003. "Crazy: The inside story." *Vancouver Sun,* 5 April, H5.

Brown, M., et al. 1991. "Comparison of outcomes for clients seeking and assigned to supported housing services." *Hospital and Community Psychiatry* 42: 1150-53.

Brown, R. 1992. "Identification and Office Management of Alcohol and Drug Disorders." In *Addictive Disorders,* ed. M. Fleming and K. Barry, 25-43. St. Louis: Mosby Yearbook.

Browne, A., et al. 2002. "On liberty for the old." *Canadian Journal on Aging* 21, 2: 283-93.

Browne, G., and M. Courtney. 2004. "Measuring the impact of housing on people with schizophrenia." *Nursing and Health Sciences* 6: 37-44.

Brunette, M., et al. 2003. "Benzodiazepine use and abuse among patients with severe mental illness and co-occurring substance use disorders." *Psychiatric Services* 54: 1395-1401.

Bryan, H. 2004. "Policing the policing of psychiatric patients." *Vancouver Georgia Straight,* 10-17 June, 41.

Bryant, T. 2003. "The current state of housing in Canada as a social determinant of health." *Policy Options* (March): 52-56.

Buccheri, R., et al. 2004. "Long-term effects of teaching behavioral strategies for managing persistent auditory hallucinations." *Journal of Psychosocial Nursing and Mental Health Services* 42: 18-27.

Bula, F. 2004. "There's no place like homelessness." *Vancouver Sun,* 24 January, B2-B3.

–, and C. Skelton. 2004. "The best strategy: Caring for the mentally ill." *Vancouver Sun,* 31 January, A1, A4-A5.

Burns, B., and A. Santos. 1995. "Assertive community treatment: An update of randomized trials." *Psychiatric Services* 46: 669-75.

Burns, D. 1989. *The Feeling Good Handbook.* New York: W. Morrow.

–. 1999. *Feeling Good: The New Mood Therapy.* New York: Avon Books.

Butters, M., et al. 2004. "The nature and determinants of neuropsychological functioning in late-life depression." *Archives of General Psychiatry* 61: 587-95.

Butzlaff, R., and J. Hooley. 1998. "Expressed emotion and psychiatric relapse: A meta-analysis." *Archives of General Psychiatry* 55, 6: 547-52.

Calgary Health Region. 2003. "New release: Phone line provides mental health access." http://www.crha-health.ab.ca/publicaffairs/news/mental_health_phone_lineApr1-03.pdf.

Calsaferri, K. and L. Jongbloed. 1999. "Three perspectives on the rehabilitation needs of consumers." *Canadian Journal of Community Mental Health* 18: 199-210.

Campbell, W. 2003. "Addiction: A disease of volition caused by a cognitive impairment." *Canadian Journal of Psychiatry* 48: 669-74.

Canadian Centre on Substance Abuse. 2004. "A national survey of Canadians' use of alcohol and other drugs: Prevalence of use and related harms." http://www.ccsa.ca/pdf/ccsa-004804.pdf.

Canadian Counselling Association. 1999. *Code of Ethics*. Ottawa: Canadian Counselling Association.

Canadian Housing and Renewal Association. 2002. *On Her Own: Young Women and Homelessness in Canada*. Ottawa: Status of Women Canada.

Canadian Institute for Health Information. 2003. "Data announcement: Hospital mental health statistics, 2000/2001." http://secure.cihi.ca/cihiweb/dispPage.jsp?cw_page=media_04feb2003_e.

–. 2004. "Drug spending in Canada still on the rise: Public sector's share increasing, reports CIHI." http://secure.cihi.ca/cihiweb/dispPage.jsp?cw_page=media_22jun2004_e.

Canadian Medical Association Journal. 2004. "Editorial: The 'file drawer' phenomenon: Suppressing clinical evidence." *Canadian Medical Association Journal* 170: 437.

Canadian Mental Health Association (CMHA). 2001. Submission to the Commission on the Future of Health Care in Canada. http://www.ontario.cmha.ca/content/reading_room/policydocuments.asp?cID=2590.

–. 2003. "Canadian and Ontario mental health statistics, 2000/2001." http://www.ontario.cmha.ca/content/reading_room/Statistics.asp?cID=3761.

Canadian Mental Health Association (CMHA), British Columbia Division. 1999. *Where Does Stigma Live?* (brochure). Vancouver: CMHA.

–. 2003. "Study in blue and grey: Police interventions with people with mental illness: A review of challenges and responses." http://www.crpnbc.ca/policereport.pdf.

Canadian Mental Health Association (CMHA), Thunder Bay Branch. 2001. "Mental health diversion program." http://www.cmha-tb.on.ca/mhdiversion.htm.

Canada Mortgage and Housing Corporation. 1999. *Best Practices Addressing Homelessness*. Ottawa: Canada Mortgage and Housing Corporation.

Canadian Psychiatric Association. 2001. "Clinical practice guidelines for the treatment of depressive disorders." *Canadian Journal of Psychiatry* 46, supplement 1: S13-S89.

–. 2003. "About CAMIMH [Canadian Alliance on Mental Illness and Mental Health]." http://www.cpa-apc.org/public/camimh.asp.

Canadian Psychoanalytic Society. 2001. "About psychoanalysis." http://www.psychoanalysis.ca/main/asp?P=84U1CCPSU1.

Canadian Study of Health and Aging Working Group. 1994. "Canadian study of health and aging: Study methods and prevalence of dementia." *Canadian Medical Association Journal* 150: 899-913.

Canadian Therapeutic Recreation Association (CTRA). 2003. "About CTRA." http://www.canadian-tr.org/about_ctra.htm.

CanWest News Services. 2004. "Mental health numbers." *Vancouver Sun*, 20 November, A7.

Caplan, P. 1995. *They Say You're Crazy: How the World's Most Powerful Psychiatrists Decide Who's Normal*. Reading, MA: Addison-Wesley.

Capponi, P. 1992. *Upstairs in the Crazy House*. Toronto: Penguin Books.

–. 1997. *Dispatches from the Poverty Line*. Toronto: Penguin Books.

–. 2003. *Beyond the Crazy House: Changing the Future of Madness*. Toronto: Penguin Books.

Carling, P. 1993. "Housing and supports for persons with mental illness: Emerging approaches to research and practice." *Hospital and Community Psychiatry* 44: 899-903.

Carrigg, D. 2002. "Double trouble." *Vancouver Courier*, 30 January, 1, 4-5.

–. 2003a. "Backpack hostel conversions blamed for homelessness." *Vancouver Courier*, 20 July, 8-9.

–. 2003b. "Registered nurses call Minoru switch to LPNs slapdash." *Vancouver Courier*, 12 November, 17.

–. 2004. "Health authority streamlining help for addicts." *Vancouver Courier*, 21 January, 23.

Carson, R. 1991. "Dilemmas in the pathway of the DSM-IV." *Journal of Abnormal Psychology* 100: 302-7.

Casey, J. 1994. *The Regulation of the Professions in Canada*. Toronto: Carswell.

Catalano, E. 1990. *Getting to Sleep*. Oakland, CA: New Harbinger Publications.

Centre for Addiction and Mental Health (CAMH). 2001. "Police and nurses team together." http://www.camh.net/journal/journalv4no2/in_brief.html.

–. 2002a. *CAMH Position on Harm Reduction: Its Meaning and Application for Substance Abuse Issues*. Toronto: CAMH.

–. 2002b. "Partnership profiles: First episode psychosis." http://www.camh.net/annual_reports/2002/first_episode_profile.html.

–. 2004. *The Mental Health and Well-Being of Ontario Students, 1991-2003*. Toronto: CAMH.

Chaimowitz, G., and G. Glancy. 2002. "The duty to protect." http://www.cpa-apc.org/Publications/Position_Papers/duty.asp.

Chamberlin, J., and J. Rogers. 1990. "Planning a community-based mental health system: Perspective of service recipients." *American Psychologist* 45: 1241-44.

Champney, T., and L. Dzurec. 1992. "Involvement in productive activities and satisfaction with living situation among severely disabled adults." *Hospital and Community Psychiatry* 44: 899-903.

Chandler, M., and C. Lalonde. 1998. "Cultural continuity as a hedge against suicide in Canada's First Nations." *Transcultural Psychiatry* 35, 193-211.

Cherland, E., and R. Fitzpatrick. 1999. "Psychotic side effects of psychostimulants: A five year review." *Canadian Journal of Psychiatry* 44: 811-13.

Chue, P., et al. 2002. "Dissolution profile, tolerability and acceptability of the orally dissolving tablet in patients with schizophrenia." *Canadian Journal of Psychiatry* 47: 771-74.

–, et al. 2004. "Client and community services satisfaction with an ACT subprogram for inner-city clients in Edmonton, Alberta." *Canadian Jounral of Psychiatry* 49: 621-24.

Clarke Institute of Psychiatry. 1997. "Best practices in mental health reform: Discussion paper." Report prepared for the Federal/Provincial/Territorial Advisory Network on Mental Health.

Cohen, C., et al. 2003. "The future of community psychiatry." *Community Mental Health Journal* 39: 459-68.

Cohen, S. 1985. *Visions of Social Control*. Cambridge, UK: Polity Press.

Commission on the Future of Health Care in Canada. 2002. *Building on Values: The Future of Health Care in Canada*. Saskatoon: Commission on the Future of Health Care in Canada.

Committee on Addictions of the Group for the Advancement of Psychiatry. 2002. "Responsibility and choice in addiction." *Psychiatric Services* 53: 707-13.

Cook, T., and D. Campbell. 1979. *Quasi-Experimentation: Design and Analysis Issues for Field Settings*. Boston: Houghton Mifflin.

Copeland, M. 1992. *The Depression Workbook*. Oakland, CA: New Harbinger Publications.

Correll, C., S. Leucht, and J. Kane. 2004. "Lower risk for tardive dyskinesia associated with second-generation antipsychotics: A systematic review of 1-year studies." *American Journal of Psychiatry* 161: 414-25.

Corrigan, P. 2003. "Towards an integrated, structural model of psychiatric rehabilitation." *Psychiatric Rehabilitation Journal* 26: 346-58.

–. 2004. "Target-specific stigma change: A strategy for impacting mental illness stigma." *Psychiatric Rehabilitation Journal* 28: 113-21.

–, et al. 2003. "Perceptions of discrimination among persons with serious mental illness." *Psychiatric Services* 54: 1105-10.

–, et al. 2004. "Stigmatizing attitudes about mental illness and allocation of resources to mental health services." *Community Mental Health Journal* 40: 297-307.

Cotton, D. 2002. "First steps toward best practices: Models for working with the mental health system." http://www.pmhl.ca/en/2002Report.html.

Coursey, R., et al. 2000. "Competencies for direct service staff members who work with adults with severe mental illnesses: Specific knowledge, attitudes, skills and bibliography." *Psychiatric Rehabilitation Journal* 23: 370-89.

Craib, K., et al. 2003. "Risk factor for elevated HIV incidence among aboriginal injection drug users in Vancouver." *Canadian Medical Association Journal* 168: 19-24.

Croghan, T. 2001. "The controversy of increased spending for antidepressants." *Health Affairs* 20: 129-35.

Cronkite, K. 1994. *On the Edge of Darkness.* New York: Doubleday.

Culhane, D., S. Metraux, and T. Hadley. 2002. "Public service reductions associated with placement of homeless persons with severe mental illness in supportive housing." http://www.csh.org/index.cfm?fuseaction=document.showDocumentListandparentID=24.

Curtis, L., and M. Hodge. 1995. "Ethics and boundaries in community support services: New challenges." *New Directions for Mental Health Services* 66: 43-59.

–, and V. Smith. 1996. "Old rules and new dilemmas: Relationship boundaries in community support services." Paper presented at the Annual Conference of the International Association of Psychosocial Rehabilitation Services, Detroit, June.

Dallaire, R., and B. Beardsley. 2003. *Shake Hands with the Devil: The Failure of Humanity in Rwanda.* Toronto: Random House.

Dalrymple, T. 2003. "In this age, a pill for every ill." *National Post,* 13 August, A17.

Daly, G. 1996. *Homeless: Policies, Strategies and Lives on the Street.* London, UK: Routledge.

D'Andrea, J. 2003. *Illness and Disability in the Workplace.* Aurora, ON: Canada Law Book.

Dannon, P., et al. 2002. "Three and six month outcome following courses of either ECT or RTMS in a population of severely depressed individuals: A preliminary report." *Biological Psychiatry* 51: 687-90.

Davies, L. 2000. "Housing is a human right: Responding to homelessness in Canada." *Visions: BC's Mental Health Journal* 10: 37-38.

Davis, L. 1997. "The encyclopedia of insanity: A psychiatric handbook lists a madness for everyone." *Harper's Magazine,* February: 61-66.

Davis, S. 1985. "The new young chronic psychiatric patient: A study in Vancouver." *Social Work in Health Care* 11, 2: 87-100.

–. 1987a. "Four conceptualizations of schizophrenia as models for treatment." *Health and Social Work* 12: 91-100.

–. 1987b. "The homeless mentally ill: A report from Vancouver." *The Social Worker* 55: 10-13.

–. 1991. "An overview: Are mentally ill persons really more dangerous?" *Social Work* 36, 2: 174-80.

–. 1992. "Assessing the criminalization of the mentally ill in Canada." *Canadian Journal of Psychiatry* 37, 8: 532-38.

–. 1994a. "Examining the impact of Bill C-30 in British Columbia." *International Bulletin of Law and Mental Health* 5: 5-9.

–. 1994b. "Exploring the impact of Bill C-30 on the handling of mentally disordered offenders." Doctoral dissertation, Simon Fraser University.

–. 1994c. "Factors associated with the diversion of mentally disordered offenders." *Bulletin of the American Academy of Psychiatry and the Law* 22, 3: 389-98.

–. 1995a. "Fitness to stand trial: A study of a change in the law concerning pre-trial psychiatric remands." *Health Law in Canada* 16, 2: 33-38.

–. 1995b. "Treating the mentally ill in British Columbia: Recent developments in policy and legislation." *British Columbia Medical Journal* 37: 400-2.

–. 1996. "The trouble with closing the asylums." *Globe and Mail,* 18 March, A17.

–. 1998. "Injection drug use and HIV infection among the seriously mentally ill: A report from Vancouver." *Canadian Journal of Community Mental Health* 17: 121-27.

–. 2000. "An analysis of suicide attempts and completions by consumers of Vancouver community mental health teams." Paper presented at the 11th Annual Conference of the Canadian Association for Suicide Prevention, Vancouver, 12 October.

–. 2002. "Autonomy vs. coercion: Reconciling competing perspectives in community mental health." *Community Mental Health Journal* 38, 3: 239-50.

–, D. Eaves, and D. Wilson. 1999. "The Interministerial Program." Presentation at the National Conference on Best Practices and Mental Health Reform, Toronto, 30 April.

Dawson, D. 1988. "Treatment of the borderline patient: Relationship management." *Canadian Journal of Psychiatry* 33: 370-74.

Deegan, P. 1988. "Recovery: The lived experience of rehabilitation." *Psychosocial Rehabilitation Journal* 11: 11-19.

Deiser, R. 2002. "A personal narrative of a cross-cultural experience in a therapeutic recreation: Unmasking the masked." *Therapeutic Recreation Journal* 36: 84-96.

Dennis, D., and J. Monahan, eds. 1996. *Coercion and Aggressive Community Treatment.* New York: Plenum.

Department of Justice Canada. 2003. "Fetal alcohol spectrum disorder and the youth criminal justice system: A discussion paper." Ottawa: Department of Justice.

Desjarlais, R., et al. 1995. *World Mental Health.* New York: Oxford University Press.

Deutsch, A. 1948. *The Shame of the States.* New York: Harcourt, Brace, Jovanovich.

Deveau, S. 2004. "City housing worker says homeless numbers way up." *Vancouver Courier,* 31 October, 9.

Diamond, R. 1996. "Coercion and Tenacious Treatment in the Community: Applications to the Real World." In *Coercion and Aggressive Community Treatment,* ed. D. Dennis and J. Monahan, 51-72. New York: Plenum.

Dickinson, H. 2002. "Mental Health Policy in Canada: What's the Problem?" In *Health, Illness and Health Care in Canada,* 3rd ed., ed. B. Bolaria and H. Dickinson, 372-88. Scarborough, ON: Nelson.

–, and G. Andre. 1988. "Community Psychiatry: The Institutional Transformation of Psychiatric Practice." In *Sociology of Health Care in Canada,* ed. B. Bolaria and H. Dickinson, 295-302. Toronto: Harcourt, Brace, Jovanovich.

Dincin, J. 2001. "The biological basis of mental illness." *New Directions for Mental Health Services* 91: 47-56.

Dineen, T. 1998. "Are we manufacturing victims?" http://tanadineen.com/COLUMNIST/Wrtings/sexualharass.htm.

–. 2000. *Manufacturing Victims: What the Psychology Industry is Doing to People.* Montreal: R. Davies Multimedia.

Dinos, S., et al. 2004. "Stigma: The feelings and experiences of 46 people with mental illness." *British Journal of Psychiatry* 184: 176-81.

Dixon, L., et al. 1991. "Drug abuse in schizophrenic patients: Clinical correlates and reasons for use." *American Journal of Psychiatry* 148: 224-30.

–, et al. 1994. "Clinical and treatment correlates of access to Section 8 certificates for homeless mentally ill persons." *Hospital and Community Psychiatry* 45: 1196-1200.

–, et al. 1998. "Severe mental illness in an outreach intervention." *Community Mental Health Journal* 34: 251-59.

–, et al. 2001. "Evidence-based practices for services to families of people with psychiatric disabilities." *Psychiatric Services* 52: 903-8.

Donnelly, M. 1996. "Financial and personal competency assessments for British Columbia seniors." *BC Medical Journal* 38: 484-87.

–. 2001. "The state of seniors' health in British Columbia." *Visions: BC's Mental Health Journal* 15: 4-5.

Dorrance, N. 2003. "Police attitudes toward mentally ill belie stereotype." *Queens Gazette,* Kingston, ON, 27 January, 8.

Douglas, K., J. Ogloff, and S. Hart. 2003. "Evaluation of a model of violence risk assessment among forensic psychiatric patients." *Psychiatric Services* 54: 1372-79.

Drake, R., et al. 1996. "Day treatment versus supported employment for persons with severe mental illness: A replication study." *Psychiatric Services* 47: 1125-27.

–, et al. 2001. "Implementing evidence-based practices in routine mental health service settings." *Psychiatric Services* 52: 179-82.

–, et al. 2003. "The history of community mental health treatment and rehabilitation for persons with severe mental illness." *Community Mental Health Journal* 39: 427-40.

Druss, B., et al. 2001. "Quality of medical care and excess mortality in older patients with mental disorders." *Archives of General Psychiatry* 58: 565-72.

Dubey, A. 1999. "Dispelling the stigma of schizophrenia: A global campaign launches in Canada." *The Journal of Addiction and Mental Health* 2: 8.

Duckworth, K., et al. 2003. "Use of schizophrenia as a metaphor in U.S. newspapers." *Psychiatric Services* 54: 1402-4.

Duncan, D. 2004. "Is 'bad parenting' the chicken or the egg?" *Visions: BC's Mental Health Journal* 2, 3: 12-13.

Dunn, J. 2000. "Why housing? A framework for housing and mental health." *Visions: BC's Mental Health Journal* 10: 4.

–. 2003. *A Needs, Gaps and Opportunities Assessment for Research: Housing as a Socio-Economic Determinant of Health.* Report prepared for the Canadian Institutes of Health Research.

Eaton, W. 2001. *The Sociology of Mental Disorders.* 3rd ed. Westport, CT: Praeger.

Eberle, M. 2001a. *Homelessness: Causes and Effects.* Vol. 1, *The Relationship between Homelessness and the Health, Social Services and Criminal Justice System: A Review of the Literature.* Victoria, BC: Ministry of Social Development and Economic Security.

–. 2001b. *Homelessness: Causes and Effects.* Vol. 3, *The Costs of Homelessness in British Columbia.* Victoria, BC: Ministry of Social Development and Economic Security.

–. 2001c. *Homelessness: Causes and Effects.* Vol. 4, *A Profile and Policy Review of Homelessness in the Provinces of Ontario, Quebec and Alberta.* Victoria, BC: Ministry of Social Development and Economic Security.

Ehlers, A., et al. 2003. "A randomized controlled trial of cognitive therapy, a self-help booklet, and repeated assessments as early interventions for post-traumatic stress disorder." *Archives of General Psychiatry* 60: 1024-32.

Ehmann, T., J. Yager, and L. Hanson. 2004. "Early psychosis: A review of the treatment literature." Research report prepared for the British Columbia Ministry of Children and Family Development.

–, and L. Hanson. 2004a. "Measuring the Effectiveness of Care." In *Best Care in Early Psychosis Intervention,* ed. T. Ehmann, G. MacEwan, and W. Honer, 99-102. London, UK: Taylor and Francis.

–, and L. Hanson. 2004b. "Pharmacotherapy." In *Best Care in Early Psychosis Intervention,* ed. T. Ehmann, G. MacEwan, and W. Honer, 37-60. London, UK: Taylor and Francis.

–, L. Hanson, and R. Friedlander. 2004. "Special Populations." In *Best Care in Early Psychosis Intervention,* ed. T. Ehmann, G. MacEwan, and W. Honer, 85-98. London, UK: Taylor and Francis.

Eisenberg, D., et al. 1993. "Unconventional medicine in the United States: Prevalence, costs and patterns of use." *New England Journal of Medicine* 328: 246-52.

Eklund, M., L. Hansson, and C. Ahlqvist. 2004. "The importance of work as compared to other forms of daily occupations for wellbeing and functioning among persons with long-term mental illness." *Community Mental Health Journal* 40: 465-77.

el-Guebaly, N. 1997. "Psychiatry 2000: Is it time for a sequel to 'more for the mind?'"http://www.cpa-apc.org/Publications/Archives/Bulletin/1997/Feb/clinical.htm.

Elliott, L. 2000. "Ontario native suicide rate one of highest in world, expert says." *Vancouver Sun,* 30 November, http://www.st-matthew.on.ca/bulletin/Jeremy/vanart.htm.

Ellis, A., and W. Dryden. 1987. *The Practice of Rational-Emotive Therapy.* New York: Springer.

Ernst, E., J. Rand, and C. Stevinson. 1998. "Complementary therapies for depression: An overview." *Archives of General Psychiatry* 55: 1026-32.

Essock, S., L. Frisman, and N. Kontos. 1998. "Cost-effectiveness of assertive community treatment teams." *American Journal of Orthopsychiatry* 68: 179-90.

Estroff, S., et al. 1994. "The influence of social networks and social support on violence by persons with serious mental illness." *Hospital and Community Psychiatry* 45: 669-79.

Evans, R. 1984. *Strained Mercy: The Economics of Canadian Health Care.* Toronto: Butterworth.

Everett, B. 1994. "Something is happening: The contemporary consumer and psychiatric survivor movement in historical context." *The Journal of Mind and Behavior* 15: 55-70.

–. 2001. "Community treatment orders: Ethical practice in an era of magical thinking." *Canadian Journal of Community Mental Health* 20: 5-19.

–, et al. 2003. "Recovery rediscovered: Implications for mental health policy in Canada." http://www.cmha.ca/english/images/recovery_Policy_Paper_National.pdf.

Fabian, E., A. Waterworth, and B. Ripke. 1993. "Reasonable accommodations for workers with serious mental illness: Type, frequency and associated outcomes." *Psychosocial Rehabilitation Journal* 17: 163-72.

Falloon, I., et al. 1993. *Managing Stress in Families: Cognitive and Behavioural Strategies for Enhancing Coping Skills.* London, UK: Routledge.

–, J. Coverdale, and C. Brooker. 1996. "Psychosocial interventions in schizophrenia: A review." *International Journal of Mental Health* 25: 3-21.

Fauman, M. 2002. *Study Guide to the DSM-IV-TR.* Washington, DC: American Psychiatric Publishing.

Fayerman, P. 2003. "New drug policy upsets seniors." *Vancouver Sun*, 18 July, B5-B7.

"Fees limit access, forum reports." 2003. *Canadian Association of University Teachers Bulletin*, May, A1.

Felker, B., J. Yazel, and D. Short. 1996. "Mortality and medical co-morbidity among psychiatric patients: A review." *Psychiatric Services* 47: 1356-62.

Fenton, W. 2000. "Evolving perspectives on individual psychotherapy for schizophrenia." *Schizophrenia Bulletin* 26: 47-72.

Fergusson, D., et al. 2005. "Association between suicide attempts and SSRIs: Systematic review of randomized controlled trials." http://bmj.bmjjournals.com/cgi/content/abstract/330/7488/396.

Fernandez, G., and S. Nygard. 1990. "Impact of involuntary outpatient commitment on the revolving door syndrome in North Carolina." *Hospital and Community Psychiatry* 41: 1001-4.

First, M., R. Spitzer, and M. Gibbon. 1995. *Structured Clinical Interview for DSM IV Axis I Disorders.* Patient edition. Version 2. New York: New York State Psychiatric Institute, Biometrics Research.

Fischer, E., M. Shumway, and R. Owen. 2002. "Priorities of consumers, providers and family members in the treatment of schizophrenia." *Psychiatric Services* 53: 724-29.

Fischer, J., and K. Corcoran, eds. 1994a. *Measures for Clinical Practice.* Vol. 1, *Couples, Families and Children.* New York: Free Press.

–, and K. Corcoran, eds. 1994b. *Measures for Clinical Practice.* Vol. 2, *Adults.* New York: Free Press.

Fisher, D. 1999. "Healing and recovery are real." http://www.power2U.org/recovery/heal_recovery.html.

Flint, A., and R. Reekum. 1998. "The pharmacological treatment of Alzheimer's disease: A guide for the general psychiatrist." *Canadian Journal of Psychiatry* 43: 689-97.

Flores, G., et al. 2002. "The health of Latino children: Urgent priorities, unanswered questions and a research agenda." *Journal of the American Medical Association* 288: 82-90.

Foucault, M. 1965. *Madness and Civilization.* New York: Vintage Books.

–. 1977. *Discipline and Punish: The Birth of the Prison.* New York: Vintage Books.

Fowler, D., P. Garety, and E. Kuipers. 1995. *Cognitive-Behaviour Therapy for Psychosis: Theory and Practice.* Chichester, UK: John Wiley and Sons.

Fox, L., and D. Hilton. 1994. Response to "Consumers as service providers: The promise and challenge." *Community Mental Health Journal* 30: 627-29.

Freidson, E. 1994. *Professionalism Reborn: Theory, Prophecy and Policy.* Cambridge, UK: Polity Press.

Frese, F. 1997. "The mental health service consumer's perspective on mandatory treatment." *New Directions for Mental Health Services* 75: 17-26.

Fuller, C. 1998. *Caring for Profit: How Corporations Are Taking over Canada's Health Care System*. Ottawa: Canadian Centre for Policy Alternatives.

Gabbard, G., and C. Nadelson. 1995. "Professional boundaries in the physician-patient relationship." *Journal of the American Medical Association* 273: 1445-49.

Gadsby, J. 2000. *Addiction by Prescription*. Toronto: Key Porter Books.

Gaebel, W., and A. Baumann. 2003. "Interventions to reduce the stigma associated with severe mental illness: Experiences from the Open the Door Program in Germany." *Canadian Journal of Psychiatry* 48: 657-62.

Galea, S., et al. 2002. "Psychological sequelae of the September 11 terrorist attacks in New York City." *New England Journal of Medicine* 346: 982-87.

Gallagher, B. 1995. *The Sociology of Mental Illness*. 3rd ed. Englewood Cliffs, NJ: Prentice-Hall.

Ganesan, S. 2000. "Mental health and disorder in recent immigrants." *Visions: BC's Mental Health Journal* 9: 24.

Garety, P., D. Fowler, and E. Kuipers. 2000. "Cognitive behavioral therapy for medication resistant symptoms." *Schizophrenia Bulletin* 26: 73-86.

Garfinkel, P., and D. Goldbloom. 2000. "Significant developments in psychiatry: Implications for community mental health." *Canadian Journal of Community Mental Health* 19: 161-65.

Garland, E. 2002. "Taming worry dragons: Empowering children and their parents to master anxiety symptoms." *Visions: BC's Mental Health Journal* 14: 29.

–. 2004. "Facing the evidence: Antidepressant treatment in children and adolescents." *Canadian Medical Association Journal* 170: 489-91.

Garofalo, R., et al. 1999. "Sexual orientation and risk of suicide attempts among a representative sample of youth." *Archives of Pediatric and Adolescent Medicine* 153: 487-93.

Geller, J., and M. Harris. 1994. *Women of the Asylum*. New York: Anchor Books.

Genova, P. 2003. "Dump the DSM." *Psychiatric Times*, 1 April, 72.

Gerber, G., and P. Prince. 1999. "Measuring client satisfaction with assertive community treatment." *Psychiatric Services* 50: 546-50.

–, et al. 2003. "Substance abuse among persons with serious mental illness in eastern Ontario." *Canadian Journal of Community Mental Health* 22: 113-28.

Gestalt Institute of Toronto. 2004. "Theory: What is gestalt?" http://www.gestalt.on.ca/site/page.php?id=29.

Gibson-Leek, M. 2003. "Client vs. client." *Psychiatric Services* 54: 1101-2.

Gilbody, S., P. Wilson, and I. Watt. 2004. "Direct-to-consumer advertising of psychotropics." *British Journal of Psychiatry* 185: 1-2.

Gingell, C. 1991. "The criminalization of the mentally ill: An examination of the hypothesis." Doctoral dissertation, Faculty of Psychology, Simon Fraser University.

Glackman, W. 1991. "The Treatment of Sex Offenders." In *Canadian Criminology*, ed. M. Jackson and C. Griffiths, 239-56. Toronto: Harcourt, Brace, Jovanovich.

Goering, P., et al. 1994. *Essential Service Ratios in a Reformed Mental Health System: Case Management*. Report submitted to the Ontario Ministry of Health.

–, and E. Lin. 1996. "Mental Health: Levels of Need and Variations in Service Use in Ontario." In *Patterns of Health Care in Ontario: The ICES Atlas*, 2nd ed., ed. V. Goel et al., 265-85. Ottawa: Canadian Medical Association.

–, D. Wasylenki, and J. Durbin. 2000. "Canada's mental health system." *International Journal of Law and Psychiatry* 23: 345-59.

Goffman, E. 1961. *Asylums: Essays on the Social Situation of Mental Patients and Other Inmates*. New York: Anchor Books.

Goldbloom, D. 2003. "Editorial: Language and metaphor." *Canadian Psychiatric Association Bulletin* 35: 3-5.

Golden, A., et al. 1999. *Report of the Mayor's Homelessness Action Task Force: Taking Responsibility for the Homeless: An Action Plan for Toronto*. City of Toronto.

Goldenberg, I., and H. Goldenberg. 1980. *Family Therapy: An Overview.* Monterey, CA: Brooks/ Cole.

Goldner, E., et al. 2000. "Evidence-based psychiatric practice: Implications for education and continuing professional development." http://www.cpa-apc.org/Publications/Position_ Papers/Evidence.asp.

–, et al. 2002. "Prevalence and incidence studies of schizophrenic disorders: A systematic review of the literature." *Canadian Journal of Psychiatry* 47, 9: 833-43.

Golier, J., et al. 2003. "The relationship of borderline personality disorder to posttraumatic stress disorder and traumatic events." *American Journal of Psychiatry* 160: 2018-24.

Gomoroy, T. 2001. "A critique of the effectiveness of assertive community treatment." *Psychiatric Services* 52: 1394.

Goodwin, D., and S. Guze. 1996. *Psychiatric Diagnosis.* New York: Oxford University Press.

Gordon, A. 1997. "Psychiatric bed levels." *Canadian Psychiatric Association Bulletin* 29: 1-4.

Gordon, R. 1993. "Out to pasture: A case for the retirement of Canadian mental health legislation." *Canadian Journal of Community Mental Health* 37: 37-52.

–, and S. Verdun-Jones. 1992. *Adult Guardianship Law in Canada.* Toronto: Carswell.

Gorman, C. 2003. "Finding a balance: Bipolar disorders." *Canadian Journal of Diagnosis* 20, 3: 93-97.

Gove, W. 1970. "Societal reaction as an explanation of mental illness: An evaluation." *American Sociological Review* 35: 873-83.

Government of Alberta. 1983. *Report of the Task Force to Review the Mental Health Act.* Edmonton: Government of Alberta.

Government of Ontario. 1999. *Making It Happen: Implementation Plan for Mental Health Reform.* Toronto: Government of Ontario.

Grant, H., and R. Oertel. 1997. "The supply and migration of Canadian physicians, 1970-1995: Why we should learn to love an immigrant doctor." *Canadian Journal of Regional Science* (Spring-Summer): 157-68.

Grant, I. 1997. "Canada's new mental disorder disposition provisions: A case study." *International Journal of Law and Psychiatry* 20: 419-28.

Gray, J., M. Shone, and P. Liddle. 2000. *Canadian Mental Health Law and Policy.* Toronto: Butterworths.

Greater Vancouver Mental Health Service Intercultural Committee. 1999. "Multiculturalism and mental health: Developing culturally competent systems of care." Vancouver: Greater Vancouver Mental Health Service Intercultural Committee.

Grech, E. 2002. "A review of the current evidence for the use of psychological interventions in psychosis." *International Journal of Psychosocial Rehabilitation* 6: 79-88.

Green, M., B. Marshall, and E. Wirshing. 1997. "Does risperidone improve verbal working memory in treatment resistant schizophrenia?" *American Journal of Psychiatry* 154: 799-804.

Green, R., et al. 2003. "Depression as a risk factor for Alzheimer disease: The MIRAGE Study." *Archives of Neurology* 60: 753-59.

Greenberg, D. 1998. "Sexual recidivism in sex offenders." *Canadian Journal of Psychiatry* 43: 459-64.

Grove, H. 1987. "The Reliability of Psychiatric Diagnosis." In *Issues in Diagnostic Research,* ed. C. Last and M. Hersen, 99-117. New York: Plenum.

Guest, D. 1980. *The Emergence of Social Security in Canada.* Vancouver: University of British Columbia Press.

Gumley, A., et al. 2003. "Early intervention for relapse in schizophrenia: Results of a 12-month randomized controlled trial of cognitive behavioural therapy." *Psychological Medicine* 33: 419-31.

Gunderson, J., et al. 1984. "Effects of psychotherapy in schizophrenia." Part 2, "Comparative outcomes of two forms of treatment." *Schizophrenia Bulletin* 10: 564-98.

–, and A. Sabo. 1993. "The phenomenological and conceptual interface between borderline personality disorder and PTSD." *American Journal of Psychiatry* 150: 19-27.

Haddock, G., and N. Tarrier. 1998. "Assessment and Formulation in the Cognitive Behavioural Treatment of Psychosis." In *Treating Complex Cases: The Cognitive Behavioural Therapy Approach,* ed. N. Tarrier, A. Wells, and G. Haddock, 176-94. Chichester, UK: John Wiley and Sons.

Hagan, J., and W. McCarthy. 1998. *Mean Streets: Youth Crime and Homelessness.* Cambridge, UK: Cambridge University Press.

Haggarty, J., et al. 2000. "Psychiatric disorders in an Arctic community." *Canadian Journal of Psychiatry* 45: 357-62.

Hall, G., and G. Nelson. 1996. "Social networks, social support, personal empowerment, and the adaptation of psychiatric consumer/survivors: Path analytic models." *Social Science and Medicine* 49: 1743-54.

Hall, N. 2000. *Pump up the Volume: A Report from the Mental Health Advocate of British Columbia.* Vancouver: Office of the Mental Health Advocate of British Columbia.

–. 2001. *Growing the Problem: The Second Annual Report of the Mental Health Advocate of British Columbia.* Vancouver: Office of the Mental Health Advocate of British Columbia.

Halstead, K. 1998. "Parental discretion advised: Gay and lesbian issues in trauma treatment." *Centering: Newletter of THE CENTER Postraumatic Disorders Program,* March-April, 4-5.

Hamid, S. 2000a. "Culture-specific syndromes: It's all relative." *Visions: BC's Mental Health Journal* 9: 6.

–. 2000b. "Overcoming 'NIMBY' in Nelson: A lesson in perseverance and resourcefulness." *Visions: BC's Mental Health Journal* 10: 27-8.

Harckham, R. 2003. "Defining and servicing mental health in a remote northern community." Master's thesis, School of Social Work and Family Studies, University of British Columbia.

Hardin, H. 1993. "Uncivil liberties." *Vancouver Sun,* 22 July, A15.

Harding, C., J. Zubin, and J. Strauss. 1992. "Chronicity in schizophrenia revisited." *British Journal of Schizophrenia* 161, supplement 18: 27-31.

–, and J. Zahniser. 1994. "Empirical correction of seven myths about schizophrenia with implications for treatment." *Acta Psychiatrica Scandinavica* 90, supplement 384: 140-46.

Hare, R. 1993. *Without Conscience: The Disturbing World of the Psychopaths among Us.* New York: Pocket Books.

–. 1996. "Psychopathy and antisocial personality disorder: A case of diagnostic confusion." http://www.psychiatrictimes.com/p960239.html.

Harris, M., and R. Fallot. 2001. "Envisioning a trauma-informed service system: A vital paradigm shift." *New Directions for Mental Health Services* 89: 3-21.

Hart, S., and J. Hemphill. 1989. "Prevalence of and service utilization by mentally disordered offenders at the Vancouver Pre-Trail Services Centre: A survey." Unpublished report prepared for the British Columbia Ministry of the Solicitor General, Corrections Branch.

–, R. Kropp, and D. Laws. 2003. *The Risk for Sexual Violence Protocol (RSVP): Structured Professional Guidelines for Assessing Risk of Sexual Violence.* Vancouver: British Columbia Institute Against Family Violence.

Hartman, A. 1994. *Reflections and Controversies: Essays on Social Work.* Washington, DC: NASW Press.

Haslam, N. 1997. "Evidence that male sexual orientation is a matter of degree." *Journal of Personality and Social Psychology* 73: 862-70.

Hay, P., et al. 2003. "A two year follow-up study and prospective evaluation of the DSM-IV axis V." *Psychiatric Services* 54: 1028-30.

Haynes, D. 2002. "Change your mind." *Trek: The Magazine of the University of British Columbia* 56, 4 (Spring): 19-24.

Health Canada. 1997a. *Economic Burden of Illness in Canada.* Ottawa: Health Canada.

–. 1997b. *Review of Best Practices in Mental Health Reform.* Ottawa: Health Canada.

–. 2000. "Economic burden of illness in Canada." http://ebic-femc.hc-sc.gc.ca/.

–. 2001a. *Best Practices: Concurrent Mental Health and Substance Use Disorders.* Ottawa: Health Canada.

–. 2001b. *National Program Inventory: Concurrent Mental Health and Substance Use Disorders.* Ottawa: Health Canada.

–. 2002a. "Housing as a determinant of health." http://www.hc-sc.gc.ca/hppb/phdd/pdef/ overview_implications/09_housing_e.pdf.

–. 2002b. *A Report on Mental Illnesses in Canada.* Ottawa: Health Canada.

–. 2002c. *Sharing the Learning: The Health Transition Fund.* Ottawa: Health Canada.

–. 2004a. "Advisory: Health Canada advises Canadians under the age of 18 to consult physicians if they are being treated with newer anti-depressants." http://www.hc-sc.gc.ca/english/ protection/warnings/2004/2004_01.htm.

–. 2004b. "Population health." http://www.hc-sc.gc.ca/hppb/phdd/determinants/index.html.

Helling, I., A. Ohman, and C. Hultman. 2003. "School achievements and schizophrenia: A case-control study." *Acta Psychiatrica Scandinavica* 198: 381-86.

Helmes, E., and J. Landmark. 2003. "Subtypes of schizophrenia: A cluster analytic approach." *Canadian Journal of Psychiatry* 48: 702-8.

Henquet, C., et al. 2004. "Prospective cohort study of cannabis use, predisposition for psychosis, and psychotic symptoms in young people." *British Medical Journal Online,* http:// bmj.bmjjournals.com/cgi/rapidpdf/bmj.38267.664086.63v1?ehom.

Herman, J. 1992. *Trauma and Recovery.* New York: Basic Books.

Hermann, Q. 2002. "Addictive and over-prescribed." *Vancouver Sun,* 1 February, A4.

Herrell, R., et al. 1999. "Sexual orientation and suicidality." *Archives of General Psychiatry* 56: 867-74.

Hewa. S. 2002. Physicians, Medical Profession and Medical Practice, in *Health, Illness and Health Care in Canada, 3rd ed.,* ed. B. Singh Bolaria and Harley Dickinson, 55-81. Toronto: Harcourt, Brace, Jovanovich.

Hewitt, P. 2000. "Perfectionism in suicide." Paper presented at the 11th Annual Conference of the Canadian Association for Suicide Prevention, Vancouver, 12 October.

Hiday, V., et al. 1999. "Criminal victimization of persons with severe mental illness." *Psychiatric Services* 50: 62-68.

Hillegers, M., et al. 2004. "Impact of stressful life events, familial loading and their interaction on the onset of mood disorders." *British Journal of Psychiatry* 185: 97-101.

Hilty, D., et al. 2003. "The effectiveness of telepsychiatry: A review." *Canadian Psychiatric Association Bulletin* 35, 5: 10-17.

Hirschfeld, R., and L. Davidson. 1988. "Risk Factors for Suicide." In *Review of Psychiatry,* vol. 7, ed. A. Frances and R. Hales, 307-33. Washington, DC: American Psychiatric Press.

Hocking, B. 2003. "Reducing mental illness stigma and discrimination – everybody's business." *Medical Journal of Australia* 178, supplement 5 (May): S47-S48.

Hodges, J., et al. 2003. "Use of self-help services and consumer satisfaction with professional mental health services." *Psychiatric Services* 54: 1161-63.

Hodgins, S., and G. Cote. 1990. "Prevalence of mental disorders among penitentiary inmates in Quebec." *Canada's Mental Health* 38: 1-4.

–, and G. Cote. 1991. "The mental health of penitentiary inmates in isolation." *Canadian Journal of Criminology* 33: 175-82.

Hoffman, B. 1997. *The Law of Consent to Treatment in Ontario.* 2nd ed. Toronto: Butterworth.

Hoffman, J., and M. Wilkes. 1999. "Direct to consumer advertising of prescription drugs: An idea whose time should not come." *British Medical Journal* 318: 1301-2.

Hogan, D., et al. 2003. "Prevalence and potential consequences of benzodiazepine use in senior citizens: Results from the Canadian study of health and aging." *Canadian Journal of Clinical Pharmacology* 10: 72-77.

Hogarty, G. 1995. "Personal therapy: A disorder-relevant psychotherapy for schizophrenia." *Schizophrenia Bulletin* 21: 379-93.

–, et al. 1997. "Three-year trials of personal therapy among schizophrenic patients living with or independent of family." Part 2, "Effects on adjustment of patients." *American Journal of Psychiatry* 154: 1514-24.

Holden, C. 2003. "Getting the short end of the allele." *Science* 301: 291-93.

Howell, M. 2004. "Order in drug court." *Vancouver Courier,* 8 December, 9.

–. 2005. "Counting the homeless." *Vancouver Courier,* 9 January, 1, 4-5.

Hucker, S. 1998. "Editorial: Forensic psychiatry." *Canadian Journal of Psychiatry* 43: 456-57.

Human Rights Watch. 2003. "United States: Mentally ill mistreated in prison." http://www.hrw.org/press/2003/10/us102203.htm.

Hume, C. 1997. "Clubhouses as rehabilitation." *Visions: BC's Mental Health Journal* 2: 9-15.

Hunkeler, E., et al. 2000. "Efficacy of nurse telehealth care and peer support in augmenting treatment of depression in primary care." *Archives of Family Medicine* 9: 700-8.

Hurlburt, M., P. Wood, and R. Hough. 1996. "Providing independent housing for the homeless mentally ill: A novel approach to evaluating long-term longitudinal housing patterns." *Journal of Community Psychology* 24: 291-310.

Hyams, K., F. Wignall, and R. Roswell. 1996. "War, syndromes and their evaluation: From the U.S. Civil War to the Persian Gulf War." *Annals of Internal Medicine* 125: 398-405.

Hyman, I. 2001. "Immigration and health." http://www.hc-sc.gc.ca.

–, M. Beiser, and N. Vu. 2000. "Post-migration stress among Southeast Asian refugee youth in Canada: Universal, culture-specific and situational." *Journal of Comparative Family Studies* 31: 281-94.

Impara, J., and B. Plake, eds. 1998. *The Thirteenth Mental Measurements Yearbook.* Lincoln, NE: Buros Institute of Mental Measurements.

International Center for Clubhouse Development. 2002. "What is a clubhouse?" http://www.iccd.org/article.asp?articleID=3.

Irwin, J. 2004. "Who's to blame for homelessness?" Vancouver, BC, *Westender,* 24-30 June, 7.

Ivan, C., et al. 2004. "Dementia after stroke: The Framingham Study." *Stroke* 35: 1264-68.

Jacobson, N., and L. Curtis. 2000. "Recovery as policy in mental health services: Strategies emerging from the States." *Psychiatric Rehabilitation Journal* 23: 333-41.

Janicak, P., et al. 2001. *Principles and Practice of Psychopharmacology.* 3rd ed. Philadelphia: Lippincott, Williams, and Wilkins.

Jeffries, J. 1996. "The Relationship with the Schizophrenic Patient: How It's Changing." In *Schizophrenia: Breaking down the Barriers,* ed. S. Holliday, R. Ancill, and G. MacEwan, 99-109. New York: John Wiley and Sons.

Jensen, P. 1998. "Ethical and pragmatic issues in the use of psychotropic agents in young children." *Canadian Journal of Psychiatry* 43: 585-88.

Jick, H., J. Kaye, and S. Jick. 2004. "Antidepressants and the risk of suicidal behaviors." *Journal of the American Medical Association* 292: 338-43.

Johnson, C. 1997. "Recovery through employment." *Visions: BC's Mental Health Journal* 2: 8.

Johnson, D. 1990. "Long-term drug treatment of psychosis: Observations on some current issues." *International Review of Psychiatry* 9: 341-53.

Johnson, G. 2004. "Double bind." *Georgia Straight,* 2-9 December, 44-45.

Johnstone, E., and R. Sandler. 1998. "Pharmacological Treatments in Schizophrenia." In *Handbook of Social Functioning in Schizophrenia,* ed. K. Mueser and N. Tarrier, 391-406. Needham Heights, MA: Allyn and Bacon.

Jones, C. 2005. "Supporting the families of the mentally ill." *Canadian Public Policy* 31, supplement: S41-S45.

Jones, D., et al. 2004. "Prevalence, severity, and co-occurrence of chronic physical health problems of persons with serious mental illness." *Psychiatric Services* 55: 1250-57.

Kane, J. 1996. "Schizophrenia." *New England Journal of Medicine* 334: 34-41.

–, and D. Mayerhoff. 1989. "Do negative symptoms respond to pharmacological treatment?" *British Journal of Psychiatry* 155, supplement 7: 115-18.

Kaufman, C. 1999. "An Introduction to the Mental Health Consumer Movement." In *A Handbook for the Study of Mental Health,* ed. A. Horowitz and T. Scheid, 493-507. New York: Cambridge University Press.

Keefe, R., and P. Harvey. 1994. *Understanding Schizophrenia.* New York: Free Press.

–, M. Arnold, and U. Bayen. 1999. "Source monitoring deficits in patients with schizophrenia: A multinomial modeling analysis." *Psychological Medicine* 29: 903-14.

Keller, M. 2002. "Long-term treatment strategies in affective disorders." *Pharmacological Bulletin* 36, supplement 2: 36-48.

–, et al. 2000. "A comparison of nefazadone, the cognitive-behavioral analysis system of psychotherapy, and their combination for the treatment of chronic depression." *New England Journal of Medicine* 342: 1462-70.

Kelly, M., et al. 2002. "Treatment delays for involuntary psychiatric patients associated with reviews of treatment capacity." *Canadian Journal of Psychiatry* 47: 181-85.

Kendlar, K. 2003. "Editorial: The genetics of schizophrenia." *American Journal of Psychiatry* 160: 1549-53.

–. 2004. "Editorial: Schizophrenia genetics and dysbindin: A corner turned?" *American Journal of Psychiatry* 161: 1533-36.

Kennedy, M. 2004. "Mental health system in a shambles, Senate says." *Vancouver Sun*, 20 November, A7.

–. 2005. "MD shortage critical." *National Post*, 27 January, A1, A9.

Kernberg, O. 1984. *Severe Personality Disorders: Psychotherapeutic Strategies*. New Haven, CT: Yale University Press.

Kesey, K. 1962. *One Flew Over the Cuckoo's Nest*. New York: Viking Press.

Kiehn, B., and M. Swale. 1995. "An overview of dialectical behavior therapy in the treatment of borderline personality disorder." http://www.mentalhelp.net/poc/view_doc.php?type=docandid=1020.

Kieseppa, T., et al. 2004. "High concordance of Bipolar I disorder in a nationwide sample of twins." *American Journal of Psychiatry* 161: 1814-21.

Kiesler, D. 1999. *Beyond the Disease Model of Mental Disorders*. Westport, CT: Praeger.

Killeen, M., and B. O'Day. 2004. "Changing expectations: How individuals with psychiatric disabilities find and keep work." *Psychiatric Rehabilitation Journal* 28: 157-63.

Kines, L. 2004. "Auditors spurred change in mental-health care." *Vancouver Sun*, 27 August, A5.

Kingdon, D. 1998. "Cognitive-Behavioural Therapy of Psychosis: Complexities in Engagement and Therapy." In *Treating Complex Cases: The Cognitive-Behavioural Therapy Approach*, ed. N. Tarrier, A. Wells, and G. Haddock, 176-94. Chichester, UK: John Wiley and Sons.

Kinzie, J.D., et al. 1990. "The prevalence of posttraumatic stress disorder and its clinical significance among Southeast Asian refugees." *American Journal of Psychiatry* 147: 913-17.

Kirk, S., and H. Kutchins. 1992. *The Selling of the DSM: The Rhetoric of Science in Psychiatry*. New York: Aldine de Gruyter.

Kirkey, S. 2004. "'Socks sign' signals problem." *Vancouver Sun*, 11 June, A8.

Kirmayer, L., L. Boothroyd, and S. Hodgins. 1998. "Attempted suicide among Inuit youth: Psychosocial correlates and implications for prevention." *Canadian Journal of Psychiatry* 43: 816-22.

–, G. Brass, and C. Tait. 2000. *The Mental Health of Aboriginal Peoples: Transformation of Identity and Community*. Report No. 10, Culture and Mental Health Research Unit, Division of Social and Transcultural Psychiatry, McGill University.

–, et al. 2003. "Cultural consultation: A model of mental health service for multicultural societies." *Canadian Journal of Psychiatry* 48: 145-52.

Kirsch, I., et al. 2002. "The emperor's new drugs: An analysis of antidepressant medication data submitted to the FDA." *Prevention and Treatment* 5, http://journals.apa.org/prevention/volume5/pre0050023a.html.

Klassen, A., et al. 1999. "Attention-deficit hyperactivity disorder in children and youth: A quantitative systematic review of the efficacy of different management strategies." *Canadian Journal of Psychiatry* 44: 1007-16.

Kleinman, A., and A. Cohen. 1997. "Psychiatry's global challenge." *Scientific American* 276: 86-89.

Kluft, R., S. Bloom, and J. Kinzie. 2000. "Treating traumatized patients and victims of violence." In "Psychiatric aspects of violence: Issues in prevention and treatment," ed. C. Bell. *New Directions for Mental Health Services* 86 (Summer): 79-102.

Komer, W., et al. 1999. "Review board outcomes for involuntary patients in provincial psychiatric hospitals." *Canadian Journal of Psychiatry* 44: 495-98.

Kondro, W., and B. Sibbald. 2004. "Drug company experts advised staff to withhold data about SSRI use in children." *Canadian Medical Association Journal* 170: 783.

Kopelowicz, A., and R. Liberman. 2003. "Integrating treatment with rehabilitation for persons with major mental illnesses." *Psychiatric Services* 54: 1491-98.

Kozel, F., and M. George. 2002. "Meta-analysis of left prefrontal repetitive transcranial magnetic stimulation to treat depression." *Journal of Psychiatric Practice* 8, 5: 270-75.

Kramer, P. 1993. *Listening to Prozac.* New York: Viking.

Kravitz, R., N. Duan, and J. Braslow. 2004. "Evidence-based medicine, heterogeneity of treatment effects, and the trouble with averages." *Millbank Quarterly* 82: 661-87.

Kruger, A. 2000. "Schizophrenia: Recovery and hope." *Psychiatric Rehabilitation Journal* 24: 29-37.

Kutchins, H., and S. Kirk. 1997. *Making Us Crazy: DSM: The Psychiatric Bible and the Creation of Mental Disorders.* New York: Free Press.

Lafave, H., H. deSouza, and G. Gerber. 1996. "Assertive community treatment of severe mental illness: A Canadian experience." *Psychiatric Services* 47: 757-59.

Laing, R. 1964. *Sanity, Madness and the Family.* New York: Basic Books.

–. 1969. *The Divided Self.* New York: Pantheon Books.

Laird, G. 2004. "The politics of homelessness." *Georgia Straight,* 5-12 February, 19-21.

Lam, D., et al. 2003. "A randomized, controlled study of cognitive therapy for relapse prevention for bipolar affective disorder: Outcome of the first year." *Archives of General Psychiatry* 60: 145-52.

Lamb, R. 2001. "Deinstitutionalization at the beginning of the new millennium." *Psychiatric Services* 49: 483-92.

–, and L. Weinberger. 1998. "Persons with severe mental illness in jails and prisons: A review." *New Directions for Mental Health Services* 90: 29-44.

Lancet. 2004. "Is GlaxoSmithKline guilty of fraud?" *Lancet* 364: 577.

Landi, F., et al. 2002. "Benzodiazepines and the risk of urinary incontinence in frail older persons living in the community." *Clinical Pharmacology and Therapeutics* 72: 729-34.

Larkin, J., and P. Caplan. 1992. "The gatekeeping process of the DSM." *Canadian Journal of Community Mental Health* 11: 17-28.

LaRoche, M. 2002. "Psychotherapeutic considerations in treating Latinos." *Harvard Review of Psychiatry* 10: 115-22.

Latimer, E. 1999. "Economic impacts of assertive community treatment: A review of the literature." *Canadian Journal of Psychiatry* 44: 443-54.

–. 2005. "Organization implications of promoting effective evidence-based interventions for people with severe mental illness." *Canadian Public Policy* 31, supplement: S47-S52.

Latner, A. 2001. "Top 200 drugs by retail sales in 2000." *Drug Topics* 6: 18.

Lauber, C., et al. 2004. "Factors influencing social distance toward people with mental illness." *Community Mental Health Journal* 40: 265-74.

Laumann, E., et al. 1994. *The Social Organization of Sexuality.* Chicago: University of Chicago Press.

Lavoie, K., and R. Fleet. 2002. "Should psychologists be granted prescription privileges? A review of the prescription privilege debate for psychiatrists." *Canadian Journal of Psychiatry* 47: 443-49.

Lawn, S., G. Pols, and J. Barber. 2002. "Smoking and quitting: A qualitative study with community-living psychiatric clients." *Social Science and Medicine* 54: 93-104.

Lechky, O. 1999. "Bringing health care to the homeless." *Canadian Medical Association Journal* 161: 13.

Lecomte, T., et al. 1999. "Efficacy of a self-esteem module in the empowerment of individuals with chronic schizophrenia." *Journal of Nervous and Mental Diseases* 187: 406-13.

–, C. Leclerc, and T. Wykes. 2001. *Cognitive-Behavioral Therapy: Clinician's Supplement.* Unpublished document.

–, and C. Lecomte. 2002. "Toward uncovering robust principles of change inherent to cognitive-behavioral therapy for psychosis." *American Journal of Orthopsychiatry* 72: 50-57.

Lee, J. 2004. "Premiers predict health care collapse." *Vancouver Sun*, 25 February, A1.

Leenaars, A. 2000. "Suicide prevention in Canada: A history of a community approach." *Canadian Journal of Community Mental Health* 19: 57-71.

Lees, R. 2004. "We've come a way, but not far enough: Supporting families with parental mental illness." *Visions: BC's Mental Health Journal* 2, 2: 4-5.

Leff, J., et al. 1992. "The international pilot study of schizophrenia: Five-year follow-up findings." *Psychological Medicine* 22: 131-45.

Lefley, H. 1997. "Mandatory treatment from the family's perspective." *New Directions for Mental Health Services*, no. 75: 7-15.

Lehman, A., et al. 1999. "Cost effectiveness of assertive community treatment for homeless persons with severe mental illness." *British Journal of Psychiatry* 174: 346-52.

Leichsenring, F., and E. Leibing. 2003. "The effectiveness of psychodynamic therapy and cognitive behavior therapy in the treatment of personality disorders: A meta-analysis." *American Journal of Psychiatry* 160: 1223-32.

Lesage, A., and R. Morissette. 2002. "Editorial: Chronic my a**." *Canadian Journal of Psychiatry* 47: 617-20.

–, et al. 2003. "Toward benchmarks for tertiary care for adults with severe and persistent mental disorders." *Canadian Journal of Psychiatry* 48: 485-92.

Leucht, S., et al. 2003. "Relapse prevention in schizophrenia with new-generation antipsychotics: A systematic review and exploratory meta-analysis of randomized, controlled trials." *American Journal of Psychiatry* 160: 1209-22.

Lev, A. 1998. "Feminism and mental illness." http://www.choicesconsulting.com/aboutarlene/articles/feminism.html.

Levine, I. 2004. "Insight: The key piece in recovery's puzzle." *Schizophrenia Digest* (Fall): 27-30.

Levitt, A., et al. 2000. "Estimated prevalence of the seasonal subtype of major depression in a Canadian community sample." *Canadian Journal of Psychiatry* 45: 650-54.

Lewis, L., and L. Appleby. 1988. "Personality disorder: The patients psychiatrists dislike." *British Journal of Psychiatry* 153: 44-49.

Li, H., and A. Browne. 2000. "Defining mental illness and accessing mental health services: Perspectives of Asian Canadians." *Canadian Journal of Community Mental Health* 19: 143-57.

Liberman, R. 1998. "International perspectives on skills training for the mentally disabled." *International Review of Psychiatry* 10: 5-8.

–, and A. Kopelowicz. 2002. "Recovery from schizophrenia: A challenge for the 21st Century." *International Review of Psychiatry* 14: 245-55.

Lieberman, J., et al. 2005. "Effectiveness of antipsychotic drugs in patients with chronic schizophrenia." *New England Journal of Medicine* 353: 1209-33.

Lin, E., and P. Goering. 1998. *The Utilization of Physician Service for Mental Health in Ontario*. Report prepared for the Institute for Clinical Evaluative Sciences.

Linehan, M. 1993a. *Cognitive-Behavioral Treatment of Borderline Personality Disorder*. New York: Guildford.

–. 1993b. *Skills Training Manual for Treating Borderline Personality Disorder*. New York: Guildford.

–, et al. 1991. "Cognitive-behavioral treatment of chronically parasuicidal borderline patients." *Archives of General Psychiatry* 48: 1060-64.

Lines, E. 2000. "An introduction to early psychosis intervention: Some relevant findings and emerging practices." http://www.cmha.ca/english/intrvent/about.htm.

Link, B., et al. 1999. "Public conceptions of mental illness: Labels, causes, dangerousness and social distance." *American Journal of Public Health* 89: 1328-33.

–, et al. 2001. "The consequences of stigma for the self-esteem of people with mental illnesses." *Psychiatric Services* 52: 1621-26.

Livesley, W.J. 1998. "Suggestions for a framework for an empirically based classification of personality disorder." *Canadian Journal of Psychiatry* 43: 137-47.

Livingston, J., et al. 2003. "A follow-up study of persons found not criminally responsible on account of mental disorder in British Columbia." *Canadian Journal of Psychiatry* 48: 408-15.

Lo, H., and K. Fung. 2003. "Culturally competent psychotherapy." *Canadian Journal of Psychiatry* 48: 161-70.

Lorentz, W., J. Scanlan, and S. Borson. 2002. "Brief screening tests for dementia." *Canadian Journal of Psychiatry* 47: 723-33.

Lott, D. 2001. "New developments in treating anxiety disorders." http://www.psychiatrictimes.com/p010946.html.

Lovell, A. 1992. "Classification and its risks: How psychiatric status contributes to homelessness policy." *New England Journal of Public Policy* 8: 247-63.

Luchins, D., et al. 2004. "Psychiatrists' attitudes toward involuntary hospitalization." *Psychiatric Services* 55: 1058-60.

McAndrew, B. 1999. "Innu suicide rate highest in the world: British report blames Ottawa, Catholic priests." *Toronto Star*, 8 November, A1, A14.

McCabe, R., and S. Priebe. 2004. "Explanatory models of illness in schizophrenia: Comparison of four ethnic groups." *British Journal of Psychiatry* 185: 25-30.

McCaldon, R., G. Conacher, and B. Clark. 1991. "The right to remain psychotic." *Canadian Medical Association Journal* 145: 777-80.

McClellan, J., and J. Werry. 2003. "Evidence-based treatments in child and adolescent psychiatry: An inventory." *Journal of the American Academy of Child and Adolescent Psychiatry* 42: 1388-1400.

McCormick, C., and S. Martel. 2003. "Funding options for students with mental illness." *Visions: BC's Mental Health Journal* 17: 37-38.

McCreary Centre Society. 1999. *Being Out: Lesbian, Gay, Bisexual and Transgendered Youth in BC: An Adolescent Health Survey.* Vancouver: McCreary Centre Society.

–. 2004. *Healthy Youth Development: Highlights from the 2003 Adolescent Health Survey.* Vancouver: McCreary Centre Society.

MacDonald, Z. 2002. "Virtually facing real fears." *Visions: BC's Mental Health Journal* 14: 20.

McEwan, K., and E. Goldner. 2001. *Accountability and Performance Indicators for Mental Health Services and Supports: A Resource Kit.* Ottawa: Health Canada.

McGlashan, T., and J. Johannessen. 1996. "Early detection and intervention with schizophrenia: Rationale." *Schizophrenia Bulletin* 22: 201-22.

McGrath, B., and R. Tempier. 2003. "Implementing quality management in psychiatry: From theory to practice – shifting focus from process to outcome." *Canadian Journal of Psychiatry* 48: 467-73.

McGrew, J., R. Wilson, and G. Bond. 2002. "An exploratory study of what clients like least about assertive community treatment." *Psychiatric Services* 53: 761-63.

–, B. Pescosolido, and E. Wright. 2003. "Case managers' perspectives on critical ingredients of assertive community treatment and on its implementation." *Psychiatric Services* 54: 370-76.

McGuffin, P., et al. 2003. "The heritability of bipolar affective disorder and the genetic relationship to unipolar depression." *Archives of General Psychiatry* 60: 497-502.

McIlwraith, R. 1987. "Community mental health and the mass media in Canada." *Canada's Mental Health* 37: 11-17.

McIntyre, R., et al. 2003. "Risk of weight gain associated with antipsychotic treatment: Results from the Canadian National Outcomes Measurement Study in Schizophrenia." *Canadian Journal of Psychiatry* 48: 689-94.

McKee, H. 2003. "Access to college and university for consumer/survivors: A national picture." *Visions: BC's Mental Health Journal* 17: 20.

MacKenzie, H. 2004. "Financing Canada's hospitals: Public alternatives to P3s." http://www.web.net/ohc/041020summary.pdf.

McLean, P., and S. Woody. 2001. *Anxiety Disorders in Adults: An Evidence-Based Approach to Psychological Treatment.* New York: Oxford University Press.

MacMillan, H. 2000. "Child maltreatment: What we know in the year 2000." *Canadian Journal of Psychiatry* 45: 702-9.

Macnaughton, E. 2000. "Cultural competence and the 'knowledge resource base.'" *Visions: BC's Mental Health Journal* 9: 14-15.

MacPhee, K. 2002. "No safe refuge: Barriers to accessing transition houses and women's shelters from a hospital emergency department." Master's graduating essay, School of Social Work and Family Studies, University of British Columbia.

MacQueen, G., and P. Chokka. 2004. "Special issues in the management of depression in women." *Canadian Journal of Psychiatry* 49, supplement 1: 27S-40S.

McReynolds, C. 2002. "Psychiatric rehabilitation: The need for a specialized approach." *International Journal of Psychosocial Rehabilitation* 7: 61-69.

Maguire, L. 2002. *Clinical Social Work: Beyond Generalist Practice with Individuals, Groups and Families.* Pacific Grove, CA: Brooks/Cole.

Malla, A., and R. Norman. 2002. "Early intervention in schizophrenia and related disorders: Advantages and pitfalls." *Current Opinion in Psychiatry* 15: 17-23.

Manassis, K. 2000. "Childhood anxiety disorders: Lessons from the literature." *Canadian Journal of Psychiatry* 45: 724-30.

Mannion, E., P. Solomon, and S. Steber. 2001. "Implementing family-friendly services." *Psychiatric Services* 52: 386-87.

Marder, S., et al. 2004. "Physical health monitoring of patients with schizophrenia." *American Journal of Psychiatry* 161: 1334-49.

Marie-Albert, J. 2002. "The psychiatrist and the clinical practice of psychiatry in an uncertain environment: Looking ahead." *Canadian Journal of Psychiatry* 47: 913-20.

Marsh, D., and D. Johnson. 1997. "The family experience of mental illness: Implications for intervention." *Professional Psychology* 28, 3: 229-37.

Marshall, M., et al. 2004. "Systematic review of the association between duration of untreated psychosis and outcome in cohorts of first episode patients." Paper presented at the 4th International Conference on Early Psychosis, Vancouver, 29 September.

Matsui, D., et al. 2003. "The trials and tribulations of doing drug research in children." *Canadian Medical Association Journal* 169: 1033-34.

Mechanic, D. 1999. "Mental Health and Mental Illness: Definitions and Perspectives." In *A Handbook for the Study of Mental Health,* ed. A. Horowitz and T. Scheid, 12-28. New York: Cambridge University Press.

–. 2003. "Policy challenges in improving mental health services: Some lessons from the past." *Psychiatric Services* 54: 1227-32.

Medalia, A., and N. Revheim. 2003. "Dealing with cognitive dysfunction associated with psychiatric disabilities." http://www.omh.state.ny.us/omhweb/cogdys_manual/CogDysHndbk.htm.

Meltzer, H., and S. McGurk. 1999. "The effects of clozapine, risperidone and olanzapine on cognitive function in schizophrenia." *Schizophrenia Bulletin* 25: 233-56.

Mendlowicz, M., and M. Stein. 2000. "Quality of life in individuals with anxiety disorders." *American Journal of Psychiatry* 157: 669-82.

Menezes, N., and E. Milovan. 2000. "First episode psychosis: A comparative review of diagnostic evolution and predictive variables in adolescents versus adults." *Canadian Journal of Psychiatry* 45: 710-16.

Mental Health Evaluation and Community Consultation Unit. 2000. *Emergency Mental Health: Educational Manual.* Vancouver: Department of Psychiatry, University of British Columbia.

–. 2002. *Early Psychosis: A Care Guide Summary.* Vancouver: Department of Psychiatry, University of British Columbia.

Mental Patients Association. 2001a. "History of the MPA." http://www.vmpa.org/history.htm.

–. 2001b. "Residence programs." http://www.vmpa.org/group.htm.

Meyer, C. 1983. "Selecting Appropriate Practice Models." In *Handbook of Clinical Social Work,* ed. A. Rosenblatt and D. Waldfogel, 731-49. San Francisco: Jossey-Bass.

Michel, K., et al. 2002. "Discovering the truth in attempted suicide." *American Journal of Psychotherapy* 56: 424-37.

Miedema, B. 1994. "Control or treatment? Experiences of people who have been psychiatrically hospitalized in New Brunswick." *Canadian Journal of Community Mental Health* 13: 111-22.

Miller, W., and S. Rollnick. 2002. *Motivational Interviewing: Preparing People for Change.* 2nd ed. New York: Guilford.

Mina, E., and R. Gallop. 1998. "Childhood sexual and physical abuse and adult self-harm and suicidal behavior: A literature review." *Canadian Journal of Psychiatry* 43: 793-800.

Minkoff, K. 2001a. "Developing standards of care for individuals with co-occurring psychiatric and substance use disorders." *Psychiatric Services* 52: 597-600.

–. 2001b. "Program components of a comprehensive system for seriously mentally ill patients with substance disorders." *New Directions for Mental Health Services* 91: 17-30.

Mintzes, B., et al. 2001. "An assessment of the health system impacts of DTC advertising of prescription medicines." http://www.chspr.ubc.ca/hpru/pdf/dtca-v4-expertsurvey.pdf.

–, et al. 2002. "Influence of DTC pharmaceutical advertising and patients' requests on prescribing decisions: Two site cross sectional survey." *British Medical Journal* 324: 278-79.

Minuchin, S., B. Rosman, and L. Baker. 1978. *Psychosomatic Families: Anorexia Nervosa in Context.* Cambridge, MA: Harvard University Press.

Mittelstaedt, M., and K. Haggart. 1999. "UK group calls treatment of Innu 'Canada's Tibet': Suicide of native spokesman's son on the eve of launch in London of damning report highlights despair in aboriginal communities." *Globe and Mail*, A3.

Moffic, H. 2003. "Managed care or ethical care: What's in a name?" *Psychiatric Services* 54: 1063.

Molnar, F. 2004. "Recovery is in the eye of the beholder." *The Bulletin: Official Publication of the Vancouver/Richmond Mental Health Network Society* 9: 7.

Monahan, J. 1992. "Mental disorder and violent behaviour: Perceptions and evidence." *American Psychologist* 47: 511-20.

Morgan, S., K. Bassett, and B. Mintzes. 2004. "An outcomes-based approach to decisions about drug coverage policies in British Columbia." *Psychiatric Services* 55: 1230-32.

Morrison, A., et al. 2004. "Delivering cognitive therapy to people with psychosis in a community mental health setting: An effectiveness study." *Acta Psychiatrica Scandinavica* 110: 36-44.

Morrow, M. 2003. *Mainstreaming Women's Health: Building a Canadian Strategy.* Report prepared for the British Columbia Centre of Excellence for Women's Health, Vancouver.

Moscicki, E. 1995. "Epidemiology of suicidal behavior." *Suicide and Life-Threatening Behavior* 25: 22-35.

Mosher, L. 1999. "Soteria and other alternatives to acute psychiatric hospitalization: a personal and professional review." *Journal of Nervous and Mental Disease* 187: 142-49.

Motluk, A. 2001. "Placebo produces surprise biological effect." http://www.newscientist.com/news/print.jsp?id=ns99991137.

Mowbray, C., et al. 1996. "Consumers as community support providers: Issues created by role innovation." *Community Mental Health Journal* 13: 163-76.

Mueser, K., and L. Fox. 2000. "Family-friendly services: A modest proposal." *Psychiatric Services* 51: 1452.

Mulvey, E., A. Blumstein, and J. Cohen. 1986. "Reframing the research question of mental patient criminality." *International Journal of Law and Psychiatry* 9: 57-65.

Murphy, L., J. Conoley, and J. Impara, eds. 1994. *Tests in Print.* 4th ed. Lincoln, NE: Buros Institute of Mental Measurements.

Murray, R. 1999. "Schizophrenia has origins in childhood, says British expert." *Psychiatric News* 9 (March 19): 31.

Mussell, B., K. Cardiff, and J. White. 2004. *The Mental Health and Well-Being of Aboriginal Children and Youth: Guidance for New Approaches and Services.* Report prepared for the British Columbia Ministry of Children and Family Development.

Myers, J., et al., eds. 2002. *The APSAC Handbook on Child Maltreatment.* 2nd ed. Newbury Park, CA: Sage.

Nasar, S. 1998. *A Beautiful Mind.* New York: Touchstone Books.

Nathan, P., J. Gorman, and N. Salkind. 1999. *Treating Mental Disorders: A Guide to What Works.* New York: Oxford University Press.

National Advisory Mental Health Council. 1993. "Health care reform for Americans with severe mental illnesses." *American Journal of Psychiatry* 150: 1447-65.

National Council of Welfare. 2004. "Welfare incomes 2003." http://www.ncwcnbes.net/htmdocument/reportWelfareIncomes2003/WI2003_e.pdf.

National Housing and Homelessness Network. 2001. *State of the Crisis, 2001: A Report on Housing and Homelessness in Canada.* Ottawa: National Housing and Homelessness Network.

National Union of Public and General Employees. 2004. "Commons committee recommends retaining controls on DTC drug advertising." *Report of the Health Sciences Association (BC),* August, 6-7.

–. 2005. "Victory in battle to end drug patent abuse." *Report of the Health Sciences Association (BC),* February, 5-6.

Negrette, J. 2003. "Clinical aspects of substance abuse in persons with schizophrenia." *Canadian Journal of Psychiatry* 48: 14-21.

Neilson, G. 1996. *Canadian Medical Association Code of Ethics, Annotated for Psychiatrists.* http://www.cap-apc.org/Publications/Position_Papers/ethicscode.asp.

Nelson, G., G. Hall, and R. Walsh-Bowers. 1997. "A comparative evaluation of supportive apartments, group homes, and board-and-care homes for psychiatric consumers/survivors." *Journal of Community Psychology* 25: 167-88.

–, G. Hall, and C. Forchuk. 2003. "Current and preferred housing of psychiatric consumers/survivors." *Canadian Journal of Community Mental Health* 22: 5-19.

Neuman, J. 2003. "Supported education Qs and As." *Visions: BC's Mental Health Journal* 17: 5-6.

Nietzel, M., D. Bernstein, and R. Milich. 1998. *Introduction to Clinical Psychology.* 5th ed. Upper Saddle River, NJ: Prentice Hall.

Niles, B. 2000. "Independent housing that works for people with mental illness." *Visions: BC's Mental Health Journal* 10: 9-10.

Norko, M., and M. Baranoski. 2005. "The state of contemporary risk assessment research." *Canadian Journal of Psychiatry* 50: 18-26.

Norman, R., and L. Townsend. 1999. "Cognitive-behavioral therapy for psychosis: A status report." *Canadian Journal of Psychiatry* 44: 245-52.

Novalis, P., S. Rojcewicz, and R. Peele. 1993. *Clinical Manual of Supportive Psychotherapy.* Washington, DC: American Psychiatric Press.

Nurnberg, H., et al. 2003. "Treatment of antidepressant associated sexual dysfunction with sildenafil." *Journal of the American Medical Association* 289: 56-64.

Nuttall-Smith, C. 2000. "Police use taser to subdue armed mentally ill man." *Vancouver Sun,* 4 July, B1.

Oakes, D. 2003. "Drug companies help fund drive for forced outpatient treatment." http://www.straightgoods.com/item341.shtml.

O'Brian, A. 2004a. "Outside probe ordered into taser-related death." *Vancouver Sun,* 6 August, A1-A2.

–. 2004b. "Why wasn't I told my daughter was suicidal?" *Vancouver Sun,* 9 July, A1-A2.

O'Connor, N. 2003. "Pharma care." *Vancouver Courier,* 3 September, 1, 5-7.

O'Donovan, C. 2004. "Achieving and sustaining remission in depression and anxiety disorders: Introduction." *Canadian Journal of Psychiatry* 49, supplement 1: 5S-9S.

Ohayan, M., et al. 1998. "Fitness, responsibility and judicially ordered assessments." *Canadian Journal of Psychiatry* 43: 491-95.

Olfson, M., et al. 2002. "National trends in the outpatient treatment of depression." *Journal of the American Medical Association* 287: 203-9.

O'Malley, K., and J. Nanson. 2002. "Clinical implications of a link between fetal alcohol spectrum disorder and attention-deficit hyperactivity disorder." *Canadian Journal of Psychiatry* 47: 349-54.

O'Neill, P. 2003. "Gay relations a crime to half of US, poll says." *Vancouver Sun*, 26 December, A5.

O'Neill, T. 1990. "Forced to take drugs." *BC Reports*, 18 June, 21.

Ontario Psychological Association. 2001. Submission to the Commission on the Future of Health Care in Canada. http://www.cpa.ca/Romanowopa.pdf.

O'Reilly, R. 1998. "Mental health legislation and the right to appropriate treatment." *Canadian Journal of Psychiatry* 43: 811-15.

–, et al. 2003. "A survey of Canadian psychiatrists' experiences and opinions on using videoconferencing for assessments required by mental health legislation." *Canadian Psychiatric Association Bulletin* 35, 5: 18-20.

Orford, J., et al. 2002. "How is excessive drinking maintained? Untreated heavy drinkers' experiences of the personal benefits and drawbacks of their drinking." *Addiction Research and Theory* 10: 347-72.

Owen, C., et al. 1996. "Housing accommodation preferences of people with psychiatric disabilities." *Psychiatric Services* 47: 628-32.

Pantony, K., and P. Caplan. 1991. "Delusional dominating personality disorder: A modest proposal for identifying some consequences of rigid masculine socialization." *Canadian Psychology* 32: 120-31.

Parent, R. 1996. "Aspects of police use of deadly force in BC: The phenomenon of victim-precipitated homicide." Master's thesis, School of Criminology, Simon Fraser University.

–. 2004. "Aspects of police use of deadly force in North America: The phenomenon of victim-precipitated homicide." Doctoral dissertation, School of Criminology, Simon Fraser University.

Paris, J. 1998a. "Does childhood trauma cause personality disorders in adults?" *Canadian Journal of Psychiatry* 43: 148-52.

–. 1998b. "Editorial: Personality disorders: Psychiatry's stepchildren." *Canadian Journal of Psychiatry* 43: 135.

–. 2005. *The Fall of an Icon: Psychoanalysis and Academic Psychiatry*. Toronto: University of Toronto Press.

–, ed. 1993. *Borderline Personality Disorder: Etiology and Treatment*. Washington, DC: American Psychiatric Press.

Parkinson, S., G. Nelson, and S. Horgan. 1999. "From housing to homes: A review of the literature on housing approaches for psychiatric consumer/survivors." *Canadian Journal of Community Mental Health* 18: 145-63.

Paterson, R., et al. 1996. *The Changeways Participant Manual*. Vancouver: Changeways Clinic.

–. 1997. *The Changeways Core Program: Trainers Manual*. Vancouver: Changeways Clinic.

–, and C. Bishop. 2000. *Sexual Orientation: Issues in Health Care*. Vancouver: Changeways Clinic.

–. 2002. *Your Depression Map*. Oakland, CA: New Harbinger.

–, and D. Bilsker. 2002. *Self-Care Depression Program: Patient Guide*. Vancouver: Mental Health Evaluation and Community Consultation Unit, Department of Psychiatry, University of British Columbia.

Patten, S. 1999. "Long-term medical conditions and major depression in the Canadian population." *Canadian Journal of Psychiatry* 44: 151-57.

–, and D. Charney. 1998. "Alcohol consumption and major depression in the Canadian population." *Canadian Journal of Psychiatry* 43: 502-6.

–, and C. Beck. 2004. "Major depression and mental health care utilization in Canada, 1994 to 2000." *Canadian Journal of Psychiatry* 49: 303-9.

Patton, S., et al. 2002. "Antipsychotic medication during pregnancy and lactation in women with schizophrenia: Evaluating the risk." *Canadian Journal of Psychiatry* 47: 959-65.

Pedersen, P. 1995. *The Five Stages of Culture Shock: Critical Incidents around the World*. Westport, CT: Greenwood.

Peen, J., and J. Dekker. 2004. "Is urbanicity a risk factor for psychiatric disorders?" *Lancet* 363: 2012-13.

Penrose, L. 1939. "Mental disease and crime: Outline of a comparative study of European statistics." *British Journal of Medical Psychology* 18: 1-15.

Peters, R. 2000. "The multicultural mental health liaison program." *Visions: BC's Mental Health Journal* 9: 19.

–, and J. Hay. 1999. *1998 Mental Health Survey: Adult Team Clients*. Report prepared for the Greater Vancouver Mental Health Service, Vancouver.

Peyser, H. 2004. "What is normal? What is sick?" *Psychiatric Services* 55: 7.

Phares, E., and T. Trull. 1997. *Clinical Psychology: Concepts, Methods and Profession*. 5th ed. Pacific Grove, CA: Brooks/Cole.

Phillips, P., and S. Johnson. 2001. "How does alcohol and drug misuse develop among people with psychotic illness?" *Social Psychiatry and Psychiatric Epidemiology* 36: 269-76.

Phillips, S., et al. 2001. "Moving assertive community treatment into standard practice." *Psychiatric Services* 52: 771-78.

Pietrini, P. 2003. "Toward a biochemistry of mind?" *American Journal of Psychiatry* 160: 1907-8.

Pitschel-Walz, G., et al. 2001. "The effect of family interventions on relapse and rehospitalization in schizophrenia: A meta-analysis." *Schizophrenia Bulletin* 27: 73-92.

Pope, M., and J. Scott. 2003. "Do clinicians understand why individuals stop taking lithium?" *Journal of Affective Disorders* 74: 287-91.

Priest, A. 2003a. "Antidepressants: Over-prescribed cure-all or life-saving tool?" *Georgia Straight*, 23 October, 21.

–. 2003b. "Middle class addicts." *Georgia Straight*, 13 November, 21-6.

–. 2003c. "The rocketing cost of drugs." *Georgia Straight*, 8-15 May, 27.

Prochaska, J., and C. DiClemente. 1986. "Toward a Comprehensive Model of Change." In *Treating Addictive Behaviors: Processes of Change*, ed. W. Miller and N. Heather, 3-27. New York: Plenum.

Pyke, J., et al. 2001. "Improving accessibility: The experience of a Canadian mental health agency." *Psychiatric Rehabilitation Journal* 25: 180-85.

Quan, H., and J. Arboleda-Florez. 1999. "Elderly suicide in Alberta: Difference by gender." *Canadian Journal of Psychiatry* 44: 762-68.

Rae-Grant, Q. 2002. "Editorial: The role of pharmaceutical companies in research and development – plaudits and cautions." *Canadian Journal of Psychiatry* 47: 513.

Rakfeldt, J., et al. 1997. "Normalizing acute care: A day hospital/crisis residence alternative to inpatient hospitalization." *The Journal of Nervous and Mental Disease* 185: 46-52.

Ram, R., et al. 1992. "The natural course of schizophrenia: A review of first admission studies." *Schizophrenia Bulletin* 18: 185-207.

Rapoport, J., and I. Ismond. 1996. *DSM-IV Training Guide for the Diagnosis of Childhood Disorders*. New York: Brunner Mazel.

Rapp, C. 1998. "The active ingredients of effective case management: A research synthesis." *Community Mental Health Journal* 34: 363-80.

Rappolt, S. 2003. "The role of professional expertise in evidence-based occupational therapy." *American Journal of Occupational Therapy* 57: 589-93.

Raune, D., E. Kuipers, and P. Bebbington. 2004. "Expressed emotion at first-episode psychosis: Investigating a carer appraisal model." *British Journal of Psychiatry* 184: 321-26.

Reding, G., and M. Raphelson. 1995. "Around-the-clock mobile psychiatric crisis intervention." *Community Mental Health Journal* 31: 179-86.

Reesal, R., and R. Lam. 2001. "Clinical guidelines for the treatment of depressive disorders: Principles of management." *Canadian Journal of Psychiatry* 46, supplement 1: 21S-28S.

Regier, D., et al. 1990. "Comorbidity of mental disorders with alcohol and other drug abuse." *Journal of the American Medical Association* 264: 2511-18.

Reidy, D. 1992. "Shattering illusions of difference." *Resources* 4: 1-4, published by the Human Resource Association of the Northeast, Holyoke, MA.

Reiling, D. 2002. "Boundary maintenance as a barrier to mental health help-seeking for depression among the Old Order Amish." *Journal of Rural Health* 18: 428-36.

Remafedi, G. 1994. *Death by Denial: Studies of Suicide in Gay and Lesbian Teenagers.* Boston: Alyson.

Rice, D., and L. Miller. 1998. "Health economics and the cost implications of anxiety and other mental disorders in the US" *British Journal of Psychiatry* 34: 4-9.

Ridgeway, P., and A. Zipple. 1990. "The paradigm shift in residential services: From the linear continuum to supported housing approaches." *Psychosocial Rehabilitation Journal* 19: 11-31.

"Risk gene identified for schizophrenia." 2003. *Psychiatric Times,* 1 March, 28.

Robertson, G. 1994. *Mental Disability and the Law in Canada.* 2nd ed. Toronto: Carswell.

Robinson, J. 2001. *Prescription Games.* Toronto: McClelland and Stewart.

Rochefort, D. 1992. "More lessons, of a different kind: Canadian mental health policy in comparative perspective." *Hospital and Community Psychiatry* 43: 1083-90.

Roesch, R. 1995. "Mental Health Interventions in Pre-Trial Jails." In *Psychology, Law and Criminal Justice,* ed. G. Davies, 520-31. Berlin: Walter de Gruyter.

Rogers, R., and C. Mitchell. 1991. *Mental Health Experts and the Criminal Courts.* Toronto: Carswell.

Rosenberg, S., et al. 2001. "Prevalence of HIV, hepatitis B and hepatitis C in people with severe mental illness." *American Journal of Public Health* 91: 31-37.

Rosenfeld, S. 1999. "Gender and Mental Health: Do Women Have More Psychopathology, Men More, or Both the Same (and Why)?" In *A Handbook for the Study of Mental Health,* ed. A. Horowitz and T. Scheid, 348-60. New York: Cambridge University Press.

Rosenhan, D. 1973. "On being sane in insane places." *Science* 179: 250-57.

Rosenheck, R., et al. 2003. "Effectiveness and cost of olanzapine and haloperidol in the treatment of schizophrenia: A randomized control trial." *Journal of the American Medical Association* 290: 2693-702.

Ross, E., A. Ali, and B. Toner. 2003. "Investigating issues surrounding depression in adolescent girls across Ontario: A participatory action research project." *Canadian Journal of Community Mental Health* 22: 55-68.

Row, C. 2003. "Hearing voices that are not real." *Visions: BC's Mental Health Journal* 18: 27-8.

Rowland, A., et al. 2001. "Studying the epidemiology of ADHD: Screening method and pilot results." *Canadian Journal of Psychiatry* 46: 931-40.

Rubin, A., and E. Babbie. 2001. *Research Methods for Social Work.* 4th ed. Belmont, CA: Wadsworth.

Ruo, B., et al. 2003. "Depressive symptoms and health-related quality of life: The heart and soul study. *Journal of the American Medical Association* 290: 215-21.

Ruskin, P., et al. 2004. "Treatment outcomes in depression: Comparison of remote treatment through telepyschiatry to in-person treatment." *American Journal of Psychiatry* 161: 1471-76.

Russell, D. 1986. *The Secret Trauma: Incest in the Lives of Girls and Women.* New York: Basic Books.

Rutman, I. 1994. "How psychiatric disability expresses itself as a barrier to employment." *Psychosocial Rehabilitation Journal* 17: 15-35.

Ryten, E., A. Thurber, and L. Buske. 1998. "The class of 1989 and physician supply in Canada." *Canadian Medical Association Journal* 158, 723-28.

Saari, K., et al. 2004. "Serum lipids in schizophrenia and other functional psychoses." *Acta Psychiatrica Scandinavica* 110: 279-85.

Sackett, D., et al. 1996. "Evidence-based medicine: What it is and what it isn't." *British Medical Journal* 312: 71-72.

–, et al. 2000. *Evidence-Based Medicine.* London, UK: Churchill Livingstone.

Sadavoy, J., R. Meier, and A. Ong. 2004. "Barriers to access for mental health services for ethnic seniors: The Toronto study." *Canadian Journal of Psychiatry* 49: 192-99.

Sadock, B., and V. Sadock. 2003. *Synopsis of Psychiatry.* 9th ed. Philadelphia, PA: Lippincott, Williams, and Wilkins.

St. Clair, D., et al. 2005. "Rates of adult schizophrenia following prenatal exposure to the Chinese famine of 1959-61." *Journal of the American Medical Association* 294: 557-62.

Sakinofsky, I. 1994. "Epidemiology of Suicide in Canada." In *Suicide in Canada,* ed. A. Leenaars, 4-29. Toronto: University of Toronto Press.

Salyers, M., et al. 2004. "A ten-year follow-up of a supported employment program." *Psychiatric Services* 55: 302-8.

Sanchez, N. 2000. "Stigmatized views of mental illness in the Latin American Community." *Visions: B.C.'s Mental Health Journal* 9: 10.

Sands, R., and B. Angell. 2002. "Social Workers as Collaborators on Interagency and Interdisciplinary Teams." In *Social Work Practice in Mental Health,* ed. K. Bentley, 254-80. Pacific Grove, CA: Brooks/Cole.

Satel, S. 1999. "Editorial: What should we expect from drug abusers?" *Psychiatric Services* 50: 861.

–, and K. Humphreys. 2003. "Mind games." http://www.aei.org/news/newsID.19270,filter./news_detail.asp.

–, and M. Zdanowicz. 2003. "Commission's omission." http://www.nationalreview.com/comment/comment-satel-zdanowicz072903.asp.

Savage, H., and McKague, C. 1987. *Mental Health Law in Canada.* Toronto: Butterworths.

Scheid, T., and C. Anderson. 1995. "Living with chronic mental illness: Understanding the role of work." *Community Mental Health Journal* 31: 163-76.

–, and A. Horowitz. 1999. "Mental Health Systems and Policy." In *A Handbook for the Study of Mental Health,* ed. A. Horowitz and T. Scheid, 377-91. New York: Cambridge University Press.

Scheidlinger, S. 1994. "An overview of nine decades of group psychotherapy." *Hospital and Community Psychiatry* 45: 217-25.

Schizophrenia Society of Canada. 1998. Recognizing schizophrenia for what it really is: a call to action. Don Mills, ON: Schizophrenia Society of Canada.

–. 2001. "A report on psychiatrist and patient attitudes and opinions towards schizophrenia." http://www.schizophrenia.ca/survey.pdf.

–. 2002-03. "Annual report." http://www.schizophrenia.ca/newpubs/annual03e.pdf.

Schmidt, G. 2000. "Structural barriers to recovery in First Nations communities." *Visions: BC's Mental Health Journal* 9: 26-27.

Scholten, D., et al. 2003. "Removing barriers to treatment of first-episode psychotic disorders." *Canadian Journal of Psychiatry* 48: 561-65.

Scull, A. 1977. *Decarceration: Community Treatment and the Deviant – A Radical View.* Englewood Cliffs, NJ: Prentice Hall.

Scully, J. 2004. "Should psychologists have prescribing authority? A great leap backwards." *Psychiatric Services* 55: 1424.

Sealey, P., and P. Whitehead. 2004. "Forty years of deinstitutionalization of psychiatric services in Canada: An empirical assessment." *Canadian Journal of Psychiatry* 49: 249-57.

Secker, J., et al. 2003. "The how and why of workplace adjustments: Contextualizing the evidence." *Psychiatric Rehabilitation Journal* 27: 3-9.

Seeman, M. 2004. "Gender differences in the prescribing of antipsychotic drugs." *American Journal of Psychiatry* 161: 1324-33.

Segal, S., and P. Kotler. 1993. "Sheltered care residence: Ten-year personal outcomes." *American Journal of Orthopsychiatry* 63: 80-91.

Seligman, M. 1991. *Learned Optimism.* New York: A.A. Knopf.

Sells, D., et al. 2003. "Violent victimization of persons with co-occurring psychiatric and substance use disorders." *Psychiatric Services* 54: 1253-57.

Sernyak, M., and R. Rosenheck. 2004. "Systemwide costs associated with second-generation antipsychotics in the treatment of schizophrenia." *Psychiatric Services* 55: 1361-62.

Shah, C. 2004. "The Health of Aboriginal Peoples." In *Social Determinants of Health: Canadian Perspectives*, ed. D. Raphael, 267-80. Toronto: Canadian Scholars Press.

Shapiro, F. 2001. *EMDR: Basic Principles, Protocols and Procedures*. 2nd ed. New York: Guildford.

Sharma, V., et al. 2000. "Preferred terms for users of mental health services among service providers and recipients." *Psychiatric Services* 51: 205-9.

Shimrat, I. 1997. *Call Me Crazy: Stories from the Mad Movement*. Vancouver: Press Gang.

Shinn, M. 1997. "Family homelessness: State or trait?" *American Journal of Community Psychology* 25: 755-69.

–, et al. 1998. "Predictors of homelessness among families in New York City: From shelter request to housing stability." *American Journal of Public Health* 88: 1651-57.

Shorter, E. 1997. *A History of Psychiatry*. New York: John Wiley and Sons.

Shragge, E., et al. 1999. "Alternative/training businesses: New practice, new directions." http://www.omd.uqam.ca/publications/telechargements/evalu.PDF.

Silberfeld, M., et al. 1993. "Assessment of financial competence in an adult with autism." *Canada's Mental Health* 41: 1-6.

–, and A. Fish. 1994. *When the Mind Fails*. Toronto: University of Toronto Press.

Simmie, S., and J. Nunes. 2001. *The Last Taboo: A Survival Guide to Mental Health Care in Canada*. Toronto: McClelland and Stewart.

Smiderle, W. 2003. "Stand up and be heard: Unified voice putting mental health on the government radar screen." *Schizophrenia Digest* (Summer): 32-34.

Smith, C. 2003. "Martin's care cure questioned." *Georgia Straight*, 23 October, 33.

Smoyak, S. 2004. "Editorial: Our choice: To be medicated or to be responsible." *Journal of Psychosocial Nursing* 42: 6-7.

Society for Neuroscience. 2004. "The prefrontal cortex and schizophrenia." http://web.sfn.org/content/Publications/BrainBriefings/schizphrenia.html.

Solomon, P. 2001. "The cultural context of interventions for family members with a seriously mentally ill relative." *New Directions for Mental Health Services* 91: 67-78.

Somers, J., et al. 2004. "Prevalence studies of substance-related disorders: A systematic review of the literature." *Canadian Journal of Psychiatry* 49: 373-84.

Spaniol, L., et al. 1987. "Families As a Resource in the Rehabilitation of the Severely Psychiatrically Disabled." In *Families of the Mentally Ill: Coping and Adaptation*, ed. A. Hatley and H. Lefley, 167-90. New York: Guilford.

Spataro, J., et al. 2004. "Impact of child sexual abuse on mental health: Prospective study in males and females." *British Journal of Psychiatry* 184: 416-21.

Spellman, J. 2000. "NAFSA: Association of International Educators, Washington, DC, May 27, 1998." http://www.indiana.edu/~overseas/lesbigay/meetings/meet_98.html.

Sperry, L. 1995. *Handbook of Diagnosis and Treatment of the DSM-IV Personality Disorders*. New York: Brunner/Mazel.

Spindel, P., and J. Nugent. 1999. "The trouble with PACT: Questioning the increasing use of assertive community treatment teams in community mental health." http://www.peoplewho.org/readingroom/spindel.nugent.htm.

Spitzer, R. 1975. "On pseudoscience in science, logic in remission, and psychiatric diagnosis: A critique of Rosenhan's 'On being sane in insane places.'" *Journal of Abnormal Psychology* 84, 5: 442-51.

Sporn, A., et al. 2003. "Progressive brain volume loss during adolescence in childhood-onset schizophrenia." *American Journal of Psychiatry* 160: 2181-89.

Srinivasan, J., N. Cohen, and S. Parikh. 2003. "Patient attitudes regarding causes of depression: Implications for psychoeducation." *Canadian Journal of Psychiatry* 48: 493-95.

Stainsby, J. 2000. "Extended leave." *Canadian Journal of Community Mental Health* 19: 152-55.

Stamm, B.H., ed. 1999. *Secondary Traumatic Stress: Self-Care Issues for Clinicians, Researchers, and Educators*. 2nd ed. Lutherville, MD: Sidran.

Statistics Canada. 2003. "Canadian community health survey: Mental health and well-being." http://www.statcan.ca/Daily/English/030903/d030903a.htm.

–. 2005. "Study: Canada's visible minority population in 2017." http://www.statcan.ca/Daily/English/050322/d050322b.htm.

Steadman, H., et al. 1998. "Violence by people discharged from acute psychiatric inpatient facilities and by others in the same neighborhoods." *Archives of General Psychiatry* 55: 393-401.

Stein, L., and M. Test. 1980. "Alternatives to mental hospital treatment: Conceptual model, treatment programs and clinical evaluation." *Archives of General Psychiatry* 37: 392-97.

Steiner, W., and E. Amir. 2003. "Depression screening day: A mental illness awareness week project." *Canadian Psychiatric Association Bulletin* 35, 4: 14-15.

Sterle, F. 2004. "Compassion by law enforcers more common than may be expected." *In a Nutshell* (Winter): 14-15, newsletter of the Vancouver Mental Patients Association.

Stern, R. 1993. "Behavioural cognitive therapy for psychiatrists." *Psychiatric Bulletin* 17: 1-4.

Stuart, H. 2003. "Stigma and the daily news: Evaluation of a newspaper intervention." *Canadian Journal of Psychiatry* 48: 651-55.

–, et al. 1999. "Mental health institute design." http://www.fcrss.ca/docs/finalrepts/HIDG/stuart.pdf.

–, and J. Arboleda-Florez. 2000. "Homeless shelter users in the post-deinstitutionalization era." *Canadian Journal of Psychiatry* 45: 55-62.

Stuart, H., and Arboleda-Florez, J. 2001. "Community attitudes toward people with schizophrenia." *Canadian Journal of Psychiatry* 46: 245-52.

Styron, W. 1990. *Darkness Visible.* New York: Random House.

Sue, D., P. Arredondo, and R. McDavis. 1992. "Multicultural counseling competencies and standards: A call to the profession." *Journal of Counseling and Development* 70: 484-86.

Sullivan, M., et al. 2004. "Defining best practices for specialty geriatric mental health outreach services: Lessons for implementing mental health reform." *Canadian Journal of Psychiatry* 49: 458-66.

Sullivan, W., and C. Rapp. 2002. "Social Workers As Case Managers." In *Social Work Practice in Mental Health,* ed. K. Bentley, 180-210. Pacific Grove, CA: Brooks/Cole.

Sundquist, K., G. Frank, and J. Sundquist. 2004. "Urbanization and incidence of psychosis and depression: Follow-up study of 4.4 million women and men in Sweden." *British Journal of Psychiatry* 184: 293-98.

Sussman, S. 1998. "The first asylums in Canada: A response to neglectful community care and current trends." *Canadian Journal of Psychiatry* 43: 260-64.

Sutherland, A. 2005. "Almost half of Canadians think homosexuality is abnormal." *Vancouver Sun,* 2 June, A6.

Swaminath, R., et al. 2002. "Experiments in change: Pretrial diversion of offenders with mental illness." *Canadian Journal of Psychiatry* 47: 450-58.

Swanson, J., et al. 1996. "Psychotic symptoms and disorders and the risk of violent behavior in the community." *Criminal Behavior and Mental Health* 6: 309-29.

Swartz, M., and J. Monahan. 2001. "Introduction" to special section on involuntary outpatient commitment. *Psychiatric Services* 52, 3: 323-24.

Szasz, T. 1974. *The Myth of Mental Illness.* Rev. ed. New York: Harper and Row.

–. 1976. *Schizophrenia: The Sacred Symbol of Psychiatry.* New York: Basic Books.

–. 1977. *Psychiatric Slavery.* New York: Free Press.

Szatmari, P. 2000. "The classification of autism, Asperger's syndrome, and pervasive developmental disorder." *Canadian Journal of Psychiatry* 45: 731-38.

Szmuckler, G., and F. Holloway. 1998. "Mental health legislation is now a harmful anachronism." *Psychiatric Bulletin* 22: 662-65.

Tee, K., and L. Hanson. 2004. "Fraser South Early Psychosis Intervention Program." In *Best Care in Early Psychosis Intervention,* ed. T. Ehmann, G. MacEwan, and W. Honer, 131-40. London, UK: Taylor and Francis.

Teplin, L. 1984. "Criminalizing mental disorder: The comparative arrest rate of the mentally ill." *American Psychologist* 39: 794-803.

–, and N. Pruett. 1992. "Police as street corner psychiatrist: Managing the mentally ill." *International Journal of Law and Psychiatry* 15: 139-56.

Thakur, A. 2003. "Culture and mental health: Not a minor matter." *Canadian Psychiatric Association Bulletin* 35: 6.

Thara, R. 2004. "Twenty-year course of schizophrenia: The Madras longitudinal study." *Canadian Journal of Psychiatry* 49: 564-69.

Thomas, L. 2000. "What 'best practices' means for mental health housing." *Visions: BC's Mental Health Journal* 10: 5.

Thomas, S. 2004. "Lines open for suicide prevention." *Vancouver Courier*, 5 September, 15.

Thomson, H. 2003. "Drug costs may soar for Canada's seniors." *UBC Reports*, 5 June, 3.

Thomson, L. 1992. *The Kohlman Evaluation of Living Skills.* 3rd ed. Bethesda, MD: American Occupational Therapy Association.

Thor-Larsen, L. 2002. "Changing the paradigm." *The Bulletin: Official Publication of the Vancouver/Richmond Mental Health Network Society* 7: 4.

–. 2003. "Conference to help debunk stigma." *The Bulletin: Official Publication of the Vancouver/Richmond Mental Health Network Society* 8: 4.

Tibbetts, J. 2003. "Physicist wins no-drug fight." *Vancouver Sun*, 7 June, A3.

Tienari, P., et al. 2003. "Genetic boundaries of the schizophrenia spectrum: Evidence from the Finnish adoptive family study of schizophrenia." *American Journal of Psychiatry* 160: 1587-94.

Todd, D. 2004. "Schizophrenia: Two steps forward, one step back." *Vancouver Sun*, 4 December, C1-C3.

Tollefson, E., and B. Starkman. 1993. *Mental Disorder in Criminal Proceedings.* Toronto: Carswell.

Tollefson, G., et al. 1997. "Blind, controlled, long-term study of the comparative incidence of treatment emergent tardive dyskinesia with olanzapine or haloperidol." *American Journal of Psychiatry* 154: 1248-54.

Tolomiczenko, G., P. Goering, and J. Durbin. 2001. "Educating the public about mental illness and homelessness: A cautionary note." *Canadian Journal of Psychiatry* 46: 253-57.

Toneguzzi, M. 2005. "Superbug takes its toll on homeless." *Vancouver Sun*, 1 April, A7.

Torrey, E. 1988. *Surviving Schizophrenia.* New York: Harper and Row.

–. 1997. *Out of the Shadows.* New York: John Wiley and Sons.

–, and R. Kaplan. 1995. "A national survey of the use of outpatient commitment." *Psychiatric Services* 46, 6: 778-84.

Torrey, W., et al. 2001. "Implementing evidence-based practices for persons with severe mental illness." *Psychiatric Services* 52: 45-50.

Tousignant, M. 1997. "Refugees and Immigrants in Quebec." In *Ethnicity, Immigration and Psychopathology*, ed. I. Al-Issa and M. Tousignant, 57-70. New York: Plenum.

Tracy, B. 2003. "Evidence-based practices or value-based services?" *Psychiatric Services* 54: 1437.

Trainor, J., and J. Tremblay. 1992. "Consumer/survivor businesses in Ontario: Challenging the rehabilitation model." *Canadian Journal of Community Mental Health* 11: 65-72.

–, E. Pomeroy, and B. Pape. 1993. *A New Framework for Support for People with Serious Mental Health Problems.* Toronto: Canadian Mental Health Association.

Treherne, J., and K. Calsaferri. 2002. *Family Support, Services and Involvement Plan for Adult Program.* Vancouver Community Mental Health Services, Vancouver Coastal Health Authority.

Tremayne-Lloyd, T. 2003. "Right to confidentiality vs. duty to disclose: The Supreme Court of Canada in Smith vs. Jones." http://www.tlpartners.ca/?pageid=15anddocid=15.

Trott, P., and I. Blignault. 1998. "Cost evaluation of a telepsychiatry service in northern Queensland." *Journal of Telemedicine and Telecare* 4, supplement 1: S66-S68.

Turbett, H. 2000. "The mental health system ... as racist?" *Visions: BC's Mental Health Journal* 9: 28-29.

Turetsky, B., et al. 2002. "Memory-delineated subtypes of schizophrenia: Relationship to clinical, neuroanatomical and neurophysiological measures." *Neuropsychology* 16, 4, 481-90.

United Kingdom ECT Review Group. 2003. "Efficacy and safety of ECT in depressive disorders: A systematic review and meta-analysis." *Lancet* 361: 799-808.

United States Department of Health and Human Services. 1999. *Mental Health: A Report of the Surgeon General*. Rockville, MD: United States Department of Health and Human Services.

University of Toronto Psychiatric Outreach Program. 2002. "Telepsychiatry: Guidelines and procedures for clinical activities." http://www.psychiatry.med.uwo.ca/ecp/info/toronto/telepsych.

Urness, D. 2003. "Telepsychiatry and doctor-patient communication: A tale of two interviews." *Canadian Psychiatric Association Bulletin* 35, 5: 21-25.

Ustun, T., et al. 2004. "Global burden of depressive disorders in the year 2000." *British Journal of Psychiatry* 184: 386-92.

Uttal, W. 2003. *Psychomythics: Sources of Artifacts and Misconceptions in Scientific Psychology*. Mahwah, NJ: Lawrence Erlbaum Associates.

Uttaro, T., and D. Mechanic. 1994. "The NAMI consumer survey analysis of unmet needs." *Hospital and Communtiy Psychiatry* 45: 372-74.

Vagnerova, P. 2003a. "Self-management of psychosis and schizophrenia." *Visions: BC's Mental Health Journal* 18: 18-19.

-. 2003b. "What BC campus disability centres can offer students." *Visions: BC's Mental Health Journal* 17: 28-29.

Valenstein, M., et al. 2004. "Benzodiazepine use among depressed patients treated in mental health settings." *American Journal of Psychiatry* 161: 654-61.

Valentine, M., and Capponi, P. 1989. "Mental health consumer participation on boards and committees: barriers and strategies." *Canada's Mental Health* 37: 8-12.

-, D. Waring, and D. Giuffrida. 1992. "Competency and treatment refusal in psychiatric hospitals." *Canada's Mental Health* 40: 19-24.

Vancouver Community Mental Health Services, Vancouver Coastal Health Authority. 2001. *Adult Guardianship Protocols*. Vancouver: Vancouver Community Mental Health Services, Vancouver Coastal Health Authority.

Vancouver/Richmond Mental Health Network Society. 2004. "Constitution." *The Bulletin: Official Publication of the Vancouver/Richmond Mental Health Network Society* 9: 16.

Van der Kolk, B. 2002. "The Assessment and Treatment of Complex PTSD." In *Psychological Trauma*, ed. R. Yehuda, 127-56. Washington, DC: American Psychiatric Press.

Van Le, C. 2000. "Stigma and mental illness in the Vietnamese culture." *Visions: BC's Mental Health Journal* 9: 9.

van Minnen, A., et al. 2003. "Treatment of trichotillomania with behavioral therapy or Fluoxetine: A randomized, waiting-list controlled study." *Archives of General Psychiatry* 60: 517-22.

Van Os, J. 2004. "Does the urban environment cause psychosis?" *British Journal of Psychiatry* 184: 287-88.

Vedantam, S. 2002. "Against depression, a sugar pill is hard to beat." *Washington Post*, 7 May, A01.

Verdun-Jones, S. 1988. "The right to refuse treatment: Recent developments in Canadian jurisprudence." *International Journal of Law and Psychiatry* 11: 51-60.

-. 2000. "Making the Mental Disorder Defence a More Attractive Option for Defendants in a Criminal Trial." In *Mental Disorders and the Criminal Code*, ed. D. Eaves, J. Ogloff, and R. Roesch, 39-75. Burnaby, BC: Mental Health, Law and Policy Institute, Simon Fraser University.

-. 2002. *Criminal Law in Canada: Cases, Questions and the Code*. 3rd ed. Toronto: Harcourt.

Viljoen, J., R. Roesch, and P. Zapf. 2002. "Interrater reliability of the Fitness Interview Test across four professional groups." *Canadian Journal of Psychiatry* 47: 945-52.

Vine, P. 2001. "Mindless and deadly: Media hype on mental illness and violence." http://www.fair.org/extra/0105/mental-illness.html.

Waddell, C. 2001. "So much research evidence, so little dissemination and uptake: mixing the pleasing with the useful." *Evidence-Based Mental Health* 4: 3-5.

–, et al. 2002. "Child psychiatric epidemiology and Canadian public policy-making." *Canadian Journal of Psychiatry* 47: 825-32.

–. 2004. *Preventing and Treating Anxiety Disorders in Children*. Research report prepared for the British Columbia Ministry of Children and Family Development.

Wahl, O. 1995. *Media Madness: Public Images of Mental Illness*. New Brunswick, NJ: Rutgers University Press.

Walker, L.E. 1992. "Battered women syndrome and self-defense." *Notre Dame Journal of Law, Ethics and Public Policy* 6: 321-34.

Wallace, C. 1998. "Social skills training in psychiatric rehabilitation: Recent findings." *International Review of Psychiatry* 10: 9-19.

–, P. Mullen, and P. Burgess. 2004. "Criminal offending in schizophrenia over a 25-year period marked by deinstitutionalization and increasing prevalence of comorbid substance use disorders." *American Journal of Psychiatry* 161: 716-27.

Wallach, H. 2004. "Changes in attitudes towards mental illness following exposure." *Community Mental Health Journal* 40: 235-48.

Wang, J., S. Patten, and M. Russell. 2001. "Alternative medicine use by individuals with major depression." *Canadian Journal of Psychiatry* 46: 528-33.

Wang, P., P. Berglund, and R. Kessler. 2000. "Recent care of common mental disorders in the US: Conformance with evidence-based recommendations." *Journal of General Internal Medicine* 15: 284-92.

Wasylenki, D., et al. 1997. "A home-based program for the treatment of acute psychosis." *Community Mental Health Journal* 33: 151-62.

–, et al. 2000. "Tertiary mental health services." Part 1, "Key issues." *Canadian Journal of Psychiatry* 45: 179-84.

Watson, A., et al. 2001. "Mental health courts and the complex issue of mentally ill offenders." *Psychiatric Services* 52: 477-81.

–, P. Corrigan, and V. Ottati. 2004. "Police officers' attitudes toward and decisions about persons with mental illness." *Psychiatric Services* 55: 49-53.

Watson, D., et al. 2005. "Population-based use of mental health services and patterns of delivery among family physicians, 1992-2001." *Canadian Journal of Psychiatry* 50: 398-406.

Webster, C., et al. 1997. *The HCR-20: Assessing the Risk for Violence*. Version 2. Burnaby, BC: Mental Health Law and Policy Institute, Simon Fraser University.

Weiner, E. 2003. "Attaining your educational dreams." *Visions: BC's Mental Health Journal* 17: 4-5.

Weiss, M., U. Jain, and J. Garland. 2000. "Clinical suggestions for the management of stimulant treatment in adolescents." *Canadian Journal of Psychiatry* 45: 717-23.

Wells, K., A. Stewart, and R. Hays. 1989. "The functioning and well-being of depressed patients: Results from the Medical Outcomes Study." *Journal of the American Medical Association* 262: 914-19.

Whaley, A. 1998. "Cross-cultural perspective on paranoia: A focus on the black American experience." *Psychiatric Quarterly* 69: 325-43.

Whitaker, R. 2002. *Mad in America: Bad Science, Bad Medicine, and the Enduring Mistreatment of the Mentally Ill*. Cambridge, MA: Perseus.

White, H., et al. 2003. "Survey of consumer and non-consumer mental health service providers on assertive community treatment teams in Ontario." *Community Mental Health Journal* 39: 265-76.

Whitten, P., C. Kingsley, and J. Grigsby. 2000. "Results of a meta-analysis of cost-benefit research: Is this a question worth asking?" *Journal of Telemedicine and Telecare* 6, supplement 1: S4-S6.

Wiggins, J., and N. Cummings. 1998. "National study of the experience of psychologists with psychotropic medication and psychotherapy." *Professional Psychology: Research and Practice* 29: 549-52.

Williams, C. 2001. "Increasing access and building equity into mental health services: An examination of the potential for change." *Canadian Journal of Community Mental Health* 20: 37-49.

Williams, J. 1994. "Psychiatric Classification." In *Textbook of Psychiatry*, ed. R. Hales, S. Yudofsky, and J. Talbott, 221-26. 2nd ed. Washington, DC: American Psychiatric Press.

Williams, L. 1998. "Personal accounts: A 'classic' case of borderline personality disorder." *Psychiatric Services* 49: 173-74.

Wilson, D., G. Tien, and D. Eaves. 1995. "Increasing the community tenure of mentally disordered offenders: An assertive case management program." *International Journal of Law and Psychiatry* 18: 61-9.

Wilson, M. 2005. "Getting there from here: Next steps." *Canadian Public Policy* 31, supplement: S69-S74.

Wilson, S. 1996. "Consumer empowerment in the mental health field." *Canadian Journal of Community Mental Health* 15: 69-83.

Wilton, R. 2003. "Poverty and mental health: A qualitative study of residential care facility clients." *Canadian Journal of Community Mental Health* 39: 139-56.

Winram, R. 2002. "Managing bipolar disorder: A patient's perspective." Presentation at the Annual Riverview Hospital Mood and Anxiety Disorders Conference, Port Coquitlam, BC, 3 April.

Witheridge, T. 1989. "The assertive community treatment worker: An emerging role and its implications for training." *Hospital and Community Psychiatry* 40: 620-24.

–. 1991. "The 'active ingredients' of assertive outreach." *New Directions in Mental Health Services* 52: 47-64.

Wittek, S. 2001. "Enough is enough: Joe Ribeiro wants the Vancouver police to stop shooting people with mental illnesses." *Terminal City*, 3-9 August, 10.

Woerner, M., S. Mannuzza, and J. Kane. 1988. "Anchoring the BPRS: An aid to improved reliability." *Psychopharmacological Bulletin* 24: 112-17.

Woo, S. 2000. "Chinese culture and mental health." *Visions: BC's Mental Health Journal* 9: 11-12.

Wood, G. 1986. *The Myth of Neurosis.* New York: Harper and Row.

Woodside, D. 2003. "Families – our most important support network." *Canadian Psychiatric Association Bulletin* 35: 6-7.

World Health Organization. 1992. *International Statistical Classification of Diseases and Related Health Problems/Tenth Revision.* Geneva: WHO.

–. 1994. *Constitution.* http://policy.who.int/cgibin/om_isapi.dll?hitsperheading=onandinfobase=basicdocandrecord={9D5}andsoftpage=Document42.

Wright, P., et al. 2003. "Intramuscular olanzapine and intramuscular haloperidol in acute schizophrenia: Antipsychotic efficacy and extrapyramidal safety during the first 24 hours of treatment." *Canadian Journal of Psychiatry* 48: 716-21.

Yager, J. 2004. "Antipsychotic medication, cardiac risk factors, and medical management: Comment." *Journal Watch Psychiatry* 10: 96.

Yates, D. 2004. "Should psychologists have prescribing authority? A psychologist's perspective." *Psychiatric Services* 55: 1420-21.

Yehuda, R., ed. 2002. *Psychological Trauma.* Washington, DC: American Psychiatric Press.

Yung, A., et al. 2003. "Psychosis prediction: 12-month follow-up of a high risk ('prodromal') group." *Schizophrenia Research* 60: 21-32.

Zacharias, Y. 2003. "Depression is a hidden, unrelenting killer." *Vancouver Sun*, 10 September, A1, A5-A6.

Ziedonis, D., and K. Trudeau. 1997. "Motivation to quit using substances among individuals with schizophrenia." *Schizophrenia Bulletin* 23: 229-38.

Ziguras, S., et al. 2003. "Ethnic matching of clients and clinicians and use of mental health services by ethnic minority clients." *Psychiatric Services* 54: 535-41.

Index

"by cop," 178
First Nations and, 297-98
hospital discharge and, 217n2, 217n12
protective factors, 195
rates of, 9, 11, 297-98
schizophrenia and, 11, 39, 194
sexual orientation as a risk factor, 308
supported education, 266-69
Swain (court decision), 285
symptom substitution, 235, 322
systematic desensitization, 234-35
Szasz, Thomas, 270-71

Tarasoff (court decision), 76
tardive dyskinesia, 201-2, 322
tasers, 179, 189n1
telepsychiatry, 131, 151-53, 322
Teplin, Linda, 177
tertiary care, 131, 322
Titicut's Follies (documentary film), 107
tolerance, 207, 322

Torrey, Edwin Fuller, 13, 20n7, 23, 271
transinstitutionalization, xvi, 106, 176, 322
trauma, as a cause of mental disorder, 27-30
treatment refusal, law concerning, 276-78

Ulysses agreements, 47, 283, 322
unemployment, 10, 253, 260
unpublished research, 100, 121-22
urbanization, 26
utility/futility, principles of, 290, 292

veracity, principle of, 289
violence, association with mental disorder, 13-16, 19

World Health Organization, 25, 41
World Psychiatric Association, 19-20

Youth. *See* children

Printed and bound in Canada by Friesens

Set in Giovanni Book and Garamond Condensed by Artegraphica Design

Text design: Irma Rodriguez

Copy editor: Robert Lewis

Proofreader: Jonathan Dore